THE LOW-FRUCTOSE APPROACH TO WEIGHT CONTROL

by George A. Bray, MD

DORRANCE PUBLISHING CO., INC.
PITTSBURGH, PENNSYLVANIA 15222

ISBN: 978-1-4349-0306-8
Library of Congress Control Number: 2008941137

Printed in the United States of America

First Printing

For more information or to order additional books,
please contact:
Dorrance Publishing Co., Inc.
701 Smithfield Street
Pittsburgh, Pennsylvania 15222
U.S.A.
1-800-788-7654
www.dorrancebookstore.com

This book is dedicated to my wife, Marilyn, and to my children, both biological and scientific.

CONTENTS

FOREWORD

A t last, a book targeting the need for sound weight-loss advice, from
the leader in obesity research, Dr. George Bray!

I am enormously grateful to George Bray for shaping my understanding
of body weight regulation. It would be difficult to overstate his impact on me
and on the field of obesity research. He has trained many, like me, and influenced virtually every scientist currently undertaking clinical obesity research.

Like most physicians of my era, when I first met George, I was operat-
ing under the assumption that overweight and obesity were easily reme-
died—that all the physician had to do to address the problem was to recommend a diet to the patient and perhaps advocate exercise in the prescrip-
tion—the "Eat Less, Exercise More" rubric. If the patient failed to lose
weight after being so instructed, then it must be a case of lack of will power
or self-control. The failure was always on the patient's part.

Of course, we now understand that overweight and obese patients are
challenged by genes that predispose them to gain weight and resist weight
loss in the current environment of plenty. Consider the environmental challenges we face. Food is cheap, readily accessible, delicious, and frequently
dense in calories. Ready access to these highly palatable and energy-dense
foods sets up and reinforces the "reward" aspects of food, making dieting a
withdrawal condition somewhat like smoking cessation. But unlike quitting
smoking, food is inescapable, since we *must* eat. The food environment is
not the only challenge, since as civilization progresses, our activities of daily
living require less and less physical activity. Furthermore, it is not just that
food availability and palatability are added on to a reduction in energy
expenditure in modern life; there may be interactive features of diet and
exercise that combine to make the problem even worse. Some of George
Bray's own research has demonstrated that being sedentary *interacts* with a
high-fat diet to further predispose to weight gain.

The bottom line: Failure to achieve and maintain weight loss is not due to a lack of willpower. Doctors should not shift the blame to the patient, but rather take responsibility for guiding and coaching patients in effective weight-loss techniques.

It is important for physicians to help their patients find tools and strategies to successfully navigate the "obesigenic" environment. In this book, George Bray does just that. He gives a recipe for successfully achieving and sustaining weight loss by avoiding high-sugar, high-fructose, and highly processed foods. This strategy will promote weight loss and weight-loss maintenance by encouraging a diet that is nutrition-dense, not calorie-dense, and which will promote satiety and diet satisfaction.

One of the keys to success in our weight-loss counseling is to "keep them coming back." We know that an encouraging, caring counselor can keep our participants engaged and committed. George Bray's tone throughout the book demonstrates that not only does he understand the biology of obesity, he also understands the psychology of the person trying to lose weight. He cares about the reader, and it shows.

This book is packed with tools for the dieter who is ready to seriously address his or her weight. I suggest the reader prepare for weight loss by reading it through. Then set a date and begin. The book can be your guide throughout the process, and you will return to different sections again and again. The book distills the career knowledge of an obesity research pioneer and a competent and caring clinician. It is the next-best thing to treatment by Dr. Bray himself.

Donna H. Ryan, M.D.
Associate Executive Director
Pennington Biomedical Research Center
Baton Rouge, Louisiana

PREFACE

P*ure, White, and Deadly.*[1] This is the title of a book about sugar written a number of years ago by a friend of mine when I was in my early training. Why such a title? The author, a famous London nutritionist named Professor John Yudkin, found a strong relationship between sugar consumption and heart disease. Unfortunately a number of other things, such as consumption of bananas, were also associated with heart disease, which made his idea about the relation of sugar to heart disease difficult to defend. Much new information has accumulated in the years since Dr. Yudkin's time. This has persuaded me that the **fructose** half of common table sugar should be a substitute for sugar as the reference for his book title.

Fructose may or may not be familiar to you, but before you finish this book, it will be. Fructose is a member of the "sugar" family, a number of sweet-tasting chemicals we find mainly in fruits and vegetables. Another principal member of this group is glucose, also known as "bloodsugar," an unfortunate confusion. Fructose, when chemically combined with glucose, is called sucrose, the common table "sugar." Fructose is the sweetest member of this group and can be found naturally in both fruits and vegetables. When eaten as part of fruits and vegetables, I will call this "good fructose" to distinguish it from the ubiquitous "bad fructose" in our diet. Most of our dietary fructose—the "bad fructose"—comes from highly refined products, primarily sugar (sucrose), produced from sugar cane or sugar beets, or high-fructose corn syrup (HFCS). "Bad fructose" has been separated from the plants in which it is found and usually comes with few other nutrients except manmade ones that are added during processing.

"Bad fructose" may be worse when combined with fat. We might call these combinations of "bad fructose" and fat the "deadly duo." In this book, I will focus on ways of eating to reduce the amount of "bad fructose" and the amount of fat in your diet. Fructose is very sweet and adds "sweetness" to our foods. In nature, sweetness is important for identifying foods that have the other important nutrients we need. Fruits and some vegetables that are naturally rich sources of vitamins and minerals can be identified from their sweet taste, usually due to fructose or sugar (sucrose).

The total amounts of good fructose in the fresh fruits and vegetables we eat, however, are much smaller than the amounts of "bad fructose" found in the refined and processed foods we buy. It is sad that sweet taste is no longer a guarantee of nutrient-rich foods; in fact, quite the opposite is true. The "bad fructose" in high-fructose corn syrup is indeed sweet, but it is also a good marker for highly processed foods, not good nutrition. High-fructose corn syrup does not exist in nature—it is man-made—so the inclusion of high-fructose corn syrup or sugar on a food label is an indication that it is a "processed" food, where other natural nutrients have often been lost. Thus reducing the intake of foods with these components will reduce energy intake and what can be called "empty calories." Since most of our pastries and other "sweets" contain fructose (HFCS or sugar), reducing "bad fructose" intake guarantees eating less of many higher-fat and highly processed foods.

Sugar and high-fructose corn syrup are sweet. Each day we eat about 80g (20 teaspoons) or about 2.7 oz of this bad fructose in added sugars, which provide 316 kcal/d or about 15% of an average individual's daily energy intake. About half of this is fructose, mostly in "bad fructose." "Bad fructose," either as HFCS or in sugar, is used as the main sweetener for soft drinks and other beverages and for most processed foods. In the United States, soft drinks are sweetened with "bad fructose"—almost entirely with high-fructose corn syrup (HFCS, called "isoglucose" in Europe). I got interested in this because the rising use of this substance in our food supply paralleled the rising prevalence of obesity.[2]

There are several elements to my Low-Fructose Approach to Weight Control. First, the listing of "HFCS," or "high-fructose corn syrup" on a food label (**NUTRITION FACTS**) is a good marker for the "bad fructose" in highly processed food. When I see it on a food label, I often try alternatives. You should use it that way, too. Second, when there is a choice, you should select less-processed foods, which are more likely to have the natural nutrients that make fresh foods more "naturally nutrient rich." Third, you should use the nutrition labels on packaged foods to find how much energy, expressed as calories, they contain. If a food product has more than 200 calories per serving, you should know that for many people this is 10% of their TOTAL DAILY energy (calorie) needs. Fourth, use food labels to get the portion size right. Sometimes the food label says "100 cal per serving," but the package actually contains two or more servings, that is, 200 calories or more. This is deceptive, in my view, since who eats half a candy bar? But that is the way labels are written right now. We can hope that more "truth" in package labeling will emerge sooner rather than later. Finally, you should reduce the fat in your diet and eat more protein, unless you have a health reason not to do so—for example, if you have kidney disease. Remember, bad fructose combined with fat may be, as Professor Yudkin said, "pure, white, and deadly."

My Low-Fructose Approach to Weight Control comes from my forty years of scientific research on the problem of obesity. It is comprised of what I have learned about treating overweight patients from my work at the Pennington Biomedical Research Center, the University of Southern California, the University of California at Los Angeles, and Tufts University Medical Center in Boston, MA. Almost all of this research has been supported by grants from the National Institutes of Health (an agency of the U.S. Government), along with a few clinical trials of anti-obesity drugs supported by industry. These are not discussed in this book, and there are thus no conflicts of interest with the statements I make. This approach to weight control describes the best techniques available to help people who want to manage their weight. In an earlier diet book,[3] published just over twenty-five years ago, I described my ideas about how to help people lose weight, which were developed from my hospital-based research in California. During my nineteen years at the Pennington Center, I have learned much more, particularly about the problem of bad fructose and overweight. The time is right for this new book, *The Low-Fructose Approach to Weight Control*. The ideas for this book have been greatly influenced by my associates and colleagues. At the Pennington Biomedical Research Center in Baton Rouge, Louisiana, I have had the wonderful opportunity to work with many dedicated people. Among them are Dr. Claude Bouchard, Dr. Catherine Champagne, Dr. James DeLany, Dr. Frank Greenway, Dr. David Harsha, Dr. Jennifer Lovejoy, Dr. Donna Ryan, Dr. Steven Smith, Dr. Donald Williamson, and Dr. David York. I am particularly grateful to Drs. Ryan, Champagne, and Greenway, who read the manuscript to help make sure I was honest and complete. Among my many associates over the years, there have been people from the University of Southern California, especially Dr. Richard Bergman, Dr. Janis Fisler, and Dr. John Nicoloff; from UCLA, Dr. Richard Atkinson, Dr. Bill Dahms, Dr. Delbert Fisher, Dr. Frank Greenway, Dr. Zvi Glick, Dr. Mark Molitch, Dr. Bill Odell, Dr. Ronald Swerdloff, Dr. Ada Wolfsen; and from Tufts University, Dr. Edwin Astwood, Dr. Henry Friesen, Dr. Tom Gallagher, and Dr. Javier Londono, along with many wonderful post-doctoral fellows. Thanks to all of you for your friendship and helpful ideas over the years. During the preparation of this book, I have been ably assisted by Ms. Carole Lachney. Without her dedicated service on many parts of this book, it would not have come to fruition.

George A. Bray, M.D.
Boyd Professor
Pennington Center
July 2008

NOTICE

As a physician, I am concerned with improving the health of all who seek my help. I know being overweight can cause health problems. I also know, however, that treatment for your weight problem by changing dietary habits or by increasing your level of physical activity may also cause difficulties for some people; therefore, I strongly urge all individuals who are planning a new diet or exercise program to do so only after consulting with their own family physician or other appropriate professional. The need for professional advice on diet and exercise is particularly important for growing children, for pregnant women, for women who are breast-feeding, for the elderly, and for people who are receiving medications from physicians.

INTRODUCTION
HOW DID AMERICANS GET SO FAT?

Have you been to your local shopping mall recently? Are you older than 20? Then you have certainly witnessed the growing girth of many Americans. The United States is now the fattest country in the world! The U.S. Government regularly surveys the American public to put numbers on the face of fatness. These surveys are called the National Health and Nutrition Examination Surveys (NHANES). Between 1960 and 1976, there was a slow rise in the number of Americans who were overweight. This slow rise was similar to the slow increase in overweight that occurred between the Civil War (in 1860) through 1976.[1] Between 1976 and today, there has been a big jump in the number of overweight and obese Americans (Figure 1). This number more than doubled between 1980 to 2002 (from 14.5% to 33.5% obese).[2] The increased rate at which people are becoming fat has led some to label this an "epidemic" (the World Health Organization (WHO),[3] the National Heart, Lung, and Blood Institute (NHLBI)[4]). To illustrate this trend, I have put the percentage of Americans who would be labeled as "overweight" or "obese" or "very obese" in each of the five NHANES surveys over the past forty-five years into a single picture (Figure 1). This graph shows the slow increase in weight until around 1980, and then the rate of weight gain takes off.

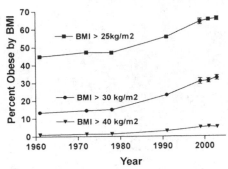

Figure 1. The increasing number of Americans who are labelled as overweight (solid line), obese (dashed line), or very obese (dash-dot line) by U.S. Government surveys from 1980 to 2004 (drawn from data in reference 2).

Nearly forty years ago, even before the "obesity epidemic" began in earnest, the plight of fat Americans became my life's work. Much of my office practice of medicine dealt with very overweight adolescents and young adults. Back in the 1960s, I was saddened and dismayed by the young people weighing more than 300 lbs who came to my office for help. The problem is much worse now. The group with a body weight greater than 300 lbs represented less than 0.1% of the American population in the 1960s; now is it over 5% and is growing rapidly. Studying this problem has provided me with many insights and personal stories about how people try to help themselves. Thirty years ago, I published my first book on obesity,[1] followed by an update in 2007[5] and twenty-five years ago, I published my first treatment program to help people conquer their weight problem.[6] Many things have changed in the intervening years. Preparation of this book has been strongly influenced by my experiences at the Pennington Biomedical Research Center in Baton Rouge, Louisiana. When I became director of this center in 1989, the current obesity epidemic was in full swing. I was proud to be director of this magnificent nutrition research facility. It gave me a new horizon and additional resources to tackle the problem that has been my life's work. This book is my effort to share with you the new ideas about weight control that I have learned through the help of many patients and professional colleagues.

Let me put my strategy of weight control forward for you and then fill in some of the details about how this approach came about. First, we know that in famines and when food is in short supply, people don't gain weight—indeed, they lose weight.[7,8] No food, no fatness. This means that food plays a key part in the problem. Focusing on food is the first step in helping you win the "battle of the bulge." Reasoning that some foods are playing a bigger role than others, we examined the data from the U.S. Department of Agriculture about changes in food supply during the twentieth century. One of the striking findings was that the epidemic of overweight occurred in parallel with the introduction of high-fructose corn syrup (HFCS) into the American food supply.[9] The association between the rapid rise in obesity and the introduction of high-fructose corn syrup (HFCS) doesn't prove that high-fructose corn syrup is the *cause* of obesity—obesity clearly has a number of causes, many of which are related to eating more food than we need. But the evidence is growing that high-fructose corn syrup (HFCS) and sugar (the sources of "bad fructose") and the rise in HFCS-containing beverage size and marketing muscle may be one contributor to the rise in obesity rates.[10]

What is high-fructose corn syrup (HFCS, called isoglucose in Europe)? It is a sweetener used in beverages and many other food products. HFCS is made from the corn starch we get from corn. In the 1960s, Japanese scientists found a way to convert the glucose found in corn starch into fructose, a molecule that is much sweeter than glucose or even sucrose (table sugar). There are more details about these sugars in Chapter 5 on "Good Nutrition." With a sweet solution that is just over half bad fructose, soft drink manufacturers and food companies that make fruit drinks and baked goods were able to replace the more expensive sucrose with lower-cost HFCS. This they did, and now almost all of our soft drinks, fruit drinks, many pastries, and many other processed foods are sweetened with HFCS. Why should this replacement of HFCS for sucrose (which also releases fructose after it enters the body) make such a difference? One difference is because HFCS makes beverages less costly; therefore, soft drink makers and food processors can make larger servings at a lower price for the consumer: a double-edged sword—sweeter but more calories for your money and more calories for your waist. The strategy I develop throughout this book is to show you how to keep your eye on the so-called "bad fructose" in your diet—from either HFCS or sucrose (sugar). Keep your eye on BOTH high-fructose corn syrup (HFCS) and sugar. When these ingredients appear on food labels, they tell you the product has been "highly processed"—something I try to avoid. Thus by focusing on reducing bad fructose in your diet—the Low-Fructose Approach to Weight Loss—you can reduce your weight and improve your nutrition at the same time. Also keep your eye on the combination of fructose and fat.

Along with this major shift in the supply of food caloric sweeteners in the American diet, a number of other changes have occurred over recent decades. Let's survey some of the changes I have observed over the past forty years. These new trends can be summed up under the five "B"s: Beverages, Burgers, Behavior, Be Active, Buyer Beware.

Beverages: You have already been introduced to beverages sweetened with bad fructose in HFCS, which makes them sweet. We will learn a lot more about the potentially harmful effects on body weight of soft drinks and sweetened fruit drinks that contain "bad fructose." At least five studies have now shown the amount of soft drinks youngsters consume predicts both their current and future weight gain.[10] To guide you through this maze, there is a chapter on beverages (Chapter 6). *Tip*: Get as much of your fluid and beverage needs as you can from water, tea, or coffee—at least six to eight 8-ounce glasses a day. *Tip*: Avoid beverages that have fructose in them if you can.

Burgers: Everyone, or nearly everyone, has eaten at one of the fast-food burger establishments. They are ubiquitous in the United States and around the world. Burgers tend to be loaded with fat—but they are "tasty." Over the past fifty years, the size of most burgers has ballooned. A single large burger meal can provide you 1000 calories, which is 50% or more of most Americans' total daily energy needs. These are problem foods for people who want to lose weight and keep it off, as well as for people who do not want to gain weight. This threat to weight control was shown dramatically in the documentary movie *Supersize Me,* where the director, Morgan Spurlock, gained over twenty-five pounds in one month while supersizing his meal every time it was offered. *Tip*: Leave the burgers in the restaurants where they are made and only eat the ones you have grilled at home without the "special" sauce.

Behavior: Eating and drinking are behaviors. One view has it that we become overweight because we have "faulty" behaviors. Whether true or not, this idea has helped a lot of people plan what they eat and with whom and where they eat to get better control over their own personal eating. The Internet is one of the most striking developments of the past decade.[11] The power of the Internet is being harnessed to use in behavioral weight management and offers promise of future successes. One of the most important concepts has been the "control" of portion size using "portion-controlled" foods. *Tip*: Use the behavioral techniques that are described later in this book to help you focus on the types of foods and beverages you choose. *Tip*: "Monitor" what you eat as often as you can.

Be Active: Be as active as you can to counteract the tendency to be inactive. Society no longer requires us to do strenuous things unless we choose to do so. Television, video games, and comfy automobiles all make the U.S. one of the most inactive societies on Earth. Inactivity is the norm. We know that overweight people sit an average of two hours more per day than do thinner people. *Tip*: Stand up while talking on your cell phone. The beauty of the cell phone is that you can talk anywhere and walk while doing so, which burns more energy. *Tip*: Use a step counter to count the steps you take, with a goal of 5,000 steps per day or more.

Buyer Beware: We are all influenced by the prices of the things we buy, including food. Price reduction and sale items get our attention. Food pricing works the same way. Special deals, such as "two for the price of one" and "supersizing," are ways of selling more for a "better deal"—a better deal for the seller, but not necessarily a better deal for you. *Tip*: Buy healthy foods, not cheap ones, and avoid beverages containing "bad fructose." Remember, you don't have to clean your plate. Put the waste in the garbage bin rather than on your own waist. Avoid combinations of "bad fructose" (HFCS or sucrose) and fat.

We will focus on reducing "bad fructose" intake, switching high-fat foods to healthy lower-fat ones, and making food choices based on health, not price.

Isn't Obesity Just a Recent Problem?

Overweight was a problem long before I finished medical school fifty years ago. I found this out when I came across a short second-hand book from the nineteenth century that traced the origins of obesity. Although it was written in French by an American who was studying in Paris—something lots of young physicians did in the nineteenth century—it opened my eyes to the long history of overweight.[12] It is hard to believe there was enough to fill a book that far back. Yet there was, and this book stimulated me to learn more about the history of obesity and when it began.[13]

Treatment for overweight has been described for more than 5,000 years[13]. These descriptions can be found in medical writings from the Egyptian, Babylonian, Chinese, Indian, Meso-American, and Greco-Roman cultures, some of which go back more than 5,000 years. Many causes were proposed and many treatments suggested long before we had any modern medicines. In spite of this long history, the problem is still with us—and getting worse, meaning we neither understand it well nor have completely effective treatments. We have greatly increased our knowledge and have much more to offer people working to control their weight, yet at this writing, the problem continues.

The first English-language books devoted solely to the subject of fatness were written in the eighteenth century, well before the American Revolution.[14,15] These were followed during the next two hundred years by books in many languages.[13] The first American book dealing with the medical side of obesity was published in 1940, just prior to World War II. By the time Rony[16] wrote this book, the basic concepts of energy balance and body metabolism had been well established. Scientific studies at the time of the French Revolution[17,18] had clearly shown that metabolism was similar to burning a candle. Some fifty years later, the Law of Conservation of

Energy[19,20] was clearly stated by two German scientists. This work in Germany stimulated Americans to develop equipment that could measure human metabolism.[21] With this equipment, they showed the idea of energy balance applied to human beings just as it did to other animals. We were metabolically part of the same evolutionary animal kingdom.

While the basic science behind fatness was developing, the first popular weight-reduction "diet" was published in London in 1863.[22] William Banting, its author, was a layman. The first edition of his small pamphlet, titled "Letter on Corpulence Addressed to the Public," was published because he was thrilled with the success he achieved using a diet given to him by his doctor.[23] It was high in protein and low in carbohydrates, and it aroused the same fervor in England at the time of our Civil War as have some of the modern popular diet books. Later in this book, I will discuss some of these diet books and how to evaluate them, since new ones appear each year.

We made a major step forward when we recognized that overweight could be caused in many ways. One type of overweight, although rare, is due to brain tumors that are often associated with impaired vision and glandular disturbances.[24,25] Shortly after this discovery, a famous American neurosurgeon, Dr. Harvey Cushing, showed in 1912[26] that a tumor in the "master gland" (the pituitary) could also produce overweight.

For more than half of the twentieth century, the life insurance industry did its best to convince Americans that being overweight was dangerous to health and tended to shorten lifespan.[27] Industry leaders knew this from the money they had to pay out to settle death-benefit claims for insurance on people who were overweight. Even modest increases in excess weight were associated with shortened lifespan.[28] From recent studies, we know that losing weight prolongs life.[29,30]

Lessons Learned about Obesity in the Past Thirty Years

Overweight as a problem came of age in the 1970s. The National Institutes of Health (NIH) are funded by American taxpayers to support basic research aimed at curing heart disease, diabetes, arthritis, cancer, and other diseases. In the late 1960s, the Fogarty International Center for Preventive Diseases at the National Institutes of Health was established to honor Congressman John E. Fogarty (1913–1967), a U.S. Congressional Representative from the state of Rhode Island, who had been a long-time and vocal supporter of expanded research at the NIH. One of the first activities of the new Fogarty Center was to organize a conference on prevention of obesity. "Obesity" was perceived, even in the 1970s, to be a major public health issue. This conference was held at NIH in 1973.[31]

The impetus for the study of overweight given by the Fogarty Center Conference on obesity was followed by the first in a series of International

Congresses on Obesity, with the first held in London in 1974.[32] Along with the development of these international meetings came the publication of the first journal devoted specifically to overweight: the *International Journal of Obesity.*

Two political events occurred at the same time at the 1973 Fogarty Center Conference. One was the development of the "isomerase" process for converting corn starch into high-fructose corn syrup (HFCS) containing bad fructose, which is cheap to make and which has displaced much of the sucrose (sugar) in foods and essentially all of the sucrose used to sweeten soft drinks in America. At the same time, and without adequate recognition at the time, agricultural policies in the United States were undergoing changes that made some food products, including corn, cheaper. As food prices fell, they represented a smaller fraction of the household budget, and this allowed more people to eat away from home and enjoy the tasty, high-energy-density foods provided by the increasing number of fast-food and other restaurants. Tucked away at the same time was the first edition of my first book about obesity, *The Obese Patient,* published in 1976.[1]

The most important advance in obesity in recent years was the discovery of leptin.[33] This peptide hormone is made predominantly in the fat cells. When leptin is absent, massive overweight occurs in human beings and in research animals. Defects in the leptin receptor, the "lock" the leptin molecule "key" fits into, are also responsible for a small number of massively overweight people.[34] In addition to derangements in the leptin genes, defects in other genes can produce obesity in human beings. One of these genes, called the melanocortin-4 receptor gene, is defective in up to 5% of markedly overweight youngsters.[34] This is one of the most frequent genetic causes for a chronic human disease yet reported. Yet collectively, these individuals are only a tiny fraction of all obese people.

Just prior to the Fogarty Center Conference in 1973, there was a landmark study showing that behavior modification could be used to treat overweight subjects.[35] As this technique was developed in detail, it became one of the "three pillars," along with diet and exercise, for the treatment of overweight people. Because of the response to behavioral strategies, overweight has been labeled a "lifestyle disease." Efforts have been made to adapt these behavioral techniques to prevent development of weight gain in larger groups of people, but they have been disappointing. Behavioral strategies are cognitive strategies, that is to say, they require you to do something active, such as dieting, exercising, or modifying the way you live. We are slowly learning these cognitive strategies do not translate into the prevention of overweight, and the weight people initially lose using them is often regained. The alternative to "cognitive" approaches is the use of "non-cognitive" approaches, that is, ways of dealing with overweight that do not require much active individual involvement. In the prevention of dental caries ("cavities"), the addition of fluoride to the water supply is a good example of a non-cognitive strategy. When our water was fluoridated, dental caries were dramatically reduced, without our intentional activity.

Recent studies have suggested several things that may help prevent overweight and don't require much effort. Taking more calcium may be one of them. People with higher intakes of calcium have lower body weight in some, but not all, studies. The use of low-fat dairy products, which are a good source of calcium, lowers blood pressure and is part of the one of the diets I describe later in this book. *Tip*: Use fruits, vegetables (sources of "good fructose"), and low-fat dairy products to take in more calcium, unless you are susceptible to kidney stones. Calcium can help your bones and may have some benefit for your body weight.

Less sleep is associated with higher body weights. Children who sleep less gain more weight in their preschool years.[5] This also applies to adults, and there is now a potential explanation for this effect in the changes of sleep-influencing hormones—changes that occur with too little sleep. *Tip*: Try to get your eight hours of sleep each night and even more sleep for your children.

Another low-effort strategy for weight loss would be to buy foods for "health," not for "price." Turning off that natural desire to get more for your money when buying food may be hard. But what you get for your money when you buy cheap food may be "bad fructose" and fat, which may simply become "waste on your waist." *Tip*: It is better to eat well than to eat cheaply.

The fat cell is much more than where fat is stored.[36] It is a cell that plays a part in the daily orchestra of life. It makes music through the chemicals it produces. Sometimes the notes are beautiful, but they can also be discordant. With the discovery that leptin is made almost entirely in the fat cell, it has become clear that the fat cell has very significant functions besides storing fat. Fat cells are part of the largest glandular (endocrine) tissue in the body. They produce numerous products that are released into the circulation and act on other cells. Among these are molecules that cause inflammation, molecules that are involved in controlling blood pressure or influencing cell growth, and molecules that regulate fat metabolism and blood clotting. What a powerhouse fat tissue is in the human body!

The past thirty years have seen the development of a plethora of new drugs for the treatment of many diseases. Some of these medications produce weight gain.[5] I will discuss these in more detail later. *Tip*: If you take medicines, ask your physician whether you are taking something that could produce weight gain. If so, s/he may be able to switch you to an alternative medication that does not cause weight gain.

The commonly called "beer belly," or "apple shape," is medically termed "central adiposity." We have learned that central adiposity is a risk to your health. This was first noted nearly one hundred years ago, but it wasn't until 1982[37] that it became widely appreciated that people with central adiposity were at high risk for diabetes and heart disease. Waist circumference has become the standard way to measure central adiposity. Increased waist circumference (more than 40 inches in men or more than 35 inches in women) is a criterion for diagnosing central adiposity. It is also one of a group of signs and symptoms related to heart disease and diabetes, including high blood pressure, high blood sugar, low levels of HDL-cholesterol, and high levels of triglycerides.

Diets can reduce your risk of disease and prove a way to treat some of them effectively. This was shown elegantly in a study comparing the effects of three different dietary patterns on blood pressure.[38,39] The first diet, the reference diet, was a standard American diet or Western type of diet, with plenty of fat, meat, and normal amounts of fruits and vegetables. The second diet, one of the two experimental diets, was called the "fruits and vegetables diet" because it was enriched with fruits and vegetables. The aim was to increase dietary intake of magnesium and potassium from fruits and vegetables to the seventy-fifth percentile of normal, that is, a level above what three out of four people would normally get in their diet. The third diet—the combination, or DASH diet—was enriched to the same degree as the second diet with fruits and vegetables. In addition, it had more low-fat dairy products to increase calcium intake and also had lowered total fat intake (27% versus 33% in the control diet), more fiber, higher protein from (18%) with the extra 3% from vegetable sources, and reduced intake of calorically sweetened beverages and other sweets. Blood pressure was significantly reduced in people eating the "fruits and vegetables diet" and reduced even more in the people eating the combination (fruits, vegetables, low-fat dairy products), or DASH diet.[38,39] *Tip*: Include a DASH-type diet—one with plenty of fresh fruits and vegetables, somewhat higher protein, and lower fat—into your eating plan.

Another large clinical trial, called the Diabetes Prevention Program, showed that weight loss with a reduction of fat and more activity could significantly reduce the risk of diabetes mellitus in people at high risk for this disease.[40] *Tip*: Modest weight loss can have important health benefits for you.

Obesity remains a stigmatized condition. Prejudice against and dislike for people who are overweight are commonplace. The efforts, particularly among women, to lose weight cost billions of dollars per year.

In addition to the health benefits from weight loss, including prolonging life,[29,30] there is an improvement in the quality of life, and for many people this is very important. Weight loss improves your ability to move and get around. When your weight loss is not sufficient to give you the cosmetic benefits and improvements in quality of life you want, from your point of view, you may not be willing to continue the effort needed to maintain your weight loss program. *Tip*: Set goals you can accomplish and take small steps toward these goals.

Surgical treatment for obesity began in the 1960s. The current popularity of these procedures is the result of the lowered risk from surgery with the use of newer, so-called laparoscopic surgeries. Using laparoscopic techniques reduces the risk and has increased the number of treated patients. It is estimated that more than 100,000 people have this surgery each year. The mortality has been reduced, and many of the complications associated with surgery have been reduced. *Tip*: Try other methods first; this is the last resort.

This book has been divided into three parts:

Part One: A Strategy for Success

The first seven chapters make up Part One of this book. Whether you are overweight or not, the tips provided here will help you help yourself with better nutrition and a more healthful life. This material is based on my experiences of the past fifty years with overweight people and their problems. Many years ago, one of my patients said, "Doc, you should write a book." Well, I have written many books for doctors and a raft of scientific articles, but none of them were designed for you, the concerned overweight individual. I hope this book fills that need.

Are you ready? This is the first question you have to answer, and it is where I start. If you are ready, then let's go. First, there are several popular and trendy ideas and issues that are important for you to understand to be successful at helping yourself lose weight. How do you know if you are overweight and by how much? What causes overweight? What are the things inside and outside of you that affect your weight? With this as a background, my next agenda item for you is think positively. It can help you help yourself to a healthy eating plan. I have illustrated the uses of positive thinking with examples from the weight-control field. Don't forget that positive thinking can be important for others you help when you help yourself. Nutrition affects all facets of life. As one person said, "We are what we eat." Nutrition is a large area. To help you master it, I have provided a road map and road signs, including ideas on the beverages we drink. Finally in this section, I discuss exercise along with nutrition and positive thinking.

Part Two: The Steps to Success

You are now ready to manage your weight problem once and for all. Can this be done? Of course it can be done, but *you* have to make it happen. I am only your guide. You are the adventurer. The first challenge is to give you some road signs for success. As more and more successful people are studied, we can give you better and better signs. When the first explorers trekked across America, they did not have road signs. They had to find their own way. Nowadays we have detailed road maps and global positioning satellite pictures.

Several strategies are available to lead you to success. Some will work better for you than others. Some will work better now than later. You choose. I know your individuality makes a difference. My job is to provide you with the choices. Yours is to choose. There are low-fat maps, portion-controlled scenarios, nutrient-density guides, suggestions for group support, and old-fashioned calorie counting. Some take the high road and some take the low road, but all roads, as they say, lead to Rome, which in this case is managing your weight.

Part Three: Maintaining Your Success
The final two chapters of this book are working manuals for some of the things you need to do to be successful. They are the components I have used in my treatment program for more than fifteen years. They served as the basis for a teaching film prepared by the American Medical Association to help other doctors treat the serious problem of being overweight. They have been continually improved to keep them up to date. They are practical approaches to menu planning, energy expenditure, nutrition, and behavioral modification. Following these, there are a number of reference materials and a bibliography for those of you who want more reading and more information.

Thank you for giving me this opportunity to share with you my long-held hopes of helping people shed unwanted pounds.

PART ONE
A STRATEGY FOR SUCCESS

CHAPTER ONE

Are You Ready?

Features of People Who Lose Weight Successfully

Helping Yourself Helps Others
Every time you eat, you help yourself to food. You make a choice to eat this or that, or not to eat this or that. In this book, I will share with you my ideas about a healthy approach to eating, with a generous dose of reading nutrition labels to make healthy food choices that help you lose weight and avoid "bad fructose." These ideas are based on theories of why some people gain weight easily while others do not. "Bad fructose," to me, is one of the best focal points. If you eliminate or markedly reduce "bad fructose" (both HFCS and sucrose), you will also reduce fat intake—remember, fructose and fat may be called the "deadly duo."

When you help yourself to a healthy lifestyle, you also help those around you who love and need you. Remember, weight loss lengthens life.[1,2] You are improving your health and your wellbeing and moving toward a longer, healthier, and more enjoyable life. Whether it is genetic or not, we know children who grow up in a family with overweight parents are much more likely to be overweight themselves. When you help yourself to healthy nutrition and a healthy weight, you are also helping those loved ones around you—children, spouse, and significant others—toward a healthier life, too. Recent studies emphasize the relation of fatness in people to fatness in other members of the family and to close friends.[3] There is, if you like, a kind of "contagiousness" about fatness.

Helping yourself to healthy nutrition also helps you to a healthier life. You will move more easily, wear smaller clothes sizes, and feel better. Are you ready to help yourself?

3

Features of Successful Weight Losers

You've probably read about other weight-loss programs. At the Pennington Center, we have tested some of these programs that allege to help people manage their weight. Perhaps you've tried one of them. For more than forty years, I've helped people manage their weight. I've analyzed why some people succeed and others don't. Throughout this book, I will share with you the experiences of both successful and unsuccessful dieters so you can learn from them and be successful yourself.

People do succeed, and you can be one of them! Experiences of successful people can motivate you and provide insight into a proper and healthy way to lose weight. I will share the strategies that have proven successful in helping my patients and others reduce their weight to where they want it and often keep it there. And most importantly, this advice is an essential tool in encouraging successful people to maintain their weight loss.

Mr. G.G. is the heaviest man I've ever treated. I didn't know him at his peak weight—some 1,100 pounds. I do know Mr. G.G.'s first recorded weight after he started his diet was 980 pounds. But a balanced 1200- to 1500-calorie/day diet, along with help and encouragement from his physicians, his friends, and his family, enabled him to drop his weight to nearly 200 pounds. I saw Mr. G.G. off and on over ten years, and while his weight has fluctuated to just over 300 pounds at times, he is still more than 800 pounds below his peak weight! And he has kept it there for more than ten years.

So you see, people do succeed. Another of my patients, Angela, was told that if she did not lose weight she would need to take insulin shots to control her diabetes. Weighing 220 pounds at the time, Angela agreed to give it a try. Prior to beginning her diet, she prepared herself using some of the ways I'll describe later. Ultimately, she brought her weight down to 170 pounds. Several years later, she has maintained that weight. Best of all, she doesn't have to take insulin shots. The basis for her success was that she learned to help herself.

Several features characterize people who successfully help themselves lose weight. First, they are more physically active. If you become more active, you are more likely to enjoy long-term success. Joan was a thirty-two-year-old nurse who brought her weight down from 200 pounds to 140 pounds and kept it there for nearly five years. Her secret was a combination of exercise and a low-fat, high-fiber diet. I was extremely impressed with Joan's commitment. She jogged for an hour during her lunch break, five days a week. Even when it rained, she would jog in the shopping mall. She kept her weight off for five years, until she became pregnant. But with the birth of her child, she quit her exercise routine and re-gained weight.

Mindset is a second major factor of successful people who help themselves. Ms. P. is a very successful businesswoman who wanted to lose 25 pounds to improve her appearance and self-image. She joined our group and began our weight-management program. As we began discussing being more active, each participant was asked how much time s/he could devote to being active. Ms. P. was fairly adamant that she didn't have time in her busy day for more activity. This was an immediate sign to me that she wasn't ready to lose weight. She didn't place a high enough priority on helping herself lose weight. It wasn't long before she quit the program, even though her initial results were promising.

If you don't have time to incorporate your weight-loss plan into your lifestyle and undertake the long-term changes necessary to succeed, you are likely to be disappointed. I often meet patients who are looking for a fairy godmother who can wave a magic wand and make them 30 pounds lighter. Unfortunately, I don't own that magic wand, nor does anyone else. The only magic I offer is the magic of helping yourself to make healthy nutrition choices based on my ideas about why you became overweight.

As you are reading this book, you are likely running some scenario or another through your mind. This internal self-talk can be beneficial, or it can be very destructive to helping you help yourself. Successful people make this self-talk work in their favor. I will focus on this internal self-talk, and in a later chapter will describe how it can help you help yourself in your efforts to lose weight and adopt healthier eating habits.

A third major characteristic of successful people is an understanding of the role good nutrition plays in helping you make healthier choices in the foods you eat and in making those choices second nature. I used to think people who came to our clinic after trying other weight-loss programs knew all there was to know about nutrition. I now know better. You need a good working knowledge of nutrition to be successful in helping yourself lose weight. The food label can be a big help. We will describe it in detail later, but it provides information on calories, portion size, and whether the product contains "bad fructose," such as high-fructose corn syrup (HFCS) or sugar, a sure sign of a highly processed food. Remember that when you see high-fructose corn syrup (HFCS) or sucrose on the label, you will do yourself a service by selecting fresh fruits and vegetables as an alternative—ones that are "naturally nutrient rich."

We know people are motivated to lose weight for different reasons. Some, like my diabetic patient, are encouraged to lose weight for the sake of their health. Others simply want to dazzle their spouse in a new bathing suit. Whatever your reason may be, it is important to me to help you help yourself reach your goal. But first, let's be clear what we mean by being overweight.

Are You Overweight?

If you didn't think so, you probably wouldn't be reading this book. This section, however, will help you understand how serious your weight problem may be and why you need to help yourself. There are several ways you can tell whether you are overweight. The simplest way is to look in the mirror in the morning before you put your clothes on. If you see too many bulges, you are probably overweight. We'll call this the "bulge test." If there are bulges where the skin seems to roll over itself, you can consider yourself overweight.

Another method is the "pinch test." If you pinch the skin on the back of your arm between your thumb and forefinger and the distance is more than an inch, you are probably overweight. The pinch test is particularly good for women; they have relatively more fat beneath their skin than men.

The "belt test" is particularly good for men. Buckle your favorite belt comfortably around your waist. If you can lower it over your hips to the floor while it is still buckled, you need to help yourself to new eating habits. If you are a man and your waist is more than 40 inches around, this also shows you have too much "central fat"—the kind of fat that carries the most health risks.

The "ruler test" is another easy one. Lie flat on the floor. Place a ruler on your stomach between the bottom of your breastbone or sternum and your pubic bone. If the stomach in between keeps the ruler from touching both the lower end of your breast bone *and* your pubic bone at the same time, you may be overweight.

You probably already know of the Metropolitan Life Insurance Company, or at least of the weight tables they provide. The life insurance people have been interested in weight for more than one hundred years.[4] They know overweight people do not live as long as people of normal weight. The relatives of overweight people collect on life insurance policies earlier than do the relatives of average-weight people. It thus costs the insurance company more to insure overweight people.

Throughout most of the twentieth century, the Metropolitan Life Insurance Company has published weight tables based on their experience. These tables use the familiar small, medium, and large frame sizes. Of course, everyone wants to use the weights associated with the "large frame." But there are few data behind the use of these frame sizes by the insurance industry. The heights and weights used to create these tables came from medical examinations performed on individuals purchasing life insurance. Height and weight were measured, but there was no determination of frame size. Nevertheless, the insurance companies divided recommended weights into frame sizes.

Table 1. Metropolitan Life Insurance Height and Weight Table of 1983 for Women (corrected for height without shoes and weight without clothes).

Height (ft & in)	Small Frame	Medium Frame	Large Frame
4'9"	99-108	106-118	115-128
4'10"	100-110	108-120	117-131
4'11"	101-112	110-123	119-134
5'0"	103-115	112-126	122-137
5'1"	105-118	115-129	125-140
5'2"	108-121	118-132	128-144
5'3"	111-124	121-135	131-148
5'4"	114-127	124-138	134-152
5'5"	117-130	127-141	137-156
5'6"	120-133	130-144	140-160
5'7"	123-136	133-147	143-164
5'8"	126-139	136-150	146-167
5'9"	129-142	139-153	149-170
5'10"	132-145	142-156	152-173
5'11"	135-148	145-159	155-176

I think there is a better way to determine whether you are overweight. This method was actually developed more than one hundred years ago[6] but has only been studied and widely used for the past twenty years. It has now been adopted by both the World Health Organization[7] and by the National Heart, Lung, and Blood Institute of the U.S. Government[8] and the National Center for Health Statistics[9] as the way to assess weight status. It is called the body mass index (BMI) and is calculated by dividing your weight by the square of your height. There are two easy ways to determine your BMI. One is with a table like the one shown below (Table 2), and the other is with a website provided by the National Institutes of Health (*http://www.nhlbi.nih. gov/guidelines/obesity/bmi_tbl.htm*). Find your height in inches on the left side and then move along that line from left to right until you find the weight closest to yours. Your BMI is listed at the top of the column where you found your weight.

The normal range of BMI is between 18.5 and 24.9 (less than 25). For most Americans, a BMI below 20 is too thin. You are considered overweight if your BMI is between 25 and 30, unless you are of Asian descent, in which case a lower value has been recommended, with a BMI above 25 being obese. For other Americans, obesity is defined as a BMI above 30. The "obesity" category is further divided into Grade I (BMI 30 to less than 35), Grade II (BMI 35 to less than 40), and Grade III (BMI is above 40).

Table 2. A Table of Body Mass Index and Risk

	Good Weights							Increasing Risk →														

BMI

Height	19	20	21	22	23	24	25	26	27	28	29	30	31	32	33	34	35	36	37	38	39	40
4'10"	91	96	100	105	110	115	119	124	129	134	138	143	148	153	158	162	167	172	177	181	186	191
4'11"	94	99	104	109	114	119	124	128	133	138	143	148	153	158	163	168	173	178	183	188	193	198
5'	97	102	107	112	118	123	128	133	138	143	148	153	158	163	168	174	179	184	189	194	199	204
5'1"	100	106	111	116	122	127	132	137	143	148	153	158	164	169	174	180	185	190	195	201	206	211
5'2"	104	109	115	120	126	131	136	142	147	153	158	164	169	175	180	186	191	196	202	207	213	218
5'3"	107	113	118	124	130	135	141	146	152	158	163	169	175	180	186	191	197	203	208	214	220	225
5'4"	110	116	122	128	134	140	145	151	157	163	169	174	180	186	192	197	204	209	215	221	227	232
5'5"	114	120	126	132	138	144	150	156	162	168	174	180	186	192	198	204	210	216	222	228	234	240
5'6"	118	124	130	136	142	148	155	161	167	173	179	186	192	198	204	210	216	223	229	235	241	247
5'7"	121	127	134	140	146	153	159	166	172	178	185	191	198	204	211	217	223	230	236	242	249	255
5'8"	125	131	138	144	151	158	164	171	177	184	190	197	203	210	216	223	230	236	243	249	256	262
5'9"	128	135	142	149	155	162	169	176	182	189	196	203	209	216	223	230	236	243	250	257	263	270
5'10"	132	139	146	153	160	167	174	181	188	195	202	209	216	222	229	236	243	250	257	264	271	278
5'11"	136	143	150	157	165	172	179	186	193	200	208	215	222	229	236	243	250	257	265	272	279	286
6'	140	147	154	162	169	177	184	191	199	206	213	221	228	235	242	250	258	265	272	279	287	294
6'1"	144	151	159	166	174	182	189	197	204	212	219	227	235	242	250	257	265	272	280	288	295	302
6'2"	148	155	163	171	179	186	194	202	210	218	225	233	241	249	256	264	272	280	287	295	303	311
6'3"	152	160	168	176	184	192	200	208	216	224	232	240	248	256	264	272	279	287	295	303	311	319
6'4"	156	164	172	180	189	197	205	213	221	230	238	246	254	263	271	279	287	295	304	312	320	328

Locate your height in inches along the left-hand column and then follow the row toward the right to the weight in pounds closest to yours. Your BMI is noted at the top of that column. For example, a person of a height of 5'6" weighing 173 pounds has a BMI of 28.

Now you know whether you are overweight, and if so, by how much. Are you ready to help yourself change? There are millions of Americans with the same problem. Caucasians, African-Americans, Native Americans, and Mexican-Americans all have the same problem: Too many of us are overweight. Whatever index you use, too many people are overweight. Look at Figure 1. It shows the percentages of Americans who are obese.

The number of obese Americans is increasing (see Figure 1 in the Introduction). Each year a sample of Americans from all fifty states are called on the telephone by their state health department and asked a number of questions about their health, including their height and weight. From these numbers the BMI is calculated, and then the percentage of people who are obese is determined. The results over the past fifteen years are shown in this map. Striking, isn't it? Each map shows a large increase in the percentage of fat Americans in each state. The Southeast tends to lead the way, with the high plateau states (Colorado, Wyoming, Utah, Montana, and Idaho) in the West having somewhat lower numbers of fat Americans. But it is the *increase* that is alarming. In 1991 only a few states were dark blue but by 1996, most states had their rates of obesity become dark blue. The progression continued with a few states showing the highest frequency of obesity (red) and most showing the next highest (tan) and the number of dark blue states receding.

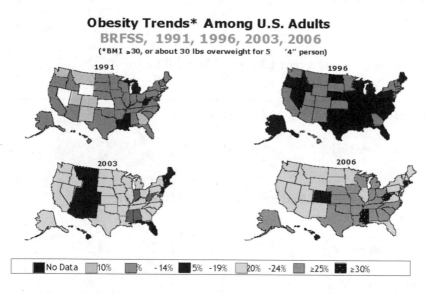

Obesity Trends* Among U.S. Adults
BRFSS, 1991, 1996, 2003, 2006
(*BMI ≥30, or about 30 lbs overweight for 5′4″ person)

Figure 1. Change in Percentage of Obese Americans from 1991 to 2006. The percentage of obese adults above age twenty has been estimated over the past fifteen years, and these maps show the changing pattern. There has been a rapid and impressive increase in the percentage of obese people, both men and women, in all of the United States. (Source: Centers for Disease Control and Prevention, *http://www.cdc. gov/nccdphp/dnpa/obesity/trend/maps/index.htm*)

Some Americans are fatter than others. The numbers below show the numbers of fat Americans by various ethnic groups. Among women, the African-Americans consistently show the highest rates, with Mexican-American women second. Among men, the only ethnic differences to note are at the highest BMI, where rates for African-American men are twice as high as for the other two groups.

Table 3. Prevalence of overweight (BMI 25–29.9), obesity (BMI > 30), and extreme obesity (BMI > 40) by various ethnic groups in men and women over twenty years of age in 2003–2004.

Category	Men	Women
Percent Overweight (BMI 25-29.9 kg/m^2)		
Non-Hispanic Caucasian	70.6	58.0
African-American	69.1	81.6
Mexican-American	76.1	75.4
Percent Obese (BMI > 30 kg/m^2)		
Non-Hispanic Caucasian	31.1	30.2
African-American	34.0	53.9
Mexican-American	31.6	42.3
Percent Extreme Obesity (BMI > 40 kg/m^2)		
Non-Hispanic Caucasian	2.8	5.8
African-American	5.4	14.7
Mexican-American	1.7	7.8

* Adapted from reference 7.

Where Is Your Fat Located?

In addition to the *amount* of fat on your body, *where* the fat is located is also important to your health. This distinction is often illustrated as "apples" versus "pears" (Figure 2). It can most easily be seen in the differences between men and women: Women tend to store fat on their hips and thighs—as "pears." With pregnancy, fat is stored in areas where it can be used when nursing a newborn baby.

Body Shape Matters!
"Central" Obesity

An Index of Abdominal versus Peripheral Obesity

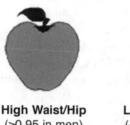

High Waist/Hip	Low Waist/Hip
(≥0.95 in men)	(<0.95 in men)
(≥0.80 in women)	(<0.80 in women)

Figure 2. "Apples" versus "Pears." This illustration presents two different body types as illustrated with the apple and pear. The difference is between upper-body fatness, depicted as the apple, where fat is located around the abdomen, and lower-body fatness, typified by the pear shape, where fat is located on the hips and thighs.

Fat on the hips and thighs is less risky than the same amount of fat on the abdomen—the so-called "beer belly"—which is typical of so many men. This is one reason women tend to live longer than men do in most cultures; they have less of this "risky" fat.

If a woman has a lot of central fat (an "apple" shape), it is just as hazardous to her health as it is to a man's. When women carry their fat in their belly, they are no longer likely to outlive men. Men generally start with more central fat in their belly, however, and this accounts for most of their early additional health problems, particularly diabetes, hypertension, gall bladder disease, and heart disease.

To determine the location of your fat, put a tape measure around your waist at its narrowest spot. If you are a man and it is more than 40 inches (102 cm) around or greater than 35 inches (88 cm) around and you are a woman, you are considered to be at a high health risk. If you have a high waist circumference, it is another reason you need to help yourself to a new healthy eating pattern.

Now that you know what is considered a normal weight and waist circumference and the category into which you fall, you probably would like to help yourself lose sufficient weight to fall into the "normal" category. For some, that is an entirely reasonable goal. But for others, it may be too optimistic to expect to do this with a single effort.

If you are young and have recently gained a few pounds but are within the normal BMI or weight range, you may be able to help yourself to a more normal weight with little trouble. Many who read this book, however, will be substantially overweight. My waist had become a bit too large for my pants and belts, so I went on a "weight-loss" program like the one described here. I did this myself by reading labels to determine the calories and learn whether there was "bad fructose" (HFCS or sugar) present, to use as a marker for highly processed foods. I then laid out a portion-controlled diet with about 300 calories for breakfast, 300 calories for lunch, and 600 to 900 calories for dinner, using the calorie values in foods. The pounds melted away at 1–2 pounds per week until I reached my goal. A reasonable weight goal is important for you. If your goal is not reasonable for you, your road to success may be frustrating.

What should you weigh? From the point of view of health, you would do well to have a BMI below 30, and even better, close to or below 25. If you are already below 25, you may still want to lose a few pounds to improve your quality of life. But from a health standpoint, there is no need to lose weight; it is mainly for your self-esteem.

For those of you with a BMI of more than 30, is it realistic to reduce it to below 25? At a BMI of 30, you are 20% overweight. If it is closer to 30 than to 35, the answer may be yes. If your BMI is above 35, your task is more difficult. The good news is you can receive substantial benefits from helping yourself lose even modest amounts of weight. For example, if you weigh 209 pounds (a BMI of 30 for someone 5' 10" tall), a loss of 20 pounds would be a tremendous benefit to your health. This would be 60% of your excess weight. It would be difficult for many people, particularly those who are older, to aim their sights on reducing that weight to 140 or 150 pounds. An unrealistic goal will get unrealistic results.

What is your weight today?   _____

What is your weight for BMI 25?   _____

How much weight loss to reach 25? _____

What is your goal weight?   _____

A goal that is more than 10% below your current weight is attainable, has health benefits, and will improve your quality of life. If you want to lose more, that is the next step. Once you establish a reasonable goal, it is also important to establish a reasonable time frame for the weight loss. Sure, you would like to be thin tomorrow. But of course, how long did it take you to gain that extra weight? I have seen an occasional patient who gained 100 pounds in a year or 200 pounds in two years. But this is very, very rare. It usually occurs a pound or two at a time over years.

Food Intake and Body Fat

We must get comfortable with a few simple truths. None of us can violate the laws of nature and get away with it. Even when you sleep, you lose weight because you burn fat. Although you are not eating, your body requires energy every minute to maintain life. When you sleep, you take this energy from the fat that is stored on your body.

Think of this fat as a fuel reservoir, like the gasoline tank on your car. The ten to twenty gallons of gasoline in your tank can take your car several hundred miles. But in the case of your body, the amount of energy in your "tank" is comparable to a tanker truck full of fuel that would supply your energy from fifty to more than two hundred days, depending on your starting weight!

You can picture how your extra weight is stored as fat by looking at Figure 3. There are two bars on the left and two on the right that show what happens to your body if you gain 66 pounds (30 kg). The bars with the four sections represent the chemical make-up of your body as water, protein, fat, and minerals at the lower weight of 154 pounds (70 kg) and again at the higher weight of 220 pounds (100 kg). The bar with the two sections represents the amount of energy (calories) that is stored in fat and protein. The difference in weight I used for these illustrations is 66 pounds (30 kg). About 75% of this extra weight is fat. But look at the tremendous difference this extra fat makes in the amount of extra fuel energy you are carrying around as fat. It nearly doubles, from 180,000 calories to 360,000 calories. This is a twelve-month supply of energy for your body rather than the six-month supply of energy at the lower weight. Body fat is like a fuel tank for heating oil in your house. It would be hard for your car to pull around that much fuel, and it is hard for your body!

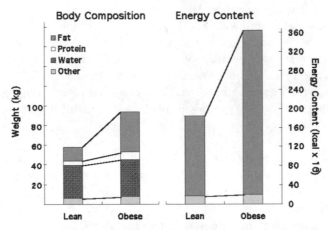

Figure 3. Body fat of a lean individual and an obese individual, who differ in weight by 30 kg (66 pounds). There are two bars for the lean individual and two bars for the obese individual. The left pair of bars are the weights of various components of the body at each weight. The right two bars are the energy or calorie values for the fat and protein that make up the body. The amount of energy in body fat nearly doubles when body weight increases by 50%—from 154 pounds (70 kg) to 220 pounds (100 kg).

Each day the energy from the food you eat is equivalent to less than 1% of the amount of energy you have as stores of fat in your fat tissue. In evolutionary terms, this was a great idea: When the food supply was short, our ancestors could live off their fat, so to speak. Even normal-weight men and women have enough fat to last several weeks with no food at all. Folks with a BMI above 40 have enough fuel in their tanks to last more than a year!

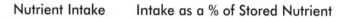

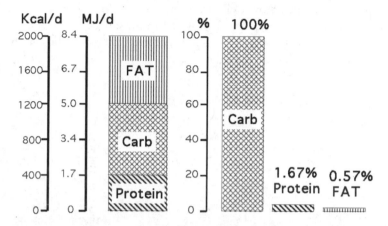

Figure 4. Your food intake in relation to the amount you have stored in your body. The left-hand column shows the calories from fat, carbohydrate, and protein in a 2000-kcal day's worth of food where 40% comes from carbohydrate (800 calories or 200 grams of carbohydrate), 40% from fat (800 calories or 89.9 grams of fat), and 20% from protein (400 calories or 100 grams of protein). In the three bars on the left, the percentage of the day's intake of carbohydrate, protein, and fat is related as a percent of the amount stored in your body. Carbohydrate each day is nearly the same as the total amount you have stored in your body, but fat is less than 1% and protein just over 1% in this illustration.

I have chosen a 2,000-calorie diet for the illustration in Figure 4. With this diet, the daily intake of carbohydrate is 40% of the total, fat was 40% of the total, and protein 20%. The amount of carbohydrate you eat each day is nearly the same as the amount of carbohydrate in your body. This has an important meaning for us. Our bodies can't convert fat (fatty acids) into the glucose (blood sugar). Thus we must eat carbohydrate or make it from the building blocks of protein (amino acids) each day. The carbohydrate our bodies need is glucose—the main sugar in starch. There is no dietary need for fructose—either for good fructose or particularly for "bad fructose." This is one reason why I am focusing on reducing the "bad fructose" in your diet to allow you to reduce calories, but to get the other important nutrients, protein, and essential fats your body needs. In contrast, your daily intake of fat is less than 1% of the amount of fat you have stored in your body, and protein is only a little more than 1% of the total amount of stored protein.

Obviously, the more fuel you have stored on your body as fat, the longer it will take to reduce this inventory. The length of time it took to put on the weight gives you a good idea of how long it will take to lose it. Figure 5 below gives a reasonable expectation for the time it will take us to help you lose your desired weight. Slow weight loss would be a half a pound a week or so, shown in the top line. Rapid weight loss would be more than two pounds per week, shown in the lower line. Almost everyone who wants to lose weight will fall within these limits.

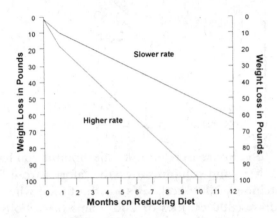

Figure 5. Expected rates of weight loss. Find the amount of weight you want to lose on the left or right vertical scale, then draw a horizontal line across the figure. The points where that line cross the "higher-rate" and "slower-rate" slopes are directly above the "months" it will take to lose that amount of weight.

Managing your weight loss is like managing your checking account. You have to keep track of your income and expenses to determine your account balance. And if you want the balance to increase, you have to either spend less or save more.

But I hardly eat anything at all! It's time to understand another one of Mother Nature's cold, hard facts: If you are gaining weight as fat, then you are eating more than your body needs. If you want to decrease your "fat checking account" balance, then you have to "spend" more energy from your fat than you are taking in.

It is easy to be mistaken about how much you actually eat. Calorie counting is challenging. Believe me, I've tried it. I'm a physician and scientist and have all the accurate equipment at my disposal to do it well. For two weeks, I took accurate balances and measuring equipment home, wrote down everything I ate, and used my calorie books to estimate how many calories each dish contained.

How did I do? I was way off. I guessed that my cereal was 1 ounce, and it was 1½ ounces. The estimates of fruit sizes were off by more than 10%, and my estimates of meat were worse. This experience taught me how difficult it is to accurately count calories. This difficulty has now been demonstrated by several scientific studies that found that overweight men and women typically *under*estimate how much they eat by at least 30%. On top of that, they also *over*estimate their daily activity levels by up to 50%.

With those figures in mind, I've learned not to place too much reliance on diet records and calorie charts. This is one test in which almost nobody can come up with the right answer. To convince myself of this, we did an experiment at the Pennington Center. We reasoned that if any group of people could keep accurate records of the foods they ate, it would be dietitians. They know food—they plan menus for a living. So we asked ten dietitians to record what they ate at each meal for a full week. During this time, and with their knowledge, we measured their total energy needs using a very accurate measurement known as the doubly labeled water technique. If done well, it gives a fool-proof answer to the question of how much energy you used. At the end of the week, we added up what they ate and how much energy they expended. The records kept by our dietitians were very close to their actual food intake. They recorded 94% of the food needed to match the energy expenditure estimated from doubly labeled water. The big shock to me was the wide range of food eaten from day to day. I show this in Figure 6. Some women varied by as much as 2000 calories from one day to the next. Yet over seven days, the amount of energy they put into their bodies was quite close to their actual energy expenditure. Obviously, we have some longer-term ways of balancing our bodies' checkbooks than single meals.

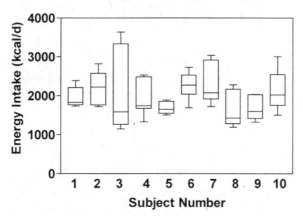

Energy Intake over 7 days

Figure 6. Daily food intake provided by ten dietitians. Energy intake during this seven-day period was very close to the total energy expended.

Note the wide day-to-day variation for each of the ten people. Variations were as high as 50% of the average intake.

This graph shows what ten different dietitians ate for one week. The line in the middle large bar is their median intake for the week in calories. The solid bars are the range from the 25th percentile to the 75th percentile during this week. What is striking is the wide day-to-day differences in food intake for a single individual who nonetheless averaged very close to their energy expenditure over the entire seven days. These bars tell us measurement of food intake for any single day for an individual has real limitations. Three days are better, but seven days seems to give a good picture of intake.

Fortunately, as I said earlier, most of us gain weight relatively slowly. And we all lose weight each and every night of our lives when we go to sleep. There are proven solutions to your weight problem that don't require a compulsion for calorie counting.

A patient of mine moved out of town and called back a few months later to tell me that his weight had gone up by 10 pounds. What was he to do? I advised him to begin the program I'll describe later to tackle the problem before it got out of hand. Like most other tasks in life, practice improves you. And continuing to practice this program and take small steps forward will make it work even better for you.

CHAPTER TWO

Get Set

Set-Point and Other Things You Wanted to Know about Being Overweight but Were Afraid to Ask

Why Do Some People Gain Weight More Easily than Others? Not everyone is overweight. Why were you unlucky? How can you change it? Good questions! We are living in a time of "epidemic obesity." Over the last fifteen years, the number of obese Americans has gone up by more than 50%.[1] You saw this in the last chapter. This epidemic is spreading worldwide.

Although the number of overweight people has gone up worldwide, not everyone gets fat. The increasing problem affects mainly those who are in the upper part of the weight curve. The thinnest people seem to be at little risk. It is the chubby children and slightly overweight adolescents and young adults who are most likely to become overweight. By helping yourself lose weight, you are also helping your family members avoid this epidemic in their own lives. There is clearly a "contagious" part to being overweight.[2] The network of relationships of people living in one small community was tracked for thirty-two years (1971–2003). Obesity spread among the 12,067 people in this network. One's chances of developing obesity (BMI>30 kg/m^2) increased by 57% if a friend became obese, by 40% if an adult sibling became obese, and by 37% if a spouse became obese. Thus you can have an important influence not just on yourself, but you can help others in your family and family network by managing your own weight.

"An ounce of prevention is worth a pound of cure." Helping yourself early may be that ounce of prevention that will help your loved ones who are not now overweight from becoming that way. It is particularly important to address small weight changes, since it is easier to make small changes than to make large ones. *Tip*: Weigh yourself regularly. Just like your bank account, which you check monthly and where you take action if it gets too low, for your weight the action needs to be taken before it gets too high. Scientific data has shown that stepping on a scale regularly helps reduce weight gain.[3]

Why do some people shift from pre-overweight to overweight and others do not? One reason is passive over-consumption of "bad fructose" and fat. Fatty foods taste so good, particularly *sweet* fatty foods—the "deadly duo." They melt in your mouth, and the waste goes to your waist, but they sure taste good. The number of overweight individuals is higher in the countries where people eat high-fat diets (such as the U.S. and Italy). This is shown in the accompanying figure. The information came from the United Nations Food and Agricultural Organization. It shows that, in general, the higher the fat intake in a country, the larger the number of people there were in that country who are overweight. In the research laboratory, giving any group of animals a high-fat diet will fatten up almost all of them.

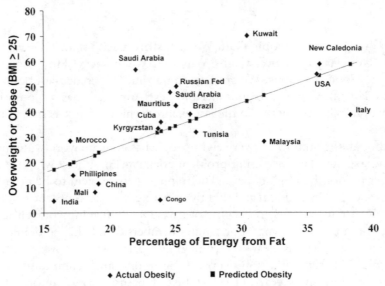

Figure 1. Relation of the percentage of energy from fat to the percentage of people in several countries who are overweight or obese, using information from the World Health Organization and the Food and Agricultural Organization of the United Nations.[4]

But why should a high-fat diet fatten some people but not others? Here is where our genes come into play. They determine how our bodies use the foods we eat. A high-fat diet is also a low-carbohydrate diet, since fat and carbohydrate are the major parts of our daily food intake. Carbohydrate can be converted to fat, but fat cannot be converted back into carbohydrate. There is a one-way street from carbohydrate to fat. To keep our body in balance, we have to burn the amount of carbohydrate and fat we eat each day, as I described in the last chapter. If we burn slightly more carbohydrate each day than we eat, we will gradually deplete the body's carbohydrate, since we can't convert fat to carbohydrate. Then your body has two choices. If you are burning more carbohydrate than you have stored up, your body can either burn less carbohydrate OR you will have to eat more food to get the carbohydrate you need to replace what your body has burned up. A high-fat diet makes less carbohydrate available so the body must burn more fat. One way to help you help yourself burn more fat is to become more active. Even moderate amounts of increased activity can increase the amount of fat you burn and conserve your body's stored carbohydrate.[5,6] Your genes provide the directions to make the body's machinery move in the appropriate direction. If your genes don't direct the body to conserve carbohydrate when you eat a high-fat diet, your brain will get a message that you need more carbohydrate, which you will get by eating more food. When this happens, you get slightly more calories from fat (9 calories per gram) than you get from carbohydrate (4 calories per gram). Thus having your "carbohydrate tank" well stocked is important for helping your body control its weight through the messages from a "full tank" of carbohydrate stores.

Another way to help yourself build your carbohydrate reserves, which exist as glycogen in your liver and muscle, is to eat more carbohydrate. This is how athletes store the glycogen in their muscles they need for physical activity. If you eat more carbohydrate, the result will be more energy for your body, but beware of the type of carbohydrate. Choose whole grains and leave the bad fructose and fat combinations on the shelf in the store. To get the same amount of carbohydrate but not increase your total energy intake, you can reduce your use of foods with fat. That is, choose lower-fat, lower-fructose foods. Foods with more fiber have a lower glycemic index and may help you feel fuller and allow you to get the carbohydrate you need. These better-carbohydrate foods are found mainly as whole-grain products, less refined foods, and food with more fiber. Here is where watching food labels for bad fructose (HFCS and sugar, particularly when combined with fat or in beverages) can help. I will help you help yourself to nutritious and healthful foods after discussing some of the other things you always wanted to know.

Set-point, brown fat, heredity, fat cells, smoking, pregnancy, carbohydrate cravings, depression, risk from being overweight, bad fructose, and uric acid. Each of these can affect your weight and has been the subject of many stories in the popular press. Let me try to demystify some of them. I will also give you my perspective on them and help clear the way for your weight-management success. Then you can decide how important they are to you.

Set-Point: Do You Have One?

What is a set-point? If you live in a cold climate, you use a furnace to heat your home. Your furnace has a thermostat. If you live in a hot climate, like I do, you use an air conditioner, which also has a temperature-control device. Thermostats and temperature-control devices are the engineers' way of turning your furnace or air conditioner on and off to regulate your environment. They work around the "set-point" of your selected temperature.

A set-point for body weight is a concept some scientists have proposed for how your brain might control food intake. No one has scientifically identified a "set-point" in you or me—it is only a way of thinking. Any good thermostat can keep your house temperature comfortable—at a temperature where you set it. If there were a good "set-point" in our body, our body weight and our body fat stores would be similarly well regulated.[8,9] During the course of a year, an adult man will eat about 1 million calories and an adult woman about 750,000 calories. During that time, most people's weight doesn't change by more than a pound or two; only the unfortunate few gain more than this. To balance this million calories of food with a one-pound gain in weight, you must burn 996,500 of these calories (a pound of fat stores about 3,500 calories). During this year, your body would have made an error of less than half percent (0.5%) in energy storage—pretty darn good, I would say. This implies an important regulatory system for weight control in most people over time intervals of several months. This is also shown in a very nice trial where a weight-loss drug was given for one year and then replaced with an inactive medicine (placebo) during the second year.[9] During the first year, there was a weight loss of about 20 pounds. When the switch was made, individuals regained weight during the second year at almost exactly the same rate they lost it in the first year—another great demonstration of a regulatory system with a set-point that works.

But we all know weight varies and some people get fat more easily than others. Thus the set-point works better in some people than in others, and any simple idea of a set-point doesn't fit very well with how we live and the fattening of America. The way I look at it is that we have a set-point, but it can go bad in some circumstances. To give it a scientific name, I call it a "homeostatic system with an hedonic override." A homeostatic system is the "set-point" we have been describing. The "hedonic override" refers to the fact that pleasurable foods can prevent the set-point system from working correctly. This was brought home to me repeatedly in studying why some animals get fat eating a high-fat diet and others do not. The ones that get fat "like their food"—it gives them a kind of pleasure, a hedonic or pleasurable feeling. This pleasure sense limits the effectiveness of the set-point—hence, "homeostatic system with an hedonic override."

One of my colleagues thinks that for people trying to manage their weight, waistbands or belts may be your most important "set-point" devices.[10] He asked several overweight people to come into a hospital program for several weeks. They were supplied with loose-fitting hospital gowns, and their own clothes were taken away so they did not have the usual "constricting" items around their waists. They could eat all they wanted. Without the external information from belts and well-fitting clothing, they all gained weight. For this study, each subject served as their own "control," since weight changes were compared before and after changing the types of clothing they wore.

You can use this belt idea yourself. Many fashion models already do. If you wear a belt regularly, make sure it remains at the same setting. If you feel you need to let it out, you know it is time to do something about your weight, unless you want to gain weight. Some fashion models wear a copper or gold waistband. Indeed, this is what gave my colleague his original idea. A simpler technique, and the one he has used, is to place a nylon string around the waist so it is snug but not too tight. Then fasten it securely and leave it in place twenty-four hours a day. When your weight begins to rise, you will know it because the cord becomes tighter.

The bathroom scale may be your best "set-point." For the subjects in the hospital (the ones wearing loose-fitting clothes) with no scales to read, there was no outside indicator of their weight. They gained weight. If used regularly, your bathroom scale can help you help yourself with clues about changes in your weight.[3] I often weigh myself in the morning after getting up and emptying my bladder and before putting on any clothes. In this way, I can catch changes in my weight before they have gotten beyond five pounds. The sooner you catch a "drift" in your weight, the easier it is to correct it. My Motto: Know thyself—know your weight, and help yourself sooner rather than later.

Brown Fat: The Furnace Within

"Brown fat" got its name from its reddish brown color.[12] It is a special kind of fat, which differs from most of your fat, which is "white." All babies have brown fat. It is a heat furnace that helps them keep warm just after birth. When it doesn't work, infants cannot maintain their body temperature very well. As we grow up, our brown fat is no longer needed and it largely disappears. In small mammals, such as rats and mice, brown fat remains an important heat furnace throughout life.

Brown fat achieved notoriety because it was found to be under-active in most forms of obesity in animals. Because it becomes inactive in human adults, it has been suggested that brown fat may play a role in why some people become fat. Activating this heat furnace in overweight adults has also been suggested as a way to treat obesity.[12] The chemicals that turn on the brown fat "furnace" keep experimental animals from getting fat. The search was on to find similar chemicals to help people. Several drugs have been developed that can turn on brown fat in animals, but none have yet been successful in human beings.[13] This may be because humans have too little brown fat or because the chemicals that turn on brown fat metabolism in animals do not work well in human beings. One advantage of the brown fat furnace is that it burns primarily fat. When this metabolic furnace is turned on, heat is produced, and fat is burned up. Heat for fat. Most of us with a weight problem would jump at this possibility. It is like exercising to lose fat without having to exercise. As I say, stay tuned.

The Genes in Your Jeans

Do you inherit fatness? We all know people who come from families in which everyone is overweight. This is nowhere more clearly stated than by the character Johnny Tarleton in George Bernard Shaw's play[14] *Misalliance*. Johnny says, "No matter how little you eat, you put on flesh if you're made that way." A great deal of work has gone into finding out how important genes are in making you overweight and how this can be used to help you help yourself in your fight against fat. Some animals are born to be fat.[15] In biological terms, they are "genetically predisposed." Both so-called dominantly and recessively transmitted types of fatness are known. Many different chromosomes influence body fat. We already know of several types of genetic obesity in human beings, but they are very rare.[16]

If your parents were overweight, you have a much higher likelihood of being overweight yourself. How much higher? To answer this question, we need to separate the environment (nurture) from genetic influences (nature). This can be done by studying adopted children who are raised with biological children in the same family. It turns out that adopted children are more like their biological parents than their adoptive parents in terms of weight status.[17] The adopted children also have body weights that are also more like their biological brothers and sisters than their adoptive brothers and sisters.

We all know twins. Identical twins are remarkably similar, but fraternal twins are often very different, being as much like the other brothers and sisters in the family as their twin.[18] These differences between types of twins provide another way to distinguish the influences of environment from those of genetics. The weights of identical twins are much closer together than those of fraternal twins. Genes are important, but don't get discouraged and blame it all on your genes. As twins get older, they become less alike in terms of weight status. Environment has a big impact, and this is where you can help yourself.

The genetic factors that influence fatness and where fat is laid down are defined by your "susceptibility" genes. These genes are the ones that make you more likely to become fat in any given family or setting. If you are susceptible, and food is available, you have a high likelihood of becoming fat. If you are not susceptible, then the presence of high-fat foods, too much bad fructose, or a culture in which we do not exercise much, is less important. The best guess is that 30 to 50% of the differences in fatness between people results from genetic differences. The FTO gene is a recent addition to the list of genes causing obesity in children and adults. People with one form of this gene may weigh 6-7 pounds more than people with another form of the gene.[20] The rest, 50 to 70%, however, is from how we live: our environment. This is where you can help yourself.

Genetic and Non-genetic Influences in Obesity

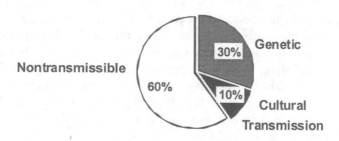

Bouchard et al Int J Obes 1988;12:205

Figure 1. Your genes and overweight. This pie chart shows one estimate of the genetic influences on body fatness. Using twins and other family members, the similarity in percent body fat was estimated and divided into the non-transmissible (not related to genetic or cultural factors) and transmissible parts. Of the transmissible part, due to genes and family culture, about 25% was genetic and 15% cultural. Clearly genetics is important, but the environment, that is the non-transmissible part, is more important.

Overweight dogs provide another example of how the environment can affect everyone in the household. Overweight dogs are becoming more common. One veterinarian did a survey of the animals that were brought to his office and compared their weights with the weights of the pets' owners. He found that overweight dogs usually have overweight owners.[21] Certainly the weight of the dog in a household in which overweight people live is not the result of genes! It must be the environment. The scraps of rich table food that are so readily available can cause weight problems for both dogs and their masters.

What should we say about genes, then? First, they are important in your *risk* of becoming overweight: Some people have genes that increase their risk of becoming fat. But even in the presence of these genes, you can help yourself and your loved ones to a healthy diet. *You* are still in charge—without food, you cannot become fat. Eating foods of the kinds and amounts that your body needs is where you can help yourself most.

Medications That Can Cause Weight Gain

Even without genes for fatness, however, you can become fat. Several diseases and medications used for other diseases can lead to weight gain.[22] The most important of these are the medicines we use to treat many major illnesses. For example, some medications used to treat depression, epilepsy, or mental illness can also cause weight gain. If you need one of these medications, ask your physician whether s/he can use one that does not aggravate your weight problem. Another example is the drugs used to treat diabetes. Many of them produce weight gain, although two of them, metformin and exenatide, actually produce weight loss. If you are taking medication to treat diabetes, talk to your physician about whether your medication is likely to affect your weight. Still other medicines used to treat asthma or allergies and that are used in preventing the rejection of organ transplants can cause weight gain. Finally, some drugs used to treat glandular problems can cause weight gain. Here again, you need to talk to your physician.

Diseases That Can Cause Weight Gain

An important problem for some girls maturing sexually is a disease called polycystic ovary syndrome, or PCOS for short. Girls who have irregular menstrual periods, weight gain, and more body hair than normal may have this problem. If you think this describes you or a loved one, you should discuss this possibility with your physician.[23]

Tumors that develop in the base of the brain and damage the regions that control appetite often produce weight gain.[24] Certain glandular diseases, particularly ones involving the adrenal gland, can produce obesity. Except for medications that cause weight gain, where you can help yourself by using alternative medicines, these other causes of overweight are fortunately quite rare.

Metabolic Rate and Weight

Does a low metabolism cause you to gain weight? I have been told repeatedly by my patients, "Doctor, everything I eat turns to fat because my metabolism is out of order." I have spent a lot of time learning about the metabolism of people who are overweight. I have measured metabolic rate. I have turned rooms into metabolic machines to be able to measure people around the clock. I have taken food records without end. Finally, I have used a new technique called doubly labeled water to measure metabolism. This test measures your metabolism twenty-four hours a day for 7–14 days while you are doing your daily activities of life. It tells us that almost everyone underreports the amount of food they eat. People who are overweight tend to underreport more than normal-weight people. To illustrate this, I have shown the results of a recent study in Figure 2. The people who volunteered kept food-intake records to the best of their ability. They also participated in a study to measure the energy they used each day. The energy their bodies actually used was 6 to 16% higher than the amount of food energy that they recorded (and there was no weight loss), so they must have under-counted calories.[25] This supports my long-standing distrust of food records to estimate your daily food intake, but calorie counting can be very useful for some people when it comes to losing weight. For those who record carefully and accurately, calorie counting can be a useful technique that we will expand below.

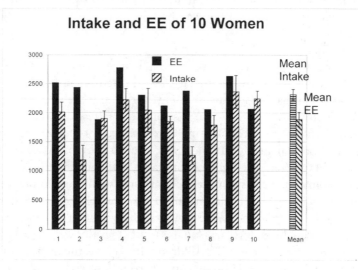

Figure 2. Underreporting of food intake. Each pair of bars shows the energy expenditure estimated from doubly labeled water (solid bar) and average from the seven days of energy intake from food-intake records for the same ten women who were depicted in Chapter 1.

For many overweight people, the dietary records they keep on their food intake are 50% or more below what they actually need to *maintain* their weight. For lean people, it tends to be closer to 10–30% too low. Why do some people underreport more than others? I don't know. What this does tell me, however, is that counting calories accurately is very hard. Some people are excellent at it, and you may be one. Most people are not. Unless you are the type of person who wants to use measuring cups and a balance at home and food labels in the store, calorie counting is probably not the way for you to help yourself.

The *heavier* you are, the *higher* your metabolism! Machines to measure metabolic rate and the doubly labeled water technique all show this. The mystery is gone. The solution for making us better observers of what we eat, however, is not yet at hand.

Overweight people have many changes in the way their bodily systems function. The list is long. Most of these changes return to normal when you lose weight, but there is one exception. It is the gatekeeper for fat storage. A key protein—an enzyme—called lipoprotein lipase (LPL)—is high when you are overweight. LPL is the enzyme that helps fat cells transfer fat molecules from the blood into the fat cell. When you lose a lot of weight, the amount of this LPL enzyme in your body seems to go even higher. When LPL goes up with weight loss, it makes it easier to get fat back into the fat cells. This may well be one factor in how easy it is to *regain* weight and why some people have trouble losing weight.

Your Fat Cells

Fat cells are where fat is at. We normally have about 40–60 billion of them[26]—nearly ten times as many fat cells in one human body as there are people on Earth! Fat cells do many things for us, but their major job is storing fat. When we are born, we are among the fattest mammals on Earth. Only baby whales are fatter! During the first year of life, we become even fatter, and body fat nearly doubles. But the number of fat cells does not increase—they merely get bigger. You can see this in Figure 3. There is a steep line connecting the size of fat cells at birth with those at one year. This is the near-doubling that occurs in the size of fat cells in babies during the first year of life. During the next 2–4 years, the *size* of fat cells decreases dramatically in lean children (black squares) but does not decrease as much in children who are overweight. In children who get fat, the *number* of fat cells begins to rise (Figure 4). This continues throughout childhood and reaches a peak in adult life. At one time, the *number* of fat cells was thought to be a major cause of fatness. No more. In most cases, people who are fat increase the number of fat cells their body, since a single cell can only get so big. To store more fat, new cells appear. The life of the fat cell has undergone a recent reexamination. There are now some data suggesting that fat cells are being born and dying at a regular rate.[27] This offers new hope of a way to control the number of fat cells you have.

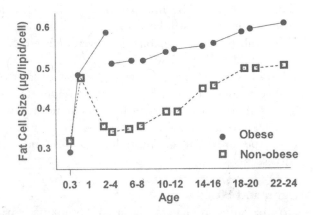

Figure 3. Fat cell growth. The changes in the size of fat cells in children who eventually became fat and those who did not are shown. Note that in the first year of life, the sizes of fat cells started at the same level and increased to the same size in both groups. After the first year, the differences in size became apparent. Fat children had larger fat cells.[26]

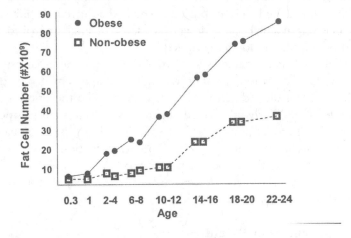

Figure 4. The numbers of fat cells are shown. Fat children have more fat cells, but this only becomes evident after 1 year of age.[26]

It is not overfeeding in infancy that increases the *number* of fat cells. The doubling of fat in the first year of life does not increase the number of fat cells but makes each cell much bigger. When babies lose this early baby fat, the number of fat cells begins to increase in children destined to become overweight. This is well after weaning. So mothers, fat children are not from your infant feeding practices. The number of fat cells seems to be programmed into these babies who will become fat. You can still help an overweight child learn healthy nutrition habits, however, and reduce the impact of childhood overweight as they grow into adults.

A fat child who has one fat parent is at higher risk of later obesity and needs to be weighed to identify this risk if his or her weight starts to increase significantly. Infants of diabetic mothers and infants of mothers who smoked during pregnancy are also at increased risk of becoming overweight.[22] Babies from any of these types of parents are more likely to become overweight as children and adolescents.

Smoking, Weight, and Health

Thirty years ago, the Surgeon General declared, "Smoking is bad for your health." Many people have given up smoking. Airline flights in the United States are now non-smoking. Yet more than 25% of adults still smoke. Many patients tell me that when they stop smoking, they gain weight. This is true: Most people who stop smoking do gain weight—an average of 5–10 pounds or more.[28] This is one reason why many people, particularly women, start smoking again. The nicotine in cigarette smoke stimulates your metabolism. When people stop smoking, food intake goes up and metabolism goes down. My wife used to smoke. She is typical of many: When she stopped smoking, she gained weight, but once she had adjusted to "life after smoking," her weight slowly came down. Her sense of smell improved, and foods tasted better. She no longer coughed.

There are many strategies to control the weight gain that usually occurs after smoking cessation. Joining a weight-management group that uses a portion-control diet (described later), which is like the one I used earlier, can be helpful. After you are through the "withdrawal" from smoking, one of the pills approved for control of smoking (bupropion, Zyban) may be helpful with your weight control, along with a portion-controlled diet that you can buy at the supermarket, drug store, or health-food store. Remember, even if you are a few pounds heavier after you stop smoking, you will have a much longer and healthier life.

Pregnancy and Your Weight

During pregnancy, a woman is growing a new life, which needs nourishment. She provides this nourishment from the foods she eats. Trying to lose weight during pregnancy is a bad idea. Keeping your weight gain in control, however, is a good idea. For most women, weight gains of 20–25 pounds are best. A few women tend to gain much more—up to 50 pounds or more. If you see this happening, seek help.

After the baby is born, most women lose weight, but on average a woman will be 2–5 pounds heavier a year after the baby is born than her pre-pregnancy weight. Small additions to your weight will probably occur with each pregnancy. Women with more pregnancies are heavier. One way to lose pregnancy weight, particularly fat from the thighs, is to nurse the baby. A recent study showed me that women who nurse their babies lose more of the fat that is stored up during pregnancy to provide energy to nourish their newborn baby.[29]

Carbohydrate Craving
Do you crave carbohydrates? Do you have a "sweet tooth?" Millions of people do. The "bad fructose" in HFCS and the sucrose molecule satisfy this sweet tooth. That is why the soft drink, sweetened fruit drink, candy, and pastry industries are so large. For some people, this is no problem. But for others, it can be.

The carbohydrate in bread and potatoes is starch that can be rapidly digested and therefore can increase blood glucose rapidly. Starchy foods that increase blood glucose rapidly are by definition called high-glycemic-index foods. Starchy foods that are digested more slowly usually have more fiber, which releases the glucose more slowly. The rise of blood glucose is slower. Some diets use this concept of glycemic index as a basis for recommending foods. The limitation of this concept is that what goes into the intestine from the stomach depends on what's in the stomach at the time. Mixing a high-glycemic-index food with other foods will change the blood glucose rise. Even with this limitation, it is good advice to eat more whole-grain foods and to leave the highly processed foods—which most often have a high glycemic index—on the shelf. Fructose, whether "good" from fruits or "bad" from HFCS or sucrose, has a low glycemic index. This is because fructose is NOT glucose and thus is not measured by the tests that measure glucose to determine glycemic index. In spite of its low glycemic index, fructose has other problems we will discuss shortly.

The problem with many of the snack foods we call high-carbohydrate foods is that they often also contain fat. Before you blame "carbohydrates" alone, make sure the so-called high-carbohydrate foods you crave do not also have a lot of fat. To do this, you will need to read the label on the package. The combination of bad fructose and fat is very tasty—and, as Yudkin said, "pure, white, and deadly."[32]

Feeling Blue Affects Your Weight
Feeling sad, discouraged? These can be signs of depression. Depression, particularly among overweight people, is common. Sleeplessness, the "blues," frequent crying spells, and thoughts of the uselessness of life are other signs.

If these are common thoughts for you and they are making it difficult for you to do your work or have fun, you may need help.

Depression sometimes occurs during weight loss. One of the best examples of diet-induced depression was reported during World War II. A group of conscientious objectors volunteered to participate in a scientific study on starvation as an alternative to combat duty.[33] They were given half the amount of food they needed to maintain their body weight. As expected, they gradually lost weight over six months. As they lost weight, they also lost interest in many other things, including companionship, women, and conversation. Their thoughts turned more and more to food. When they had lost the *planned* amount of weight, they could think about nothing but food. This increase in hunger often happens to overweight people, too, when they have lost a lot of weight. It can be a major problem in a program for losing weight. If it occurs to you, you may need to seek additional help beyond what I can provide through this book.

Overweight Is Risking Fate

One slogan says, "Overweight is risking fate." We already defined overweight and how to measure it, and you already know whether you are overweight. If you are overweight, it makes you more liable to get diabetes, heart disease, gall bladder disease, high blood pressure, and some kinds of cancer.[34,35] This is illustrated in Figure 5. The road map for nutrition (Chapters 4 and 5) and the chapters on successful ways to eat will help you reduce these risks

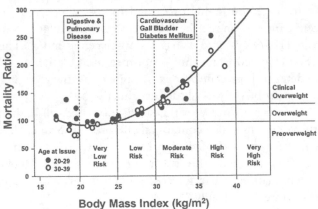

Figure 5. Increasing body weight increases your health risks for many diseases and your risk of mortality. These data are from the life insurance statistics. The "age at issue" refers to the age at which the

insurance policies were issued. The diseases listed in the right upper box are those associated with overweight (BMI >25) and those in the left-hand box with underweight (BMI <20). The lowest risk of disease occurs when the BMI is between 20 and 25 and increases thereafter with higher body mass index (BMI). This is indicated by the vertical dashed lines.

Good Fructose, Bad Fructose, and Uric Acid

Dietary fructose comes from several sources. It is present in fruits and is particularly plentiful in dates, raisins, figs, grapes, apples, pears, persimmons, and blueberries. In these fruits and others with lesser amounts, it serves as a pleasurable reward for eating something that also contains many other nutrients, including vitamin C. The high amount of fructose in apples and grapes is why the concentrates of these juices, which contain basically only the "fructose," are used to blend "fruit drinks." The fructose in whole fruits I call "good fructose" because it contains these other important nutrients. Dietary fructose also comes from high-fructose corn syrup, sucrose (fructose is one half of this molecule), and from fruit juice concentrates, which are little other than the fructose and other sweeteners from the initial fruits, stripped of most of the other nutrients. These I call "bad fructose" because the foods in which they are used usually have little else than "calories"—they are bereft of most if not all of the other nutrients that were originally present in the plant.

Fructose, both good and bad, is absorbed into the body from our digestive track. As I said earlier, fructose, both good and bad, has a low glycemic index because it is not measured as "glucose." Both good and bad fructose, however, have calories. Fructose is burned mainly in the liver. When this happens, the processes in the liver can produce an end product called uric acid. The higher amounts of fructose we are eating as a result mainly of high use of bad fructose in HFCS and sucrose produce more of this uric acid and may help explain part of why there is a relationship between uric acid and heart disease.

Several studies now suggest that ingesting fructose, most of which is from bad fructose, increases our risk of disease and ill health. Drinking large amounts of soft drinks (which are sweetened primarily with high-fructose corn syrup or sucrose) is related to risk of the metabolic syndrome.[36] This syndrome is usually present if you have a large waist measurement along with an increase in blood pressure, an increase in blood glucose, or abnormalities in two of the circulating blood fats (high triglycerides or low high-density lipoprotein-cholesterol (HDL-cholesterol)). Individuals consuming one or more soft drinks per day were more likely to have the metabolic syndrome, and if they didn't have it, they were at higher risk of developing the metabolic syndrome over four years. In a study of Swiss children, those with the higher intake of fructose had more of the "bad" form of cholesterol: low-density lipoprotein-cholesterol (LDL-cholesterol).[37] Finally, drinking increased amount of soft drinks, most of which have bad fructose in the sweetener, is associated in men with a higher risk of developing a joint disease called gout, which is a very painful swelling of the joints.[38]

Yo-yo Dieting

Have you been on a diet before? Surveys of Americans find that more than 50% of us have dieted at one time or another.[39] Adolescent girls and young women frequently go on diets. The months just after the holiday season in the winter are the peak times for diets. The lure is thinness before the summer season. You don't want to have bumpy and flabby thighs or a pouching stomach when the summer season comes.

Fashion also dictates dieting. In our culture, thin women are thought to be more attractive. This is different from the preferences in earlier centuries. One college survey indicated that men would prefer to marry a drug-addicted woman rather than a fat one. Thus there is great pressure for a slim, trim, thin you.

Bulimia, or gorging and purging, can be one consequence of this cult of thinness. It is one of the concerns about the risks of frequent dieting, particularly in adolescents. When I was in medical school, bulimia was almost unheard of. During the 1970s, this problem became more frequent. Now it is a clinical disease in the list of major psychiatric diseases. Purging, vomiting, gorging, and the use of laxatives are hallmarks of bulimia. Learn what is involved in successful control of weight and put these strategies into your everyday life, making healthy weight loss your goal. This will reduce the risk of bulimia.

So you have been on a diet before—maybe more than once. Since many diets don't teach permanent lifestyle changes, most people who go on a diet regain weight once they stop the diet. They go on a diet a second time, lose weight, and regain it. This up-and-down pattern of losing and regaining weight is called weight cycling. Other names are "yo-yo dieting" and "the rhythm method of girth control." You may have had this experience yourself.

What is wrong with yo-yoing or weight cycling? Several years ago, reports began to suggest that weight cycling might be bad for you. One report suggested that after a weight cycle, you tended to become more overweight. Another suggested that you might be more resistant to losing weight a second time after the first weight cycle. Still other reports suggested that yo-yo dieting might be bad for your health. One of these studies showed that losing and regaining weight was particularly bad for people of normal weight as compared to more overweight people. I have reviewed these data. The people with weights at the upper level of normal showed more risk of ill health as they gained or lost more weight. People who were slightly overweight also showed some risk to their health. But the people who were most overweight showed the least effects on their health of gaining and losing weight.

How bad is weight cycling? The reports described above have been widely publicized by the popular press. Unfortunately the popular press is not held to rigid guidelines of peer review. Rather, it is the sensationalism of the story that sells magazines, and this is what gets published. Since these early reports, a lot of other studies have been done, including some of my own. In addition, the National Institutes of Health have reviewed this information on your behalf and published a critique of the studies.[40] They concluded that "The currently available evidence [about weight cycling] is not sufficiently compelling to override the potential benefits of moderate weight loss in significantly obese patients." They go on to encourage individuals with weight problems to choose programs that emphasize long-term changes in eating behavior, diet, and activity. That is exactly what I emphasize here.

The sensationalism given to weight cycling by our magazines and newspapers was overdone. Until more data become available, I subscribe to the position of the expert panel from the NIH. This book is designed to help you lose the weight you want to lose, and by learning about your weight problem at the same time, it is designed to help you select what works best and to keep using it.

Older people have a lower metabolism and may be less active. Thus you might think they would have more trouble losing weight. Not so. One large study that used techniques like those described later in this book for changing eating behavior actually found that the older overweight people were more successful.[41] Maybe they have more time. Maybe they are more committed. Whatever the reason, they can do it. We have learned that individuals who are at high risk for diabetes can delay or prevent its onset by losing an average of 7% of their initial body weight. Just think of the advantages of delaying or avoiding insulin injections or other treatments for diabetes, just by losing a little weight and keeping it off!

Lose Weight, Live Longer

We noted earlier the relation of increasing weight to an increased risk of dying early and to having diabetes, heart disease, gall bladder disease, bone and joint diseases, and some kinds of cancer. Does losing weight lengthen your life? This missing link in our understanding of obesity has now been found. Several studies show that lowering body weight and keeping it lower over a period of years can increase the length of life. [42,43] Good news for all of us who work to control our body weight!

CHAPTER THREE

Think Positively about Losing Weight

Words are powerful. They help you help yourself gain the power you need to manage your weight successfully. Words are an invaluable tool in helping you set your goals and finding the path to help you reach your goals. Most importantly, words will help you reap the rewards of your efforts. We will use words to learn to think positively. In turn, thinking positively will make your goals appear closer at hand and motivate you to continue the pursuit of your goals to manage your weight. "Fructose," as in high-fructose corn syrup (HFCS) and in sugar, is an important word I use over and over again. To distinguish fructose in fruit I have used "good fructose" from the highly purified type of fructose made in factories, I have used the words "bad fructose." By adding the words "good" and "bad," I have given them a more powerful meaning and way to distinguish them in your mind. Words are powerful.

The way you *feel* is influenced by the way you *think*. Thinking positively can help focus your thoughts. When you walk, sit alone, shop, or drive your car, you continually "talk" to yourself. These internal conversations often involve your feelings about the way you would like things to be done versus the manner in which they are actually being done. For example, you are driving to the store and find yourself in the left lane when you need to make a right turn. The car in the right lane refuses to allow you to move over unless you slow down. You let up on the gas, curse the driver to yourself, and then switch lanes and make the right turn.

Anything Is Possible
One response you might have is to say to yourself, "Why doesn't that jerk let me in?" Another is to give the driver a visible sign of your displeasure. A

third approach is to talk to yourself about why you didn't think ahead and get in the right lane earlier or how maybe the other driver doesn't even realize you want to merge. We need to think positively and learn to put things in their proper perspective. Having to wait a couple of moments to move safely into the right-hand lane isn't really that big a deal, is it? Don't waste your time stewing over trivial and unimportant events. The stress it produces in you isn't worth it. Adopt a "live and let live" attitude. Change the things you can change, and don't worry yourself about the things you can't change.

Thinking positively means having positive conversations with yourself on a regular basis. You may find yourself at a lunch where most of the guests are better dressed than you. One approach is to criticize yourself for not calling ahead and asking the host what you should wear. But a better way to look at it is to forget about what you're wearing and think positively about what you will contribute to the gathering. Your attire isn't important; what is important is that you were invited to the lunch.

Thinking positively means avoiding the negative. Think about the things you do in a positive light. Don't focus on how you should have done them differently. In the case of the drive to the store, don't beat yourself up over failing to move over more quickly to make the right turn. Rather, focus on how you might have better accomplished your goal. Talk to yourself about step-by-step solutions to daily problems. Thinking positively means classifying these problems into small steps and taking one step at a time.

Believe you can take these steps. But if things don't always work out the way you planned, don't think of yourself as a failure. Stuff happens. Change the things you can change. The things you can't change are minor bumps in the road. The fact that you didn't change them today gives you a challenge for tomorrow.

Maintaining enthusiasm for your goals and objectives is an essential part of a positive approach to helping yourself. Everyone likes praise and enjoys recognition for their accomplishments. Take the same approach when having these private conversations with yourself. Give yourself a pat on the back when you've done something well. Use such descriptive words as "terrific," "magnificent," "wonderful," "great job," and "outstanding" when describing both your own accomplishments and those of others. If you are an enthusiastic and positive person outwardly, this can't help but reflect on your inner self.

Learn to relax and allocate time to release your boundless internal energy. Thinking positively can help you rejuvenate yourself. Relaxation can provide an extra boost during a long day. One technique I use and recommend to my patients is to sit quietly with your hands in your lap and your eyes closed. Think about the place you would most like to be: a quiet beach, a mountain, or any place in which you find peace and contentment. Imagine yourself in that place, completely relaxed. Let the tension out of your arms, back, stomach, and legs. Think about the positive things you have accomplished using the positive words you have introduced into your life. This will help you help yourself relax.

The old glass-and-water analogy is a wonderful way to illustrate the difference between positive and negative thinking. If you take a glass and fill it halfway to the brim with water, it can be viewed two ways: The positive thinker will say it is half full, with room for more water. The negative thinker will say it is half empty. Viewing life as a half-full glass with plenty of room for more new experiences allows you to expand your horizons and embrace a new and broader range of interests and activities, which helps you and those around you.

Here are my steps toward positive thinking. First, put a positive spin on everything you do. Remember, your feelings are controlled by the way you think. To feel good, you must have good thoughts. It is through your sense of sight, taste, smell, and hearing that you perceive the world around you. You also experience your environment through internal senses of position, location, and muscle movement. By activating your brain through one of these senses, the direct experience produced by light, sound, taste, or smell is accompanied by an emotion. This provides the flavor or feel of the experience. As a result of the perception and accompanying emotion, you act.

Before you commit to any given action, you want to think through the positive consequences that will help you from the experience. These thoughts themselves breed an emotional sensation. It is these emotions and thoughts we want to frame in a positive and optimistic way. Here are words that help you help yourself think positively: *It is possible to do what I want; I can succeed; I can relax; I can maintain enthusiasm through the use of positive words.*

Of course you can. You didn't learn to walk in a day, Rome wasn't built in a day, and developing your powers of positive thinking won't happen in a day, either. But you did learn to walk, Rome did become one of the great cities of human history, and you can learn to help yourself think positively. Thinking positively means you believe anything is possible. You can do what you want to do. Tell yourself it is possible, rather than "there's just too many things that can go wrong, too many barriers." We all know people who have overcome major obstacles and excelled in their chosen fields. Beethoven wrote his final great works after he became deaf. After major back surgery, football great Joe Montana was told he would never play football again. He later came back to win two Super Bowls. Both were able to accomplish their goals because they helped themselves and moved forward.

A well-known song titled "Accentuate the Positive" sums up this way of thinking very nicely: *You've got to accentuate the positive and eliminate the negative.* We all experience sickness, sorrow, financial difficulties, hardship, and frustration. Unfortunately, we cannot wipe these things from our lives. But their significance in our lives and the manner in which we deal with such events can be changed. The ability to fail, learn from our mistakes, and then move on is a key to this outlook on life. When things go wrong, don't panic. Think how to help yourself to achieve the outcomes you want and obtain the strengths you need to have, and how to maintain the faith to keep you going. If you devote the appropriate diligence and skill to a task, few things are impossible. But it is up to you to develop diligence and the skill of helpful thinking through continuous practice. A friend of mine, Dr. Peter Lindner, says, "What the mind conceives, it can also achieve."[1] He made me more positive, and I want you to be more positive, too.

Maintain a focus on the important things in life. By focusing on the things that are important, you won't get bogged down in trivial matters. If you didn't mow your lawn today, so what? It'll be there tomorrow. Other matters were more important. This outlook helps you keep your eyes on the goals ahead—to change the things you can change and recognize the others that don't really matter in the longrun. Remember, life will go on. The events that are upsetting you now are over with, and you may not even remember them in a few weeks. This approach will help you help yourself.

Each day we need to renew ourselves. This renewal is essential to helpful thinking. Use positive words such as "fantastic," "exhilarating," "marvelous," "amazing," "dynamic," "delightful," "great job," and "superb." These are words that help you feel good about yourself and will make others feel good when you use such words to describe their actions. Keep a list of the descriptive words you use in talking to yourself. Every week or so, write down the words you have used in the last few days. Examine those that are helpful as compared to those that are not helpful. As you become more sensitive to the words you are using, you can control the flow of these words, accentuating the helpful and eliminating the others.

A helpful attitude will change your view of the lane-change decision from "If only I had pulled into the right lane earlier, if only that driver had let me in, if only I had thought ahead, I would not have had to go around the block," to the more positive approach of "Next time I will plan my trip further ahead. I will make my lane change earlier and take things one step at a time."

The power of helpful thinking allows you to reach your goal through a step-by-step approach. If you believe you can accomplish each of these steps, the rest is easy. You need to repeat these reinforcing words on a daily basis. Think of the glass as half full, not half empty. We all make mistakes. But mistakes are not as important as what we learn from them. Every time something goes wrong, it gives you the opportunity to practice your helpful attitude.

Avoiding Manipulation

We all get tired. But much of that fatigue is a feeling rather than actual physical exhaustion. It is the way your brain reacts. But you control your brain. If you use positive words and have positive feelings, the words "fatigue" and "tired" will rarely enter your vocabulary. The relaxation exercise we used earlier is a great way to overcome fatigue. Boredom is also a symptom of negative thinking. One way to avoid boredom is to develop new activities. It may sound corny, but take up a new hobby. Pick up that musical instrument you played in high school. Get out that old stamp or coin collection and start working on it again. Softball, volleyball, bicycling, swimming, and jogging are great hobbies. The library is full of great plays, poetry, novels, and DVDs. There are new languages to learn, new websites to explore. There's no place for boredom. Developing new activities is an important part of helpful thinking and creating a new and improved attitude toward things around you.

If you think this way, nothing can keep you down! You will always be filling the glass to the brim. You believe you can solve any problem by dividing the problem into its many component parts. Another skill you need to help you help yourself is to learn not to be manipulated. You must say no when you mean no and not be manipulated into saying yes.

The following example is one from a professional colleague and friend, Dr. Peter Lindner, who used it in his practice.[1]

There is a knock at your door and a high school student skilled in the art of manipulating you is standing there in front of you. S/he introduces her/himself and offers to sell you a box of candy to benefit the school or church. This is the conversation that might take place:

Student: I am sure you will enjoy a box of this delicious candy. The money goes to a good cause.

You: I understand. But I am not interested in buying any candy today. Thank you.

Student: I am certain that other members of your family will really enjoy this candy.

You: I understand. But I am not interested.

Student: You should consider the underprivileged children will benefit from the money we receive from your purchase of this delicious candy.

You: I understand. But I am not interested in buying any today.

Student: Don't you care about those underprivileged children from your own neighborhood?

You: I care very much about them. But I am not interested in buying any candy today.

Student: All of your neighbors on this block have bought at least one box of candy. If we can get a whole solid block to buy candy, we get an extra bonus that we also plan to donate to the needy children.

You: That's very nice. But I am not interested in buying any today.

Student: You would not want to be the one to keep us from earning that extra reward, would you?

You: I understand how you feel. But I am not interested in buying any candy today.

Student: Let me ask you just a few questions. How old are your children?

You: I understand. But I am not interested in buying any.

Student: Won't you even tell me how old your children are?

You: I understand how you feel. But I am not interested in buying any today.

Student: How come you keep repeating the same words over and over again?

You: I know how you feel. But I am not interested in buying any today.

Student: You are the only one who has not bought any candy from us.

You: I don't doubt that. But I am not interested in buying any today.

Student: Do you know how many of these underprivileged children will be able to go to summer camp?

You: I understand. But I am not interested in buying any.

Student: I have been walking all day. Could I come in and get a drink of water?

You: I understand how you feel. But I am not interested in buying any today.

Student: Do you think perhaps you could give some of this candy to your friends or relatives?

You: I understand how you feel. But I am not interested in buying any today.

Student: Do you ever eat candy?

You: I am really not interested in buying any today.

Student: If you bought one box of candy, since it is my last stop, I could give you five boxes free.

You: I don't doubt that. But I am not interested in buying any today.

Student: Is there anyone else in the house who might be interested in buying candy from me?

You: There might be. But I am not interested in buying any.

Student: Don't you want the rest of your family to enjoy this delicious candy? You do care about the rest of your family, don't you?

You: That's true. I do care about them. But I am not interested in buying any today.

Student: If you don't talk to me, I will leave.

You: I understand. But I am not interested in buying any today.

Student: You sure are stubborn.

You: You are right. But I am not interested in buying any today.

Student: Well, I'm sure glad the other people in the neighborhood aren't as stubborn as you.

You: I am sure you are. But I am not interested in buying any.

At this point the student leaves. It is a case of a manipulator at work using the weapons at his or her disposal to get you to do something he/she wants you to do. The defense used is a simple technique of persistent repetition of the same answer without having to apologize or justify your actions.

You are surrounded by people who want to manipulate you. One of the principal techniques of manipulation is to make you feel guilty. Notice that the student was trying to make you feel guilty for not supporting underprivileged children. You need to gain control over your feelings if you are going to control the situation. You need to assert yourself. Being assertive doesn't mean being aggressive. Notice that in the previous conversation, there was nothing aggressive about the responses to the student. Assertiveness simply means making up your mind and then standing your ground without feeling guilty. Aggressiveness means attempting to invade someone else's territory. The aggressive person tends to overreact, can be belligerent, and can alienate those around him or her.

Let's look at some of the small steps you can take to become assertive. Just as in positive thinking, small steps are important. To become assertive, you need to practice the principles used here.

The Right to Make Mistakes

The word "should" is a major pitfall on the road to helping yourself. In describing his response to "should," one of my colleagues says, "Don't 'should' on me." It is your right to act as you like and take the responsibility for those actions. To say you were merely following orders is running away from responsibility for your own actions. You are the final judge of your behavior. No one has the right to manipulate you. Forget about the notion that you should do something simply because the person who told you to is wiser than you. When you are assertive, you stick to the facts as you see them and as you wish to act on them.[2]

When you go to a cocktail party, you have the right to drink club soda instead of an alcoholic beverage. You also have the right to provide no explanation of your choice. Even if others attempt to pressure you into having a drink, you have the right to say, "No, thank you," without feeling guilty or insecure.

Each of us also has the right to make mistakes. I certainly know I make plenty of them. But when we make choices, we also accept the responsibility for the outcome of those choices. You have the right to change your mind without a need to justify the change. Your definition of what you want to be is for you, and only you, to decide. Our actions are rarely either right or wrong. They usually lie somewhere in between. Since nobody is perfect, you have the responsibility to meet your needs as best as you can and accept the goodwill of others if they wish to offer it.

Taking Charge

One of the methods of controlling yourself is the parrot technique. This approach was used in our earlier exchange with the student selling candy. You simply assert and reassert your position, and that's that. The goal is to reach mutually agreeable solutions. To accomplish that, however, several different approaches may be needed.

Your ability to be assertive depends on your skill at sensing the emotional state of the person with whom you are talking. You do not need to respond to all questions. But the responses you offer should take into consideration the feelings of the other person. This may provide an opportunity to shift the conversation to your own benefit. When you talk to a friend or business associate, it is important to pick up clues to how the other person feels from the words that are spoken. What is really being said, and how does the person feel about what he or she is saying?

For example, when the host of a cocktail party offers you a drink you don't want, you can say, "No, thanks. I don't care for a drink." To change the subject, you might then comment on how nice that person looks today. Or you might comment on what a magnificent home your host has. You can say that you appreciate the offer but you do not care for drink. You then add the party is wonderful and you appreciate being invited.

Another technique is identifying and agreeing with the truth of an appropriate criticism. To use this approach, you must listen carefully. You must respond to the exact words being used—not to what you imply from the statement. Your spouse might say you have overdrawn the checking account again, and you should know how bad that is for the family's credit rating. You have several choices of how to respond.

You could say, "I don't have the ability to keep track of the finances." Or, "Why don't you just take over the checkbook? I can't handle the responsibility." Another approach is to counter the criticism: "Well, you were overdrawn last month. People in glass houses shouldn't throw stones."

But a better approach is to acknowledge the criticism. "You're right. I was overdrawn again." In this case, you responded to the truth of the statement rather than the implication that you have ruined the family's credit rating due to financial incompetence. As we said, very few things in life are right or wrong. Most things fall into shades of gray. Everybody makes mistakes. When you agree with a criticism, you remove one of the ways in which people may be attempting to manipulate you.

Another technique is to draw out your critic in order to identify his or her true agenda. This sets the stage for developing mutually acceptable compromises that are often the best solution to settling a difference of opinion.

Prompting the critic to elaborate on the basis of the difference may allow you to accept responsibility for some errors you may have made.

When you apply these positive approaches to your everyday life, some of the issues related to weight concerns may be easier for you to solve and control.

Good luck in mastering your skills for dealing with the world positively!

CHAPTER FOUR

The Roadmap to Good Nutrition One: The Big Picture

Let's Read the Map Together
Our focus is on eating less "bad fructose" and using the presence of high-fructose corn syrup (HFCS) and sugar (sucrose) on food labels as a guide to avoiding processed foods. I have already given you an introduction to the reason for this approach. Now we need to identify the places we find good and bad fructose and how to reduce it. Once you have begun to lower your "bad fructose," I will give you more background on the scientific rationale for a lower-fructose approach. Since fructose pops up in many places and in many foods, I will review the different kinds of foods we eat using the Food Pyramid guide.

Food Groups and Food Pyramids

Most of us eat several times a day. In fact, we often eat without even thinking about it. What our bodies get from this food is nourishment, derived from the nutrients in the food. As children, we need nutrients to grow up to be active, healthy adults. As adults, we need food and nutrients to maintain our health and provide the energy we need for everyday activities. Helping yourself to good nutrition also helps those around you. Remember, there is a "contagious" part about the spread of fatness.[1] If you become fatter, your close friends and relatives may do so, too—a double reason to control your weight: Help yourself and help others.

For centuries, physicians and scientists have offered advice about the proper foods to eat. From the famous Greek doctor Hippocrates[2] 2500 years ago to Nobel Prize laureate Linus Pauling,[3] many strategies have been promoted to cure and restore our bodies through diet. Indeed, until the beginning of the twentieth century, most medications were derived from plants believed to possess healing properties.[4] Today modern medical science has a greater understanding of the role nutrition plays in helping you to good health. Our foods contain, in addition to the basic proteins, carbohydrates, fats, vitamins, minerals, and many other compounds that can affect health. Food can be both nutritious and health-promoting. This chapter is a guide to helping you understand the importance of the foods you choose to eat, whether you have a weight problem or not. It will also be your guide in the first steps in identifying where you find good and bad fructose in the store.

All foods are not created equal.[5] Some come from plants and others from animals. In addition to the basic foods harvested from the fields, there are a myriad of modified foods that are made by the food-processing industry to make these products easier to prepare, easier to store, and more convenient. The industry may also try to make you believe that some of these processed foods are "healthier." But be careful of foods that say on the label "contains high-fructose corn syrup." This, to me, is a dead giveaway that it is a highly processed product, and if I can find an alternative that does not say this, I buy it instead. Remember, there is no HFCS in nature—it is all manmade.

Fresh fruits and vegetables, green, yellow, red, or orange, do not contain HFCS, a source of bad fructose, because they are not processed. Fruits do contain fructose and sugar (sucrose), but this fructose I label "good fructose," since it is associated with all of the other nutrients that are naturally part of the whole fruit. They should be an important part of your diet. Some foods are white and almost colorless, others are dark. They can be liquid or solid, chewy, crunchy, crispy, sweet, sour, bitter, or salty. They can dissolve in your mouth or stick in your throat. Canned fruits and vegetables often have "additives." For fruits these can be "heavy syrup," which contains bad fructose either as HFCS or sugar (sucrose). Buy water-packed or light syrup, although light syrup may also be "bad fructose." For canned vegetables, salt is one of the principal additives. Frozen fruits and vegetables may be a better buy for your health.

Believe it or not, the first guidance about foods from the U.S. Government (USDA) appeared more than one hundred years ago (1894).[6] During World War I, nutrition scientists began to organize foods into groups to help you choose a healthy diet. These 1917 recommendations established five food groups: 1) meat, milk, fish, poultry, eggs, and meat substitutes; 2) vegetables and fruits; 3) bread and cereals; 4) butter and wholesome fats; and 5) simple sugars (which may not be so "simple" after all). During the Depression years, the USDA tried to help poverty-stricken people get adequate nutrition through twelve major food groups. In 1941, at the beginning of World War II, the government released the first Recommended Dietary Allowances, which were brought up to date regularly through the 1970s. A wartime version of nutrition included the Basic Seven food groups. To simplify things, the "Basic Four" food groups (milk, meat, fruits and vegetables, and grains) was released in 1956. As we got smarter about nutrition and the problems of heart disease and obesity began to replace undernutrition, a series of "Dietary Guidelines" were prepared beginning in 1980. In the 1990s came the Dietary Pyramid and its modified version a few years later. We will come to these in a bit.

Table 1 lists five food groups and their major contributions to our diet. Milk, for example, is one of the major sources of calcium. Meat, fish, and poultry are good sources of protein and many vitamins and minerals. Fruits are a very good source of vitamin C, and fruits and vegetables provide many of the other vitamins we need. In the sections below, I will provide more detail about these food groups.

The Great Pyramid

After completion of the Dietary Guidelines in 1990, the U.S. Department of Agriculture replaced the four-food-group system with a Food Pyramid.[7] The Dietary Guidelines prepared in 2005 recommended including exercise in the pyramid.[8] So the USDA introduced a new pyramid called MyPyramid. You can obtain information from the government using the website www.mypyramid.gov. This system uses a six-food-group approach. I have provided both of these pyramids below for you. The advantage of the earlier one is the depiction of the important food groups. The newer pyramid only has "colors," which you need to further identify with specific food groups. It was anticipated that the MyPyramid would be an improvement. Except for adding exercise, I find the newer one with just colored lines leading upward less useful than the earlier one, so I give you both to choose.

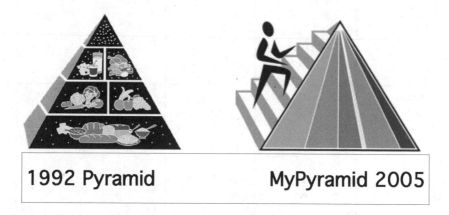

1992 Pyramid　　　　**MyPyramid 2005**

Figure 1. The 1992 Pyramid and the 2005 MyPyramid. This figure shows both food pyramids from the U.S. Department of Agriculture. In MyPyramid, exercise was added along the left side (indicated by the individual climbing stairs). The food groups were then represented as lines running up the front of the pyramid.

Table 1. Food Groups

Food Group	Examples	Serving Size*	Kcal/ Serving	Major Nutrients
Vegetables	Cooked/ canned vegetables	½ cup	25-100	Vitamins; Minerals; Fiber
	Raw salad greens	1 cup	20	
Fruits	Raw orange Apple Banana	1 medium	70-95	Vitamins; Minerals; Fiber
	Grapefruit	½ medium	40	
	Cantaloupe	¼ medium	30	
	Cooked/ canned fruit	½ cup	30-100	
Bread & Grains	Bread	1 slice	60-100	B vitamins; Fiber
	Bun (Hot dog or hamburger)	½ bun	50-80	
	English muffin	½ muffin	70	
	Dinner roll	1 roll	60-120	
	Pancake	1 (4 inch)	70-105	
	Cooked cereal	½ cup	65-100	
	Rice, noodles	½ cup	65-100	
Milk & Cheese	Whole milk	1 cup	140	Calcium; Vitamin D; Protein;
	2% milk	1 cup	120	
	Skim milk	1 cup	90	
	Ice milk	2/3 cup	135-140	
	Yogurt	1 cup	90-150	
	Cheese	1-11/3 oz	80-120	
	Cottage cheese	2 oz	60	
	Ice cream	1-1/3 cup	340-500	
Meat, poultry, fish & beans	Lean meat, Fish, poultry	2 oz	50-125	Amino acids; vitamins; minerals
	Hot dogs	2	250	
	Luncheon meats	2 oz	120-190	
	Tuna fish oil pack	2 oz	120	
	water pack	2 oz	75	
	Eggs	2	160	
	Dried beans or peas	1 cup cooked	160-230	
	Nuts	½ cup	400-600	
	Peanut butter	4 tbsp	345	

*Serving Sizes depend on whether you are male or woman and your age.

The amount of food recommended for each group in MyPyramid is shown in Table 2.

Table 2. Food Groups and Servings from the New Food Pyramid (MyPyramid)

Food Group	Servings	Comments
Grains	7 servings (Men)	Emphasize whole-grain bread, pasta, and brown rice. Be careful with white bread, white pasta, and white rice because refined grains are linked to higher risk of type 2 diabetes.
Vegetables	3 Cups	Emphasize variety. Be careful about fried potatoes because these are the leading vegetable with more fat.
Fruits	2 cups	Emphasize variety with plenty of blue and red fruits. Moderation with bananas due to calories. Emphasize 100% fruit juices. Limit juices and punches made from concentrate, since "concentrate" is another name for sugar.
Meat and Beans	6 ounces	Emphasize fish, poultry (skinless), beans, and nuts. Fish can be a good source of omega-3 fatty acids. Trim meats of fat and eat less red meat to reduce saturated fat intake.
Dairy Products	3 cups	Emphasize skim milk and low-fat yogurt. If you don't drink milk, take calcium and vitamin D supplements. Be careful with ice cream, butter, and cream.
Oils	6 teaspoons	Liquid vegetable oils without trans fats that are high in monounsaturated fats are preferred. Avoid products with trans fats because they are linked to high rates of heart disease.

Adapted with comments from the MyPyramid.gov website.

For good nutrition, you should eat: 7 servings of grain products; 3 cups of vegetables; 2 cups of fruits; 6 ounces of meat, poultry, or fish, or replace some of this with beans and some nuts; and 2–3 cups of dairy products or equivalents. Fats, oils, and sweets should be eaten very sparingly with as little "bad fructose" as possible.

So how does this help you reduce your "bad fructose" intake? Fructose appears in processed grain products (including most cereals), in fruits packed in syrup, in processed meats, and in some processed yogurts. The fact that you have a weight problem means you probably need to make some adjustments in the way you eat. Being overweight does not necessarily mean you are well nourished. It is possible to be both overweight and yet poorly nourished at the same time. Regardless of how much you weigh, you still need to eat. But the quality of your diet is more important as you reduce the amount of food you eat.

Don't think an old dog can't learn new tricks. You can help yourself to new ways of eating. I know this from experience. I grew up in a "meat and potatoes" family in the Midwest. My mother cooked some of the best roast beef, lamb, pork chops, and hamburger dishes that ever crossed your lips. She occasionally prepared chicken, but I don't remember laying eyes on fish at our dinner table while growing up.

All that has changed. I went off to college and tasted new foods: Oriental dishes, Italian pastas. I even tried fish for the first time (I hated it!). But the biggest change in my eating habits came when I began working on government nutrition programs in Washington, D.C. As I learned more about the relationship of nutrition to good health, I observed a gradual change in the foods I chose to eat. I was helping myself to better nutrition. Eggs almost disappeared from my diet. Hot dogs vanished. I actually learned to like fish. Crunchy vegetables became a regular part of both lunch and dinner. Italian pastas often replaced potatoes on my plate.

Beverages have been one of the biggest changes. I grew up in the days before there was homogenized milk. The fresh milk delivered to our doorstep had the cream on the top. It was delicious. But as I began to recognize the health issues associated with the saturated fat, I moved to 2% milk, then to 1%. Now I don't even like the "richness" of whole milk. Now I help myself to 1%, ½%, or skim milk.

In the old days of my youth, we bought soft drinks in 6.5- or 8-ounce bottles. Remember that an 8-oz HFCS- or sugar-sweetened beverage has about 100 calories. Now you can hardly find a soft drink with only 8 ounces—12 to 20 ounces is the norm (containing about 150 to 250 calories each). With the increase in the amount of "bad fructose" from the HFCS that has replaced sugar, and often with a generous dose of stimulating caffeine, these modern beverages provide an abundance of calories. One of the easiest food categories in your diet to reduce is "soft drinks" that contain "bad fructose"—a major source of fructose and calories but not much else. Replacing some or all of your soft drinks with water, diet soft drinks, or flavored fizzy water (which has zero calories and is one of my favorites) puts you on the right path.

If I can help myself make significant changes in what I eat, you can help yourself do the same. I made these changes as the evidence mounted linking major illness to diet. What we eat has a major impact on the killer diseases of modern man: heart disease, cancer, diabetes, and obesity. These findings have been confirmed many times. The Surgeon General reported in 1988 that "for the two of three adult Americans who do not smoke or do not drink excessively, one personal choice seems to influence long-term health prospects more than any other: what we eat."[9] This is one place you can help yourself. This was also the year when the Diet and Health Report was published by the National Research Council.[10]

Prior to this profound statement by the Surgeon General, the Senate Select Committee on Nutrition made the following dietary recommendations: Americans should eat less fat, more complex carbohydrates and natural sugars, and less refined sugar.[11] In other words, eat less "bad fructose" and things that contain it. That was part of the message, with a modern twist, that came from this report. The left-hand side of Figure 2 shows the estimates of the American Diet in the 1960s, when over 40% was from fat, about 12% from protein, and the remainder from carbohydrate. The bar on the right shows a pattern that many experts at the time thought was moving in the right direction. The bar has less fat, reduced from over 40% to 30%, maintains the protein about 12%, although many Americans eat more than that, and reduces fat intake, particularly saturated fat. The findings that led to these recommendations have been confirmed many times over. In addition to my focus on reducing "bad fructose," one of the other important guidelines is to reduce the total amount of fat you eat to less than 30% of your total calories. It is harder to get fat on a low-fat diet. Reduce *saturated* fat in your diet to less than 10% because saturated fat is one of the major factors linked to heart disease.[12] Dietary cholesterol should also be reduced because it is one of your two sources of cholesterol—the other is what is made in your own body. We need to help ourselves to increased amounts of fruits and vegetables, along with moderately higher levels of protein, which can reduce blood pressure.[13,14] There will be more about that later. Salt intake should be limited, and alcohol should only be consumed in moderation. We need to be sure to include enough calcium, preferably from the food we eat. Fluoride in toothpaste and drinking water is also recommended to prevent cavities in our teeth. No single food can provide a complete diet, so we eat different foods two or three times a day to get the variety of foods we need for a nutritious diet.

Current Diet and Dietary Goals

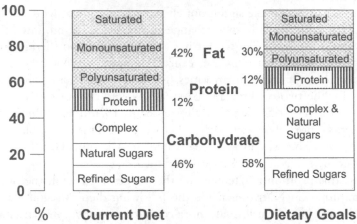

%   **Current Diet**   **Dietary Goals**

Figure 2. United States Senate Select Committee on Nutrition Recommendations for modification of the American Diet.[11]

In addition to reducing the "bad fructose", that is used in soft drinks and fruit drinks and eating a wide range of foods, another important principal is moderation. Portion control is one strategy I use, and this strategy will help you moderate your food intake. All foods have something to contribute to our diet. But eating too much of any one food can create problems, particularly for those of us trying to manage our weight. For example, shrimp is a very good low-fat source of protein. But shrimp also contains significant amounts of dietary cholesterol. So shrimp is a wonderful addition to your diet, as long as you enjoy it in moderation.

The Beauty of Breakfast

While many of us eat three "square" meals per day, others skip breakfast or are too busy to eat lunch. Eating breakfast is one way to help you help yourself.[15] Breakfast is the beginning of the day for most of us. We often wake up tired and hurry off to get to school or work. Breakfast is an easy meal to skip or overlook. But skipping meals, especially breakfast, isn't such a good idea. A careful study in children showed that school performance was improved during the weeks that children ate a good breakfast. The parents in the school were asked to participate by providing a good breakfast to their children each day for one week and then a poorer breakfast each day during a second week. The teachers did not know which kids were on which schedule. Each week on Thursday, the children were given a test as part of their regular routine. Not surprisingly, the week the children ate a good breakfast, they did much better on the test.

Breakfast for your children (and you) can also help them maintain a healthy weight. In adolescence, the children who ate breakfast cereal regularly had a lower risk of gaining weight over the years than the ones who did not.[16] So the message is clear, Mom: Sit the kids down to breakfast, and don't forget to eat breakfast yourself!

The benefits of breakfast are not limited to children. In another study, a group of factory workers were told they were participating in a taste study. During the next few weeks, the type and variety of foods they were offered for breakfast was changed. The effects that go along with heightened attention and awareness were monitored, and productivity was measured. During the weeks the workers were given good foods to choose from, and in those who chose them, productivity improved. When breakfast was of poor quality, productivity was reduced. What is a good breakfast? Aim for no more than 25% of your daily energy needs: 400–600 calories for most people. So much for breakfast. Make sure you and your children eat a healthy one, and avoid the "bad fructose" in HFCS and sugar (sucrose).

What about lunch? Lunch is also important. In another study, the performance of secretaries was found to improve during the days they had a good lunch, as compared to days when they had a poor lunch or no lunch at all. For all of us, eating a healthy breakfast and lunch can improve our daily performance and help us maintain a positive approach to our weight loss. My advice is to eat at least three balanced meals per day and avoid the foods that have "bad fructose" hidden in them. What is a good lunch? Soup (100 calories) and salad (easy on the dressing), half a sandwich (a slice of bread has about 100 calories), and fruit (small apple, banana, or berries).

What about dinner? This is the largest meal for most people. Families who eat dinner together share both food and the day's happenings. If you have used 300–400 calories for breakfast and 400–500 calories for lunch, and you only need 1600 calories per day, you will have 700–900 calories remaining for dinner. Here is where the planning that is described below can help. Beware of large serving sizes. Use smaller plates; tall, thin glasses for beverages; and no serving dishes on the table. Dinner can be a problem for some. Leaving serving dishes in the kitchen, cooking only enough for the family, and shifting to lower-energy foods we discuss in detail later (Chapters 11 and 12) could also be useful.

Your Nutrition Quotient

Now that we know when to eat, the next step is to decide what to eat. This is where a good working knowledge of the general principles of nutrition is vital. Please take a moment to help yourself by taking the following test. If you get most of the questions right, you can reward yourself by only skimming through the remainder of this chapter. If you miss a lot of questions, this chapter is essential.

Your Nutrition Quotient[17]
Instructions: Matching Test: Select the letter of the word or phrase in Column II that best describes or defines each item in Column I. Write that letter (a, b, c, etc.) on the blank line.

Column I   Column II

1.   The major nutrient in milk which   a. protein

     makes it indispensable in human   b. starch

     diets._____   c. saturated fat

2.   Building blocks of proteins._____   d. dextrose

3.   Major type of fat in corn oil._____   e. fiber

4.   Vitamin in strawberries._____   f. calcium

5.   Cellulose._____   g. Vitamin C

6.   Major component in human   h. cholesterol

     body._____   i. water

7.   A measure of heat._____   j. calorie

8.   The major nutrient in meat._____   k. amino acids

                                                l. Vitamin B

                                                m. none of the above

Instructions: Multiple Choice Test: Select the best answer for each question and circle the letter.

9.   A pound of human fat contains _____calories.
        a. 1500   b. 2500
        c. 3500   d. 4500
        e. 5500

10.   The resting metabolism of men is _____women.
        a. the same as

b. higher than
c. lower than

11. A major source of Vitamin C is _____.
    a. liver
    b. green vegetables
    c. citrus fruits
    d. lean meats
    e. bread and grains

12. Vegetable fats are usually _____.
    a. saturated fats low in cholesterol
    b. unsaturated fats low in cholesterol
    c. saturated fats high in cholesterol
    d. unsaturated fats high in cholesterol

13. Fiber in the diet is mainly _____.
    a. carbohydrate
    b. protein
    c. fat
    d. water

[Answers: 1= f; 2= k; 3=m; 4=g; 5=c; 6=i; 7=j; 8=a; 9=c; 10=b; 11=c; 12=b;13=a]

Food Groups
Bread, Cereal, Rice, and Pasta

Since agriculture became an integral part of society thousands of years ago,[18] bread, cereal, rice, and pasta have been among the principal sources of food in most parts of the world. These foods are a major source of energy, vitamins, and fiber, and may also contain a significant amount of protein. The grains used in making bread, cereal, rice, and pasta contain both a kernel and a shell. The kernel contains starch and is the source of some of our vitamins and minerals. Most of the vitamins, however, are in the shell, which may be removed in milling (the process used to make white or refined grains). Eating polished or milled white rice was a major cause of the vitamin deficiency called beri-beri.[19] To prevent this and some of the other rare nutritional deficiencies, refined grain products are now fortified by adding B vitamins, folate, and iron to the flour and other grains.

Fiber is the other component of the shell of grains. For this reason, whole-grain, bran, and germ products have more fiber than those that are refined. Whole-grain products are good sources of B vitamins, energy, fiber, and iron. The MyPyramid recommends 7 servings a day for men. A serving in this group consists of 1 slice of bread, 1 ounce of ready-to-eat cereal, or ½ cup of cooked cereal, rice, or pasta.

Table 3. Recommendations for Eating Better from the Bread, Cereal, Rice, and Pasta Group

EAT MORE OFTEN	EAT LESS OFTEN	EAT RARELY
Bread, bagels, pita	Egg breads, such as challah and egg bagels; French toast; pancakes; waffles	Bread stuffing; croissants
Muffins, biscuits, or rolls with 2 or fewer grams of fat (e.g., English muffins, hamburger buns)	Muffins, biscuits, and rolls with 3-4 g of fat	Muffins, biscuits, and rolls with more than 4 g of fat each
Unbuttered, air-popped popcorn, pretzels, rice cakes, bread sticks		Oil-popped and/or butter popcorn
Corn tortillas	Flour tortillas	
Crackers with 1 g or less of fat per ½ oz; melba toast, matzoh, flatbread, saltines	Crackers with 2 g of fat per ½ oz, such as graham crackers	Crackers with 3 or more g of fat per ½ oz such as Ritz crackers
Cold cereals with 2 or less g of fat and 6 or less g of sugar or HFCS per serving (Cheerios, corn flakes, shredded wheat, grape nuts)	Cold cereals high in HFCS or sugar or fat - especially both, such as granola	
Hot cereals Rice, barley, bulgur wheat, couscous, kasha, quinoa		
Pasta	Egg noodles	

Examples

Item	Serving Size	Calories	Grams of fat
Bread, Whole Wheat	1 slice; (1.5 oz)(43 g)	100	2
Bread, White	2 slices (1.6 oz)(46 g)	110	1.5
English muffin	1 (2.0 oz)(57 g)	260	1.0
Bagel	1 (3.5 oz)(99 g)	260	1.0
Hamburger roll	1 (1.4 oz)(39 g)	100	1.5
Oatmeal	½ cup (dry)(40 g)	150	3.0
Cheerios	1 cup (28 g)	100	2.0
Wheaties	¾ cup (27 g)	100	0.5
Special K	1 cup (31 g)	120	0.5
Raisin bran	1 cup (59 g)	190	1.5
Shredded wheat	1 cup (49 g)	170	1.0
Rice, white	¼ cup (dry)(45 g)	150	0.5
Pasta, Linguine	2 oz (dry)(56 g)	200	1.0
Pasta, Elbow	2 oz (dry)(56 g)	210	1.0
Crackers, Ritz	# 5 (16 g)	80	4
Crackers, Saltine	# 5 (15 g)	60	1.5
Crackers, Club	# 4 (14 g)	70	3.0

Grain products all provide starch, which our bodies turn into glucose, one of the "sugars" described earlier. In the test tube, this glucose can be converted into "bad fructose," which we are using as a guide to highly processed foods. We want to eat as many of the "naturally nutrient-rich" foods as possible in our diet. HFCS on the Nutrition Label is one way to recognize highly processed foods we want to avoid. The rate at which dietary starch from the plant foods we eat is turned into glucose in our body and the rate at which this glucose is absorbed varies from one starch product to another, and what the starch is eaten with. We measure this increase in glucose level and call it the Glycemic Index (GI). For example, potatoes are rapidly digested and absorbed and quickly produce high glucose levels in your body (a high glycemic index). Other bread products, cereals, rice, and pasta products that contain more "fiber" may be digested into glucose more slowly. Those foods, such as white bread, white rice, and potatoes, which are rapidly digested and absorbed, are said to have a high glycemic index. Foods that are more slowly digested and absorbed, such as legumes and whole grains, have a lower glycemic index, largely because of the fiber. This is why they are preferred. Table 4 below gives some examples of high-glycemic-index and low-glycemic-index foods as well as glycemic load.[20] The glycemic load provides a better gauge for total readily absorbed glucose because it takes both the rapidity of absorption and the total amount of that carbohydrate into account. You can help yourself by choosing foods with more fiber, which usually have a lower glycemic index. These foods, in addition to being absorbed more slowly, tend to have more fiber and are "bulkier" or more filling than higher glycemic index foods. They may also retain more of the other nutrients often lost in processing. In one study, overweight children who had lost weight maintained their weight loss better when eating a low-GI diet as opposed to a high-GI diet. The data for adults are mixed, but even if the lower glycemic index doesn't help with management of your weight, it can improve some of the associated metabolic factors. The fiber is another positive asset.

Table 4. Table of Glycemic Index Values for Various Foods

Food Item	Glycemic Index	Glycemic Load
Instant Rice	91	24.8
Baked potato	85	20.3
Corn flakes	84	21.0
White bread	70	21.0
Rye bread	65	19.5
Banana	53	13.3
Spaghetti	41	16.4
Apple	36	8.1
Lentil beans	29	5.7

Adapted from Ludwig et al JAMA 2002;287;2414–2423.

Fruits

This group has much to offer. It is a rich source of complex carbohydrates and fiber and contains a wide variety of vitamins and minerals. The sweetness of fruits comes from the small amounts of good fructose from the sugar (sucrose) that is in the native fruit. The "good fructose" in fresh fruits and vegetables is present in small amounts. Many fruits have low levels of fructose (lemons, limes, passionfruits, prunes, most melons, most berries, cherries, nectarines, peaches, oranges, and bananas). High levels of fructose are found in apples, grapes, apricots, pears, watermelon, and mango. It is the higher concentrations of fructose in apple juice and grape juice that make them widely used in "blending" fruits drinks and some "fruit juice blends." Most vegetables have no fructose or very little. A few exceptions with levels near the middle of the fruit range are sweet potatoes, eggplant, and peas. Grains have little fructose as do cereals, unless it is added as "bad fructose" during processing. Meat, milk, and cheese have very little fructose. For example, to get the amount of fructose you get from a glass of apple juice, you would have to eat nearly a dozen apples. *Tip:* It is better to eat the whole fruit than to drink the juices. If you drink fruit juices, use 100% juice and try to avoid those from "concentrate," which is another word for sugar. The so-called "fruit drinks" have little fruit juice (around 10% to 15%) and lots of "bad fructose," where HFCS or sugar (sucrose) are used to beef up the sweetness. See the chapter on beverages.

Fruits are sometimes considered as a separate group because they are rich in vitamin C and contribute good fructose and fiber to the diet. Fresh fruits are low in sodium and have little or no fat and no cholesterol. Fruits are also fair sources of many of the B vitamins and vitamin A. According to MyPyramid, we should eat 2 cups of fruit each day. A serving is one medium apple, banana, or orange; ½ cup of chopped, cooked, or canned fruit; or ½ cup of 100% fruit juice (not fruit drinks). One word of caution: Canned fruits are often packed in syrups that contain a considerable amount of "bad fructose" (HFCS or sugar (sucrose)). Always read the label and preferably buy the fresh or frozen fruit.

Table 5. Recommendations for Eating Better with the Fruit Group

EAT MORE OFTEN	EAT LESS OFTEN	EAT RARELY
All fresh fruit (except avocado and olives)	Dried fruits, fruit juices	Avocado, olives
	Canned fruit in its own juice	Canned fruit in heavy syrup
Applesauce, unsweetened		Sweetened applesauce

Examples

Item	Serving Size	Calories	Grams of fat
Avocado	¼ cup mashed	70-100	6.5-7.5
Apple	1 medium	72	0
Banana	1 med (7-inch)	105	0
Grapes	10 Fresh	36	0
Orange	1	60-70	0
Applesauce (unsweetened)	½ cup	50	0
Applesauce (sweetened)	½ cup (126 g)	100	0
Orange, Mandarin Light syrup	5.5 oz (156 g)	80	0
Pear halves in juice	½ cup	50	0
Pineapple slices	2 (114 g)	60	0
Juice, Apple	1 cup	120	0
Juice, Apple Juice Punch	1 cup	120	0
Juice, Cranberry Apple cocktail*	1 cup	140	0
Juice, Grape	1 cup	170	0
Juice, Juicy Juice	1 cup	120	0
Orange, 100% not from concentrate§	1 cup	110	0
Tropical Punch *	1 cup	110	0
Juice, V-8	1 cup	50	0

* Contains HFCS § My preference

Vegetables

Like fruits, vegetables have much to offer. They provide many vitamins and minerals, and they have fiber and are a good source of food starch—the long glucose molecules, which when digested readily enter the body to provide your needs for glucose—sometimes called "quick energy."

Table 6. Recommendations for Eating Better with the Vegetable Group Recommendations

EAT MORE OFTEN	EAT LESS OFTEN	EAT RARELY
Fresh vegetables or frozen vegetables without sauce or salt	Canned vegetables, vegetable juices	Frozen vegetables in sauce

Examples

Item	Serving Size	Calories	Grams of fat
Beans, green, canned	½ cup	20	0.2
Corn, whole kernel, canned	½ cup	60	1.0
Lettuce	1 head (6 oz)	20	0
Peas, sweet, canned	½ cup	110	0.5
Potato, baked w/skin	1 (6.5 oz)	220	0.2
Potato, baked w/o skin	½ cup	60	0
Potato, boiled	½ cup	70	0.1
Potato, French fried	3 oz	190	3.6
Potato, Hashed brown	½ cup	170	4.8
Potato, salad	½ cup	180	8
Squash, acorn cooked	½ cup	40	0.1
Squash, zucchini, sliced, raw	½ cup	10	0.1
Squash, zucchini, cooked	½ cup	15	0.1

Sweet potatoes, carrots, and spinach and other leafy green, yellow, and orange vegetables are excellent sources of provitamin A or beta carotene and other important carotenoids. They also provide other essential nutrients, such as vitamin C, iron, folacin, magnesium, and calcium. Dark green leafy vegetables are fair sources of such B vitamins as riboflavin (vitamin B_2), thiamin (vitamin B_1), pyridoxine (vitamin B_6), pantothenate (vitamin B_5), and biotin. Other vegetables also contain such B vitamins as pyridoxine, pantothenate, and biotin but are low in thiamin and riboflavin.

MyPyramid recommends 3 cups of vegetables each day, with a serving being defined as 1 cup of raw leafy vegetables, ½ cup of other cooked or chopped raw vegetables, or ¼ cup of vegetable juice.

Milk, Yogurt, and Cheese

This food group is a major source of high-quality protein and calcium. But we have to approach this group with caution because it can also provide a considerable amount of saturated fat. To help yourself make the best choices, you should always read the label and choose low-fat dairy products. Proteins in milk can be readily digested by most of us. Milk also has one of the essential amino acids that complement the protein in rice and wheat. This means the combination of the two can provide our daily protein needs. Some recommendations for eating better from the milk, yogurt, and cheese group are shown in Table 7.

Table 7. Recommendations for eating better from the milk, yogurt, and cheese group
Recommendations

EAT MORE OFTEN	EAT LESS OFTEN	EAT RARELY
Skim and 1% milk	2% milk	Whole milk
Buttermilk made with skim or 1% milk	Buttermilk made with 2% low-fat milk	
Yogurt made with skim or 1% low-fat milk	Yogurt made with 2% milk	Yogurt made with whole milk
	Hot cocoa or chocolate milk from skim or 1% milk	Hot cocoa or chocolate milk from 2% milk
1% low-fat or dry-curd cottage cheese	2% cottage cheese	Creamed or regular (4% fat) cottage cheese
Cheeses with 2 or fewer grams of fat per ounce	Cheeses with 3-5 grams of fat per ounce	Cheeses with more than 5 grams of fat per ounce
Frozen dairy desserts with 2 grams of fat or less per item or per ½-cup serving	Frozen dairy desserts with 3-5 grams of fat per item or per ½-cup serving	Ice cream and frozen dairy desserts with more than 5 grams of fat per item or per ½-cup serving
	Puddings made with skim or 1% milk	Puddings made with 2% or whole milk

Examples

Type of Dairy Product	Portion Size	Calories	Grams of fat
Milk, skim or non-fat	1 cup	90	0
Milk, 1% (low-fat)	1 cup	110	2.5
Milk, 2% (reduced-fat)	1 cup	130	5
Milk, whole	1 cup	150	8
Milk, chocolate	1 cup	230	5
Yogurt, light	6 oz	80-100	0
Yogurt, 99% fat-free with fruit	6 oz	170	2
Yogurt, plain, non-fat	1 cup	130-150	0
Cheese, cheddar, natural	1 oz	110	9
Cheese, Monterey jack	1 oz	100	8
Cheese, Mozzarella, part skim	1 oz	80	6
Cheese, Ricotta part skim	1 oz	45	2.6
Cheese, Cottage fat-free	½ cup	80	0
Cheese, Cottage (4% fat)	½ cup	110	7
Ice cream, Dreyers	½ cup	150	8
Ice cream, Dreyers Slow-Churned	½ cup	120	4
Ice milk	½ cup	100	3
Frozen yogurt	½ cup	110	2

Because milk is fortified with vitamin D, it provides one of the major dietary sources of this vitamin. Sunlight acting on our exposed skin can provide most of our necessary vitamin D. When the skin is almost completely covered, as by some women in the Middle East or during long winters in the northern climates, vitamin D deficiency can occur. Sunscreen of the highest level may also reduce the production of vitamin D in your skin. Some experts think that we need more Vitamin D than we normally get. This is particularly true for the elderly.[22]

Estimates are that milk provides up to 75% of our daily calcium needs, nearly 40% of riboflavin, and 22% of magnesium and protein. Milk and milk products are good sources of niacin and other B vitamins, vitamin A, vitamin E, and vitamin K.

The downside of whole milk is its saturated fat content. The "butterfat" in milk is a major source of saturated fat. For this reason, I recommend low-fat milk (½ or 1% fat) and skim-milk products as substitutes for whole milk. Yogurt is also a good addition, but watch out for the added "bad fructose" (HFCS or sugar (sucrose)) to the diet. For African-Americans and Asian-Americans who may have a difficult time digesting the lactose in milk, yogurt is more readily tolerated. Ice cream should be reserved as a special treat, since it contains substantial amounts of calories, saturated fat, and total fat. Cheeses also need to be selected carefully, since many have high amounts of calories and saturated fat. MyPyramid recommends that we eat 2–3 cups of milk-group foods each day, with a serving being 1 cup of milk or yogurt, 1½ ounces of natural cheese, or 2 ounces of processed cheese.

A diet high in fruits and vegetables and in low-fat dairy products has recently been shown to lower blood pressure in normal-weight people even more than fruits and vegetables alone.[13,14] You can help yourself to this diet, which will give you added amounts of potassium, magnesium, and calcium. This goes by the popular name of the DASH diet, and there is a book describing it available in your book store.

Fish, Poultry, Meat, Dry Beans, Eggs, and Nuts

This group is a major source of dietary protein, an essential nutrient in our diets. For practical purposes, it is probably best to divide this group into animal and vegetables sources of protein. The differences between the two are the quality of the protein and the associated fats. Some suggestions for improving your nutrition from this group are summarized in the next table.

Table 8. Recommendations for eating better from the fish, poultry, meat, dry beans, eggs, and nuts group
Recommendations

EAT MORE OFTEN	EAT LESS OFTEN	EAT RARELY
Beef: eye of round	Beef: Tip or bottom round; sirloin, chuck, arm pot roast, top loin, tenderloin, flank, T-bone steak	Beef: Porterhouse steak, brisket, chuck blade roast, rib-eye, ribs, short ribs, ground beef, pastrami, bologna, frankfurters
Veal: All cuts except loin, rib, and ground	Veal: Loin, rib chop or ground	
Pork: Tenderloin	Pork: Sirloin chop, top or center loin chop, rib chop, ham, Canadian bacon	Pork: Blade steak, bacon, pepperoni, sausage, frankfurters, bologna, salami
Lamb: Foreshank	Lamb: Shank half, leg, sirloin half, loin chop	Lamb: Rib chop, arm, blade, shoulder, ground lamb
Chicken breast without skin, turkey breast or leg, turkey wing without skin, ground turkey without skin	Chicken breast with skin, chicken leg, thigh, or wing without skin, turkey wing with skin	Chicken leg, thigh, or wing with skin, chicken liver, ground turkey with skin, duck and goose, poultry, frankfurters
	Poultry cold cuts with 2 grams of fat per ounce	Poultry cold cuts with 3 or more grams of fat per ounce
All fresh fish and shellfish	Smoked fish	
Canned fish, water-packed and drained	Canned fish, oil-packed and drained	
All dried beans, peas, and lentils	Soybeans & tofu	Nuts, peanuts, and other nut butters
Egg whites	Egg substitutes	Whole eggs or yolks

Examples

Type of Meat or Meat Substitute	Portion size	Calories	Grams of fat
Lean meat, poultry, fish, cooked	3 oz	175	6
Ground beef, lean, cooked	3 oz	235	16
Chicken, with skin, fried	3 oz	215	13
Bologna, 1 slice	1 oz	90	8
Beef frankfurter (1)	45 g	130	12
Egg	1 (50 g)	70	4.5
Baked beans	½ cup (1 oz)	140	1 g
Peanut butter	2 tablespoons	190	16
Nuts	39 pieces	160-170	14

Meat, poultry, fish, and eggs provide proteins whose components (amino acids) are similar to the protein components in our own bodies. Dried beans and nuts also provide good sources of protein, but the proportion of different amino acids is different from the proteins in our bodies. Consequently, vegetarians must pay close attention to eating the proper combination of vegetable proteins to receive adequate amounts of all the essential amino acids for good nutrition. Soy protein, in its various forms, is a good source of vegetable protein.

A diet containing wheat, corn, or rice as well as milk will provide an adequate mix of protein. Combining corn with legumes also provides a complete supply of the essential amino acid building blocks. Corn, wheat, or rice with eggs is another good complementary combination.

The drawback to some of the foods in the meat group is the amount of fat they contain. Red meat is a major source of saturated fat and cholesterol in the human diet. Consumption of saturated fats, in particular, is associated with a greater risk of developing heart disease and some kinds of cancer. Over the last twenty years, Americans have been eating less meat, and the consumption of chicken and fish increased. Not surprisingly, this decline in red meat consumption has been accompanied by a drop in the rate of heart attacks.

For this reason, you can help yourself by choosing lean cuts of meat and trimming off all visible fat to reduce the intake of fat and the associated calories and cholesterol. You can also help yourself by replacing as much red meat in your diet as possible with poultry, fish, and legumes, which have lower levels of both total and saturated fat. Some of the red-fleshed fish, such as salmon and mackerel, also have moderate levels of fat. But these fish and others caught in cold ocean waters are good sources of omega-3 fatty acids, which are "good fats." Scientists believe a diet high in cold-water fish that contain these fatty acids explains the lower risk of heart disease among Native-American Alaskans.[23]

Eggs are one of the most complete foods and are good sources of protein and other nutrients. Their drawback is the cholesterol found in the yolk. One strategy is to remove and discard the egg yolk, which contains essentially all of the cholesterol. As an alternative, I recommend several preparations on the market that have removed the cholesterol. The drawback to these products is that the salt content has been increased in these products, so if you are on a restricted-sodium diet, you can help yourself by avoiding these egg substitutes. The American Heart Association recommends that we eat less than four egg yolks per week.

In addition to protein, meat also provides a good source of the B vitamins niacin and cobalamin (vitamin B_{12}). Among strict vegetarians, supplements of cobalamin may be needed, since meat is practically the only dietary source of this vitamin. Red meat is also a good source of iron, whereas fish and chicken are not. Since you want to control your weight, eating a generous amount of protein can be helpful. Protein serves to increase our metabolism more than calorically similar amounts of other food groups. Proteins can also serve to "tune up" our vegetative nervous system, and this may explain in part why proteins increase energy expenditure. Thus a generous-protein diet is in your best interests for helping yourself manage your weight. We normally select a diet that contains about 15% protein. To help you help yourself to better weight control, I would suggest increasing your protein: Aim for 20–25% protein along with your lower intake of fructose.

Although some Americans may get more protein than they need, if you are working to manage your own weight or are an older American, you may benefit from more protein. Protein is also typically among the most expensive items in the supermarket, so this means we are often spending more on food than necessary in order to fulfill our basic nutritional requirements. MyPyramid recommends 6–7 ounces from this group, with a serving being 2–3 ounces of cooked lean meat, fish, or poultry; 1–1/2 cups of cooked dry beans; or 2–3 eggs.

Fats, Oils, and Sweets: The Miscellaneous Group

Fats and Oils
You can help yourself by eating less of these high-calorie foods in MyPyramid. Fats and oils come from both animal and plant sources. Butter,

lard, and tallow are from animals, and margarine and cooking oils are from plants. Many vegetable oils have been hydrogenated—that is, treated to make them partially solid for commercial purposes. There is currently a serious debate about this "hydrogenation" process, since it can produce the so-called *trans*-fatty acids that carry health risks.[24] Because of these risks, foods now must be labeled with *trans*-fat content and most companies are reducing or removing them. If the label indicates the presence of *trans* fats, I would move on to the next item on the shelf. I recommend cutting back on the amount of oil when cooking or making salad dressings. Ask for your salad dressing to be put on the side so that YOU get to choose how much to put on. When fats are required, I suggest olive oil or canola oil. Table 9 shows the amount of calories and fat in various members of this group, which you should avoid or use sparingly. And remember, it is the combination of "bad fructose" (HFCS or sugar (sucrose)) with fat that makes the most irresistible confections and are thus the ones on our list to avoid.

Table 9. Fats and Sugar (AVOID OR USE SPARINGLY) Examples

Item	Portion Size	Calories	Grams of fat
Butter or margarine	1 tbsp (14 g)	80-100	8
Mayonnaise	1 tbsp (13 g)	90	10
Salad dressing (Ranch)	2 tbsp (30 g)	150	16
Salad dressing (Ranch Light)	2 tbsp (32 g)	80	6
Salad dressing (Ranch nonfat)	2 tbsp (32 g)	50	0
Sour cream	2 tbsp	60	6
Cream cheese	1 oz	100	10
Chocolate bar (Hersey)	1.45 oz	220	12
M&M's Dark Chocolate	1.50 oz	220	12
Sherbet, Orange	½ cup	120	1.0
Fruit sorbet	½ cup	90-130	0
Cola	12 oz	150	0
Jam (Several)	1 tbsp (20 g)	40-80	0
Honey	1 tbsp (21 g)	60	0
Gelatin Dessert (1/8 dry pkg)	½ cup	80	0

Sweets

Here is where "bad fructose" comes to the foreground. Sweets include sugar (sucrose), sweeteners, and other products that contain high amounts of "bad fructose" (high-fructose corn syrup, HFCS) as well as products that are primarily fat and "bad fructose," such as many pastries. The problem with these foods is that they supply energy but usually few other essential nutrients. In fact, most of the sweets we enjoy are comprised of fat, "bad fructose," or sugar (sucrose) and little else. You can help yourself by severely curtailing the amount of "bad fructose" (HFCS or sugar (sucrose)) in your diet in foods, particularly those that mix fat and "bad fructose." "Bad fructose" is a particular problem because it is sweet and has energy (calories) in it. While it is not the sole cause, the increased amount of "bad fructose" (HFCS) found in foods today is a factor in the increasing number of Americans who are overweight. Several studies show the more soda and fruit drinks children consume, the more calories they get and the higher their weight and the greater their risk of further weight gain.[25] When I go to the store, I read the labels. If it has "bad fructose" (HFCS and sugar (sucrose)), I move on to the next item where this is possible.

Have you heard of nutrient density? It sounds like foods that would sink, doesn't it? Well, that's not it at all. Nutrient density indicates how nutritious a food is by providing information about nutrients per 100 grams of food. To compare the nutrient density of different foods, a single unit of energy is used. This is usually 100 calories (about 20 teaspoons of table sugar (sucrose) or 8 ounces of soda). The more vitamins and minerals a food has per 100 calories, the more "nutrient dense" it is. The problem with "bad fructose (HFCS and sugar (sucrose)) along with fats is that they have no other nutrients, unless fortified. Corn, for example, has protein, starch, vitamins, minerals, and corn oil. When you eat corn oil alone, you lose the other nutrients. This is why we recommend that you eat a variety of foods that will give you the nutrients you need. The more nutrient-dense foods are, the better they are for you. When shopping, I look for foods that are naturally nutrient-rich. This means they have the nutrients they came with—no need to add nutrients to them. These are the healthy choice whether or not you are on a "diet." Processed foods are often deprived of their natural nutrients. One of the key strategies of this diet plan is to help yourself to nutrient-dense foods with a low glycemic index.

Now let's wrap up this broad picture of your roadmap to nutrition. We have been focusing on the calories, fat, and good and bad fructose in foods. Table 10 is a sort of summary table that can help you select lower-fat options in place of the higher-fat options. For example, with lower-fat cheeses that you can identify from the Nutrition Label, you can reduce your fat by 50% compared to the full-fat option. Higher-fat cuts of meat make ground beef with more fat, compared to the lower-fat lean shoulder cuts. Skim milk has one-third less fat than whole milk. In the bread group, breads have lower fat than muffins, rolls, or croissants. There is similarly a large variation in the amount of fat, and thus the amount of calories, among frozen desserts.

Table 10. Comparison of full- and lower-fat options

Food Item	Full-Fat Option		Lower-Fat Option	
	Saturated Fat (g)	Energy (kcal)	Saturated Fat (g)	Energy (kcal)
Cheese (1 oz)	6.0	114	1.2	49
Ground Beef (3 oz cooked)	6.1	236	2.6	148
Milk (1 cup or 8 ounces)	4.6	146	1.5	102
Breads (Medium Croissant vs Medium Bagel)	6.6	231	0.2	227
Frozen Dessert (Regular ice cream vs Low-fat Frozen Yogurt (½ cup)	4.9	145	2.0	110
Table Spreads (Butter vs Soft Margarine with zero trans fat)	2.4	34	0.7	25
Chicken (Fried chicken leg with skin vs roasted chicken breast no skin (3 ounces)	3.3	212	0.9	140
Fish (Fried fish vs Baked fish 3 ounces)	2.8	195	1.5	129

CHAPTER FIVE

The Roadmap to Good Nutrition Two:
The Picture Magnified

Nutrients
The foods we eat contain more than forty essential nutrients. These nutrients consist of water, proteins, carbohydrates, fat, vitamins, and minerals. The energy we need each day is provided by the proteins, carbohydrates, and fats we eat in our diet and the energy stores in fat and protein. Keep the arithmetic of weight gain in mind as you read—we only need an extra 50–150 calories per day to gain 10 pounds in one year! I will present energy first. Then I will discuss proteins, carbohydrates, and fat. Vitamins and minerals will follow. Water and alcohol will be discussed in a separate chapter on beverages (Chapter 6).

Energy

Energy heats our homes, lights our football stadiums, moves our cars along the freeway, and drives the computer on which I'm writing this book. It also keeps our hearts beating and allows us to take an evening stroll around the block. When we "burn" the cereal we ate for breakfast, we use the energy produced to grow, run, think, and do all the other wonderful things our bodies are capable of doing. More than two hundred years ago, scientists learned the energy obtained when our bodies burn the food we eat is comparable to that produced by burning a candle. In fact, resting in a chair you are putting out as much heat as a 60-watt lightbulb.

That's why we usually describe the energy obtained from food in terms of calories: A *calorie* is actually a measurement of heat. In order to determine how many calories are in a particular food, chemists burn the food and measure the *heat* it gives off. This translates into the same amount of heat that will be produced by the foods we eat after our bodies have burned them.

Here's my first law of calories: the higher the water content and the lower the fat content of food, the lower the energy or calorie content of the food. That's because there are no calories in water but 9 calories in every gram of fat and 4 calories in each gram of carbohydrate or protein.

Let's take a look at what that can mean to our diet by comparing several foods in terms of the amounts needed to provide the same number of calories. Table 1 shows you the amount for size of several food items that when burned in your body will provide you with 100 calories. It takes four complete heads of lettuce to provide 100 calories because lettuce has lots of water and very little fat. It takes five cups of shredded cabbage and forty spears of asparagus (no Hollandaise sauce, please!) to generate 100 calories of heat.

Table 1. Amounts of Food with Approximately 100 Calories

Apple	2¾ inch diameter
Applesauce	1¼ cup unsweetened
Bacon	2 slices, fried crisp
Butter	1 Tablespoon (14 g)
Hershey's milk chocolate bar	⅔ ounce
Pepsi Cola	8 oz (250 cc)
Cookies	2 chocolate chip (commercial)
	6 ginger snaps
	6 vanilla wafers
Green beans, fresh	3¼ cups
Lettuce	4 heads
Asparagus	40 spears (no Hollandaise or butter)
Shredded cabbage	2½ cups
Ham	1½ oz fresh, lean, marbled, cooked
Pork chop	1 oz
Roast chicken:	
Breast	1½ oz
Light meat without skin or bones	2 oz

At the other extreme of the calorie scale, it takes about one ounce of a pork chop and about 1½ ounces of chicken breast to provide 100 calories. As you can see, you can eat lettuce and cabbage almost to your heart's content and receive very few calories as a reward. But a couple of pork chops or chicken breasts add up the calories very quickly. Burgers are even worse. Is it any wonder that it is hard to gain weight eating lettuce and easy when you have burgers with that special sauce? You can help yourself by selecting foods with fewer calories.

One implication of this comparison is that all calories are the "same" (one calorie produces an exact amount of heat when burned), but the amount of calories in a given amount of food can vary. In one way this is true, but here is one problem: if the calories in some foods make it easier to stop eating than the calories in other foods, then all calories are NOT the same. For example, the calories from "bad fructose" in soft drinks are harder for our body to recognize than those in solid food. This is another reason for avoiding "bad fructose" (HFCS or sugar (sucrose)) in beverages. By avoiding "bad fructose," you avoid HFCS (high-fructose corn syrup) in beverages as well as in solid foods, most of which are highly processed and not "naturally rich in nutrients." When we drink soft drinks, the calories in them from "bad fructose" (HFCS), or for that matter sugar (sucrose), are not as well recognized by the body as they are when they are present in solid foods. They just sort of "slip in between the cracks." The same is not true for most other beverages—such as soup—and we will return to the issue of beverages in the next chapter. For now, remember another reason to avoid "bad fructose"—it just slips into those little fat cells without being easily noticed!

This is an important lesson for our effort to lose weight while getting good nutrition. The caloric values of food give you clues to which ones to select. These are displayed on all packaged foods. Remember: Those foods that melt in your mouth are usually loaded with fat and calories. Help yourself to foods that are chewy and do not melt in your mouth.

We can look at the same principle another way. A 3½-ounce portion of lettuce provides only 14 calories. The same 3½ ounces of butter, mayonnaise, or salad dressing (7 tablespoons) would give you between 700 and 850 calories. Likewise, a 3½-ounce serving of whole milk has 66 calories, as compared to only 36 in the same-size serving of skim milk. The difference is in the fat. Help yourself to low-fat dressing on the side, or better yet, to balsamic vinegar or lemon juice.

Cooking can also affect the number of calories you get. Consider the standard apple, which contains about 70 calories. Make it into applesauce by adding sugar, and the number of calories increases to about 185 per serving. Bake the apple in brown sugar, and the count rises to 225. How about a slice of apple pie? The calories mount to even more than 350. Wouldn't a scoop of ice cream on top be nice? The calorie bill for your dessert is now 440 calories, or 20% of your total daily needs for energy! Help yourself to fresh fruits and vegetables without sugar or ice cream—better nutrition for fewer calories!

Let's consider the noble potato. A medium boiled potato has about 90 calories. Mashing that potato and adding a teaspoon (1 pat) of butter increases the calories to 120. Baking it and adding 1 pat of butter also comes to about 120 calories. Let's turn that potato into golden, crisp French fries, the most widely consumed vegetable in America! We're now looking at 155 calories. The lesson is clear: Food preparation is critical in keeping the calorie value low.

Carbohydrates

Carbohydrates are the sugars, starches, and fiber in our food, and they provide one of the body's main sources of energy. Let's begin with a little survey of the types of carbohydrates. To repeat from earlier, plants produce two major kinds: digestible starch and indigestible (or only partially digestible) fiber. The fiber serves to give "stiffness" to plants so they can "stand up." In contrast, starch is stored mainly in seeds to provide energy for the new seedling as it begins to grow. Starches are composed almost entirely of units of "glucose," which is the major sugar in the body. Nature also produces other carbohydrate units, such as malt sugar (maltose), table sugar (sucrose), and milk sugar (lactose). Each of these sugars has two units. Glucose is one part and in the case of maltose both parts. In table sugar (sucrose) and milk sugar, glucose is only half—fructose is the other half of sucrose and galactose the other half of lactose.

When I first found the strong parallel between the epidemic of obesity and the rising use of "bad fructose" (HFCS), it raised some interesting questions about man's history with fructose. Other than honey and a few fruits, concentrated sources of fructose in nature are uncommon. For some reason, nature preferred glucose, the quantity of which is very tightly regulated in the human body. No nonsense for glucose—the body keeps it within a very narrow range, unless you develop diabetes, when it can go completely whacky. Since starch doesn't have fructose and fruits have only small amounts, it means that during most of human evolution, there was precious little fructose in our diet. This may explain why the ways for handling fructose in the body are so limited when compared to glucose metabolism.

The bad fructose in high-fructose corn syrup (HFCS) is now widely used in beverages and foods. It is not a natural product, having been developed by food chemists just over forty years ago. Before the advent of HFCS, sugar (sucrose) was the major sweetener in the human diet. But even sugar (sucrose) is a product of the agricultural revolution, appearing in New Guinea and then moving to India about 2500 years ago. It took the slavery-based economies of the Caribbean and the southern United States and a few other countries, however, to make production of cane sugar and beet sugar inexpensive and thus commercially profitable.

Cane- and beet-sugar production increased rapidly from the 1500s through the twentieth century. Then in 1967, an effective and inexpensive process for converting the glucose in corn syrup into high-fructose corn syrup was discovered. It is an enzymatic process that breaks down glucose to form fructose. The resulting corn syrup contains over 90% fructose (it would normally be 50% in sugar (sucrose)), hence the name "high-fructose corn syrup" (HFCS). Before it is used commercially, HFCS is diluted with glucose from corn syrup to give 55% or 42% fructose in HFCS. Thus HFCS, in my opinion, is not a "natural" product, for it has been highly processed to get from corn starch to high-fructose corn syrup.

There is no biological need for dietary fructose. When ingested by itself, fructose is poorly absorbed and can produce diarrhea. There is almost no fructose circulating in the blood. For comparison, glucose circulates at more than five hundred times the level of fructose. Glucose stimulates insulin release—fructose does not. Most cells keep fructose out because they lack the machinery to take it into cells. The liver is one of the few organs that fructose can readily enter. Once inside the liver cell, fructose enters the pathways that make fat in the body. Recent reports suggest that dietary fructose may predict future ill health. In a small group of children, dietary fructose was the only dietary factor related to one of the circulating fats (LDL-cholesterol).[3] Studies in rodents, dogs, and monkeys eating diets high in fructose or sugar (sucrose) consistently show increased blood fats.[2] In addition to the detrimental effects on blood fats, other research has led to the hypothesis that fructose intake may relate to risk of heart disease.

Excess dietary glucose, usually from dietary starch, is stored in the liver and muscle as glycogen and may be turned to fat if it is not needed. There are many dietary sources of starch and its breakdown product: glucose. Starch is the main constituent in most grains and grain products. Rice, corn meal, and whole-wheat flour are 25–75% starch (glucose). Pasta contains 20–30% carbohydrate, and many root vegetables and tubers, such as potatoes, carrots, and onions, have 7–33% carbohydrate. Legumes range from 14–26% and fresh fruits from 3–15% carbohydrate. In fruits, this is usually good fructose. Commercially prepared baked goods such as bread, cakes, and cookies can contain from 50–80% carbohydrates—often as "bad fructose" (HFCS and sugar (sucrose))—and fat: beware.

The average amount of sugars available for consumption has increased dramatically in the last eighty years. Before World War I, it was the equivalent of 31 teaspoonfuls of table sugar (sucrose) per day per person (130 g/d or 520 kcal/d). It is now more than 40 teaspoonfuls per day per person (168 g or 672 kcal/d), and there is no indication that the American sweet tooth is going away. Simple sugars provide energy but often have few other nutritional benefits, and they also have a high glycemic index. Table 2 brings together a number of foods to show you the carbohydrate, fiber, and energy you get when you eat them. There will be differences, for example, in the number of calories in a slice of bread, depending on how big the loaf is and how thin (or thick) the slice is.

Starches are complex carbohydrates. In unprocessed foods, starches come with vitamins and minerals. Starches are usually molecules of glucose welded together chemically. Your digestive system breaks them down into a simple form called glucose. There does not appear to be an absolute requirement for carbohydrates, providing you eat sufficient protein and fat in your diet to provide all the energy, essential amino acids, and essential fatty acids you need. The body can convert some amino acids from protein into glucose. But you do need to eat complex carbohydrates (starch) in order to get enough calories *without* too much fat. You need the unrefined carbohydrates to get all of the vitamins and minerals you need. Milling grains to separate the kernel and outer shell can remove some or all of the vitamins. For this reason, all processed wheat products are now fortified with selected vitamins and minerals, but you are better off getting them from natural, unrefined foods.

Current recommendations, as shown in MyPyramid, are that you obtain more than 50–65% of your day's food energy from carbohydrate (glucose) sources. In selecting carbohydrates, keep in mind that grains and fruits come with many other nutrients as well. They have a higher "nutrient density." Selection of a variety of breads, cereals, fruits, and vegetables provides good nutrition with little fat and good fructose. One tip that I use myself in buying packaged foods is to read the label and ingredients. If it has "bad fructose" (HFCS or sugar (sucrose)) in the ingredients list, I know it is highly processed and I usually move on to something else. Labels can be confusing sometimes. In the main part of the label, they must provide "sugars," which is good, and "bad fructose" sugar (another word for sucrose or table sugar) and several other sugars.

Fiber

Fiber, like starch and table sugar (sucrose), is made up of simple sugar units, but it is difficult or impossible for the intestine to digest fiber due to the way nature put it together. Fiber is found in the seeds, skins, and pulps of fruits and in vegetables and grains. Raw vegetables and whole-grain products are the best sources of fiber because refining and processing often destroys the fiber. Table 3 contains the recommended amount of fiber for adults.

Table 3. Summary of Recommended Intake of Total Dietary Fiber for Men and Women Older than Nineteen Years of Age

Age	Men	Women
19-50 years	38 g/d	25 g/d
> 51 years	30 g/d	21 g/d

Adapted from the Dietary Reference Intake (p 389)[5]

There are two major types of fiber: soluble and insoluble. Soluble fibers, found in fruits and vegetables, hold water and are an effective bulking agent. Insoluble fibers are more dense and do not retain water but also provide bulk. The beauty of a high-fiber diet is that it increases the bulk of the foods we eat (and how full we feel) without providing unwanted calories. A detailed list of fiber and energy density for a number of foods is provided at the back of this chapter.

Fiber serves a useful purpose because it provides bulk to help in the digestive process. This is believed to help reduce bowel diseases by preventing waste from remaining in the bowel for long periods. A list of some foods and their fiber contents are shown in the next table. Help yourself by choosing high-fiber foods, which usually have a low glycemic index.

Table 4. Energy and Fiber in Selected Foods.

Table 4. Energy and Fiber in Selected Foods.

Food	Energy (kcal)	Total Fiber (g)
Fruits		
Banana	109	2.8
Grapefruit (½)	38	1.4
Grapes (½ cup)	57	0.8
Apple (1 medium)	81	3.7
Fruit juice (1 cup)	104	0.4
Vegetables		
Tossed Salad (1 cup)	16	1.5
Broccoli (1 cup)	27	3.0
Carrots, (12 medium baby raw)	51	3.6
Grains, Bread and Cereals		
Cereal (1 cup ready-to-eat shredded oats)	112	3.0
English muffin (1 white)	134	1.5
Crackers (6)	109	0.9
Roll (1 medium whole wheat)	89	2.5
Cornbread (1 piece)	173	1.3
Pretzels (1 oz)	108	0.9
Fig bar cookies (2)	111	1.5

Milk		
Milk (1% 1 cup)	102	0
Cheddar cheese (1.5 oz)	171	0
Ice cream (½ cup)	98	0.3
Meat, Beans, and Nuts		
Turkey sandwich	344	1.2
Peanut butter sandwich	138	1.3
Chili with beans & beef (1 cup)	273	6.5
Salmon in soy sauce (3.5 oz)	169	0.2
Miscellaneous		
Cola (12-oz can)	153	0
Margarine (2 tsp)	68	0

Protein

After water and fat, protein is the third most plentiful substance in the body.[6] Protein is the major component of the body's cells and is essential for repair and replacement of muscles, blood, skin, hair, nails, brain, and other cells in the nervous system.

The protein we eat in meat, fish, poultry, eggs, nuts, and dairy products provides the essential amino acid building blocks needed for your body to produce its own protein for building and repairing cells. An adequate supply of protein is essential during growth and development, and a lack of sufficient protein in childhood can lead to serious health problems. These problems are rare in the U.S. but are still seen in developing countries.

In the American diet, more than half of our protein comes from meat, fish, poultry, and eggs. Another 25% or so comes from dairy products, and about 20% comes from grain and cereal products. The remaining 5% comes from a wide range of various foods that contain protein, for example vegetables and legumes.

The Dietary Guidelines[5] and MyPyramid recommend that you eat at least 50 to 60 grams of protein per day, with two-thirds being from animal sources. Most Americans eat more than the recommended levels. As a weight watcher, you may prefer an even higher amount of protein. A 3-ounce serving of meat, fish, or poultry provides about half the recommended levels, so two 3-ounce servings a day are more than adequate.

When we eat meat, fish, poultry, or other foods containing protein, the enzymes in our stomachs and intestines break down the protein into its building blocks: the amino acids. There are more than 20 amino acids, and nine or 10 are *essential*, which means your body cannot produce these amino acids, so you must eat them in your diet.

One of the benefits of animal proteins is that they contain all the essential amino acids in approximately the same ratio as found in our own body protein. In contrast, many vegetable proteins have low levels of one or more of these essential amino acids. For this reason, people who are strict vegetarians must take great care to mix the proper vegetables to ensure they obtain all the essential amino acids. For example, corn and beans complement each other. The addition of milk and eggs to a vegetarian diet will substantially increase the level of essential amino acids. Vegetarians, and particularly vegans, who eat no animal products, have to mix and match a wider variety of foods. Vegetarians and vegans tend to weigh less, and this book may be of less value to them.

You may already have heard of tryptophan. It is one of the essential amino acids. It caused a lot of trouble when a defective lot made in Japan was sold in the U.S. and caused muscle pains. Pure tryptophan is an interesting amino acid for several reasons. In the early part of the twentieth century, diets with a lot of tryptophan prevented pellagra (a disease caused by niacin deficiency) because the tryptophan can be converted to the vitamin niacin.[7] Tryptophan is also used in the brain to make one of the essential messengers between cells, the neurotransmitter serotonin. Changes in serotonin are related to a number of behavioral problems, particularly depression, in which sleeplessness is one symptom. Tryptophan in large doses can help produce sleep. For this reason, some people have advocated tryptophan as a mild sedative. Foods that are particularly rich in tryptophan include cheddar cheese, peanuts, the light meat of chicken or turkey, tuna, meats, and cottage cheese. Table 6 provides you with more information about sources of tryptophan in the diet.

Table 5. Tryptophan Content of Selected Foods

Food	Tryptophan mg per 100 g	Calories per 100 g
Cheddar cheese	341	398
Peanuts, roasted	340	585
Turkey, light meat, roasted	340	176
Tuna, canned in oil	285	197
Chicken, roasted	250	290
Beef, chuck	217	327
Cottage cheese, 4% fat	179	106
Milk, skim	49	36
Milk, whole	49	65
Yogurt	20	61

Fats

The old adage is that "oil and vinegar don't mix." The same goes for fat and water. That would seem to be a problem for the human body, which needs to transport fats through a blood stream that is 90% water. When we eat fat, it is broken down in the intestine to form fatty acids, monoglycerides, and glycerol. After digestion and absorption, the fatty acids are reattached to a glycerol "backbone" and covered with a thin coat of protein. Because fat and water don't mix, our bodies have developed this carrier system to transport fat in our blood. In this form, the fats in our diet and those made in the liver can circulate in the bloodstream and reach other parts of the body. Cholesterol and fat-soluble vitamins (A, D, and E) also circulate in the blood as part of these protein-covered particles.

Dietary fat can be divided into three major types that are shown in the next table. Saturated fats are usually solid at room temperature. They are readily found in animal fat, such as meat and milk. Mono-unsaturated fats are liquid at room temperature. Olive oil and canola oil are abundant sources of these fats. Most plants provide amounts of polyunsaturated fats. These can also be found in marine fish and are known as fish oils.

Table 6. Types of Fats. Comparison of Three Major Groups of Fats

Type of Fat	Physical Appearance	Sources	Effect on Blood Cholesterol
Saturated	Usually firm or solid at room temperature	Lard (Pig fat)	Raises blood cholesterol
		Tallow (Beef fat)	
		Red meat	
		Fish	
		Dairy products (milk)	
		Egg yolks	
		Coconut oil	
		Cocoa butter	
		Palm oil	

Monounsaturated	Liquid or extremely soft at room temperature	Olive oil	No effect on blood cholesterol
		Canola oil	
		Peanuts & peanut products	
		Avocados	
		Some nuts, including pecans	
		and almonds	
Polyunsaturated	Liquid or extremely soft at room temperature	Corn oil	Helps to lower blood cholesterol
		Cottonseed oil	
		Sunflower oil	
		Sesame oil	
		Soybean oil	
		Some fish	

As you probably already know, there is a strong relationship between heart disease and the cholesterol that is transported through the bloodstream on the back of some of these particles. We know cholesterol can appear in two forms. High-density lipoprotein cholesterol, or HDL-cholesterol, is considered your "good cholesterol" because high levels are associated with a lower risk of heart disease. Low-density lipoprotein cholesterol (LDL-cholesterol), called your "bad cholesterol," is the one to be concerned about. High levels of this cholesterol, particularly when in small, dense particles, are strongly linked to increased risk of heart disease.[8] Elevated LDL-cholesterol can come from the cholesterol you eat or from the cholesterol that is made in your body.

Foods that already have high levels of cholesterol can increase blood cholesterol levels further. A much more important dietary factor in increasing levels of bad (LDL-) cholesterol, however, is the presence of high levels of saturated fat or *trans* fats in the diet. Don't be confused by products promoted as "cholesterol free." These products may still contain high levels of saturated fat, or even more *trans* fats, both of which promote high blood cholesterol levels far more than does cholesterol in the food we eat.

Fats derived from animals, such as butter, lard, and red meats, contain saturated fat. Margarine and salad oils tend to be made from vegetable fat, so they often have little or no saturated fat. Some cheap margarines, however, were once a source of those unwanted *trans* fats. Watch the nutrition label, where manufacturers are now required to list *trans* fats in food. There are, however, two major exceptions. Those wonderful tropical islands are a great vacation getaway, but the oils produced in paradise should be avoided. Even though they are derived from vegetable sources, the fats from coconuts, palm seeds, and palm kernels (coconut oil and palm oil) are high in saturated fat.

You can help yourself by reducing the fat in your diet and replacing as much saturated fat as possible with yet another form of fat called monounsaturated fat. Olive oil and canola oil are excellent sources of monounsaturated fat.

I will focus on fats a great deal because reducing the amount of fat along with "bad fructose" in the diet can help you help yourself in your efforts to manage your weight. Over 34–37% of your calories probably come from fats. Pound for pound, fats contain more than twice as many calories as do proteins (4 cal/g), glucose, sugar (sucrose), or starch (4 cal/g). Fats contain 9 calories/gram. Fats, oils, and butter and margarine (except the reduced-calorie types) have 80–85% of their weight as fat. Mayonnaise and salad dressings range from 50–78% fat and nuts from 46–71%. Chocolate has 36–53% fat. With meat, the cut and type make a significant difference in the fat levels. With beef, for example, shoulder cuts and carefully trimmed cuts are lower in fat than lower-quarter cuts or most steaks. You can help yourself by choosing lower-fat types of meats, mayonnaise, or salad dressing.

Figure 7. Percentage of calories from fat in various foods

>50% calories from fat	Cream Cheese
	Hot dogs (Wieners)
	Peanuts and peanut butter
	Most cheese and cheese spread
	Regular Ground beef
	Salmon, tuna (canned in oil)
	Pork loin and butt
	Pork lunch meats
	Granola
40-50% calories from fat	Chicken with skin (roasted)
	Beef - porterhouse, T-bone, round rump
	Lean ground
	Kidney
	Pork - fresh & cured ham & shoulder
	Lam - shoulder, rib
	Salmon - red sockeye, canned

	Ice cream
	Cream cheese sandwich
	Peanut butter sandwich
30-40% calories from fat	Beef - sirloin, arm, flank & heart
	Turkey - flesh & skin, dark meat
	Lamb - leg & loin
	Pork - heart & kidney
	Chicken - dark meat, roasted flesh
	Creamed cottage cheese
	Lunch meat
	Chicken spread sandwich
20-30% calories from fat	Beef - heel or round & pot roast
	Liver - pork, chicken lamb, beef
	Fish - bass, ciscoe oysters, salmon (pink)
	Chicken - roasted, light meat broilers without skin
<20% calories from fat	Fish - haddock, cod, tuna (water packed), ocean perch, halibut, smelt, sole
	Shellfish – most
	Porridge
	Bread
	Most peas, beans and lentils
	Skim milk cheese
	Uncreamed cottage cheese
	Skim milk
	Most breakfast cereals (except granola types)

* Adapted from NutriScore by Fremes and Sabry[9]

Fats are so important to you and your health that I want to run the risk of overkill by repeating myself.

1. *Saturated fats* are the ones that can raise your cholesterol and increase your risk of heart disease. Animal and dairy products are high in saturated fats. That is why I recommend you buy lean cuts of meat and trim the visible fat before cooking them. To get lean hamburger, ask the butcher to grind shoulder cuts that YOU choose. You can also help yourself to lower-fat hamburger meat by browning the meat and then putting it in the refrigerator covered with water. The solid fat will congeal on top and can be discarded. A second major source of hidden saturated fat is the coconut oil and palm kernel oil that is used in many of our baked goods. Beware! Processed foods are often cheap and have "bad fructose" (HFCS or sugar (sucrose)) and fat in abundance but may not be worth the cost to your health. Meat, too, must carry a label, and this can provide a good guide to what you are buying.

2. *Monounsaturated fats* are the good guys. Olive oil and canola oil are particularly rich sources. They are also common in some vegetable oils. They do not raise or lower your cholesterol.

3. *Polyunsaturated fats* are found in many plant oils such as corn oil, soybean oil, cottonseed oil, and safflower oil. They are liquid at room temperature. Fish oils are another type of polyunsaturated fat that may reduce the risk of heart disease. The final answer is not yet in, but I do not favor eating more of these polyunsaturated fats than recommended by the National Research Council until we know more about their overall effects.

4. *Stanols* are plant-derived substances (steroids) that reduce entry of cholesterol into your body from the intestine. They help lower cholesterol and are now included in some margarines.

Trans Fatty Acids

Why all this concern about *trans* fatty acids? *Trans* fatty acids are among the nutritional "bad guys." Eating foods containing *trans* fatty acids can increase your risk of heart attacks. Indeed, fats containing large amount of *trans* fatty acids may be more hazardous to your health than saturated fats. Nature doesn't make many *trans* fatty acids, but manufacturers do. They make *trans* fats by taking polyunsaturated fats and "partially hydrogenating" them. Read your food labels to select foods (mayonnaise, peanut butter, salad dressing) that do not have *trans* fats. Recently, New York City banned the use of *trans* fats in restaurants. This along with other pressures has gradually reduced the amount of *trans* fats that are used in the food supply and will be more so in the near future.

Cholesterol

As with fat content, cholesterol content varies widely. To give you some idea, Table 8 summarizes the cholesterol content from a variety of foods you can buy at the store or eat in restaurants. Milk provides a good example of what happens when the butter fat is removed. An 8-ounce glass or 1 cup of whole milk has about 150 calories. An 8-ounce glass of milk with 2% fat, so-called reduced-fat milk, has 120 calories. This is not really low, when compared to the 90 calories in skim milk, in which all of the fat has been taken off. Similarly, one cup of whole milk has 34 mg cholesterol, while skim milk has only 5 mg. Some shellfish have fairly high levels of cholesterol. Shrimp have 130 mg of cholesterol in only three ounces. But the same amount of oysters or clams has only 40–55 mg. The light meat from chicken and turkey is slightly lower in cholesterol than beef, pork, lobster, and dark meat from chicken or turkey. The important difference, however, is that beef and pork typically contain more saturated fat, unless they are trimmed closely. At the extreme end of the cholesterol spectrum is organ meat (excluding brains) and eggs, with 230–680 mg per 3-ounce serving.

Table 8. Cholesterol Content of Selected Foods

FOOD	AMOUNT	CHOLESTEROL (MG)
Brains	3 oz raw	>1700
Kidney	3 oz cooked	680
Liver beef, calf, hog, or lamb	3 oz cooked	370
Egg	1 yolk or whole egg	250
Heart (beef)	3 oz cooked	230
Shrimp	3 oz cooked	130
Lamb, veal, or crab	3 oz cooked	85
Beef, pork, chicken, turkey (dark meat), or lobster	3 oz cooked	75
Chicken, turkey (light meat)	3 oz cooked	67
Tuna, halibut, and clams	3 oz cooked	55
Salmon and oysters	3 oz cooked	40
Butter	1 tablespoon	35
Milk, whole	1 cup	34
Cheese, cheddar	1 oz	28
Ice cream (10% fat)	½ cup	27
Cream, half & half	¼ cup	26
Cottage cheese, creamed	½ cup	24
Cream, light table	1 fluid oz	20
Lard	1 tablespoon	12
Cottage cheese, uncreamed	½ cup	7
Milk, skim	1 cup	5

There are several important messages about fat. The first is that a diet lower in fat—less than 30% of total calories and preferably 25%—can improve your long-term control of your weight. The National Weight Control Registry collects information from many Americans who have lost weight and kept it off.[10] A key feature these successful people claim to use is to eat a low-fat diet. Remember, fat and fructose make a bad combination—the "deadly duo." You want to lower both.

Second, the foods you choose are important when you want to help yourself reduce fat and cholesterol in your diet. Substitute fish, turkey, and chicken (skim or low-fat milk and vegetables, for vegetarians) for red meat and pork. Trim fat off all meat before cooking. Select shellfish judiciously. Use 1%, ½%, or skim milk, and choose high-quality margarine that has no *trans* fats instead of butter. When cooking or salad oil is needed, choose canola or olive oil. Use lemon juice and balsamic vinegar instead of high-fat salad dressings. In restaurants, have the waiter put the dressing on the side so that you, not the chef, decide how much you use. The way you cook your food is also important. Use low-fat cooking methods such as broiling, baking, or poaching instead of frying or sautéing.

The National Cancer Institute recently examined the relationship of a low-fat diet to the risk of breast cancer in women. In performing the study, they also found that women eating a low-fat diet ate less fat and lost more weight. Over the seven years they regained weight, but the women who ate the least fat maintained the most weight loss. Not only is it difficult to become fat on a low-fat diet, it is hard to keep weight up. You can help yourself by eating low-fat foods in portion-controlled amounts. Low-fat diets alone won't cure your weight problems—but then no other diet does, either. Since successful dieters report that they usually stick to a low-fat diet, my tip to you is follow their advice. Keep the fat in your diet low, and make it good fat.

Another law: The fat you eat is the fat you wear, OR don't eat the fat you don't want to keep, OR eat only the fat you can burn. These statements bring us back to fat. Fat easily slips into your fat cells. Unlike glucose and amino acids, which can mix with water, fat cannot. During evolution, it was important to have a source of energy that could be carried around easily, was compact, not bulky, and might provide some insulation and protection. Fat fits the bill perfectly. It has more than twice the number of calories per gram as do protein or carbohydrate. Fat is stored without water. It is flexible—note the dimpling when you push it in. In eons past, fat was an ideal source of energy in the human diet.

For our modern-day society, however, fat is no longer so ideal. If you are genetically susceptible to gain weight (see Chapter 1), dietary fat is not your friend. If you eat more fat than you need, you either burn it or store it. Without the right genes, you store it. Adding butter to a piece of bread does not increase your metabolism.[12] Unless this butter decreases your desire for other food, you will store the extra fat in your fat cells. Thus beware of the lure of fat. Eat only the fat you burn. The extra fat you eat is the fat you will wear. Fat mixed with sweet-tasting "bad fructose" (HFCS or sugar (sucrose)) may be a particular problem.

Vitamins

The drugstore shelf isn't the only place to find vitamins. In fact, vitamins are available in great abundance in the foods we eat. Vitamins are chemical compounds—when they are lacking, we can get such diseases such as beriberi, scurvy, pellagra, and rickets.

Most of us eat sufficient amounts of vitamins in our diet to prevent these deficiency diseases. But there is a growing feeling among both the general public and the scientific community that vitamins may also help cure and prevent certain diseases.

There are two broad groups of vitamins. The water-soluble group includes the B vitamins, vitamin C, and folate. Fat-soluble vitamins include vitamins A, D, E, and K.

Deficiencies in the B vitamins were once common among poor people in this country. Sharecroppers got pellagra from eating diets composed largely of cornmeal, which does not have enough tryptophan or niacin. People living in urban areas eating white bread with all the B vitamins stripped out by processing also developed deficiencies in such B vitamins as thiamin and riboflavin. But the government ordered millers to put these B vitamins back into flour and cornmeal, making B vitamin deficiency rare.

Most of our thiamin is provided by cereal products, but meat, fish, and poultry also provide thiamin, as do fruits and vegetables. Dried legumes are a very good source, but the vitamins can be lost if the legumes are soaked for a long period of time in water that is then discarded. Pork is among the richest foods in thiamin, but orange juice, lima beans, and whole-grain or enriched flour are also good sources.

Riboflavin is provided by dairy products, meat, fish, poultry, and eggs. Of individual foods, liver is among the best sources, as it is for many other vitamins and minerals. Next in line is broccoli, with milk, yogurt, and cheese also being good sources.

A deficiency of niacin causes pellagra, a once common disease in parts of the southern U.S. Meat, fish, poultry, and eggs provide nearly half of the dietary supply of this vitamin, with cereals accounting for another large part. In addition to occurring naturally in foods, niacin can also be synthesized by the body from tryptophan, one of the amino acids in protein. As a result, foods high in protein and some enriched grain products provide good overall sources of niacin. Liver leads the list, with peanut butter running a close second.

Pyridoxine is a key player in processing protein. Meat and eggs provide nearly half our supply of this B vitamin. Fruits and vegetables provide approximately 25%. Once again, liver leads the list, with bananas coming in second. Meats, salmon, lima beans, spinach, potatoes, and strawberries also provide pyridoxine.

Pantothenic acid is another essential vitamin. It is part of all living creatures, so it is found in a variety of meat and vegetable sources. Liver is the best source, but most fish and whole-grain products are also very good sources.

Folacin, or folate, is important in the formation of blood and many other bodily functions, including neural tube development in the fetus. By far, liver is the best source. Other major sources of this vitamin are fruits and vegetables. Meat, fish, poultry, and eggs provide just over 20%, and dry beans, peas, and nuts provide slightly less. But folacin is also available through asparagus, bread, potatoes, raw cabbage, orange juice, rice, peas, eggs, and bananas. Grain products are now fortified with folate. During pregnancy, you need folacin to help the baby you are carrying be as healthy as s/he can be. Lack of folacin can result in neural tube defects (for example, spina bifida) in your developing fetus. Grains are now fortified with folacin because of this critical need for folacin during pregnancy. I have provided a table with the folic acid content of some foods.

Table 9. Some sources of folic acid.

Food Items	Serving	Micrograms of folic acid
Cereals		
Total	1 cup	466
Grape Nuts	1 cup	402
All-Bran	1 cup	301
Bran flakes	1 cup	173
Wheaties	1 cup	102
Vegetables and Legumes		
Lentils, cooked	½ cup	179
Spinach, cooked	½ cup	131
Black beans, cooked	½ cup	128
White beans, cooked	½ cup	123
Asparagus, cooked	½ cup	121
Spinach, cooked, raw	1 cup	108
Turnip greens, cooked	½ cup	86
Collard greens, cooked	½ cup	65
Fruits		
Orange juice	1 cup from concentrate	109
Raspberries, frozen	1 cup	65
Pineapple juice, canned	1 cup	58

Orange sections	1 cup	55
Papaya	1 cup	49
Meats, Poultry, and Nuts		
Chicken liver, cooked	¼ cup	269
Beef liver, cooked	4 oz	162
Peanuts	1/3 cup	117
Sunflower seeds	1/3 cup	109
Trail mix	½ cup	54

Vitamin B_{12}, or cobalamin, was the last vitamin to be discovered and synthesized. Deficiency of this vitamin causes serious mental and blood problems. Strict vegetarians may risk deficiency of this vitamin, since it is only found in meat, fish, poultry, eggs, and dairy products. They may need to take a supplement of vitamin B_{12}. Liver and oysters are among the richest sources, but all meats, fish, poultry, eggs, and dairy products supply it.

Most animals produce their own vitamin C, but human beings and guinea pigs must get it from food. A deficiency of vitamin C causes scurvy with its internal bleeding. Vitamin C has also been credited with a wide range of other benefits. Some very well-known scientists believe vitamin C can reduce the risk of cancer.[13] These claims are being studied but are not yet substantiated. Others believe it reduces the frequency of the common cold, although I have not yet seen any convincing evidence that it does so.[13] Vitamin C is a water-soluble vitamin, meaning it cannot be stored by the body. We should get a dose of vitamin C almost every day. The recommended daily allowance is 30–75 milligrams per day, or the amount that is available in one orange. But there is no risk associated with somewhat higher levels, so I usually include more than 100 milligrams in my diet. Fortunately, there is a wide range of foods that are high in vitamin C. Broccoli, Brussel sprouts, collards, kale, turnip greens, sweet peppers, and parsley all contain healthy amounts. Guava and black currants have very high levels of vitamin C, while oranges, lemons, papayas, strawberries, cabbage, cauliflower, kohlrabi, mustard and turnip greens, spinach, and watercress are good sources. Surveys show that Americans generally receive more than their daily allowance of vitamin C in their diets. In addition, a 100-milligram pill would do no harm. Extremely high levels of vitamin C, however, do carry a risk of kidney stones. The table below shows a list of some good sources of vitamin C.

Table 10. Vitamin C Content of Selected Foods

Food	Serving Size	Vitamin C (mg)
Fruits		
Blackberries	½ cup	15
Blueberries	½ cup	10
Cantaloupe	½ cup	25
Cherries	½ cup	10
Grapefruit	½ cup	38
Grapefruit juice	¾ cup	45
Honeydew melon	½ cup	23
Lemon juice	¾ cup	85
Orange	1 medium	90
Papaya raw	½ cup	40
Strawberries, sliced	½ cup	70
Tangerine	1 large	31
Vegetables		
Broccoli	½ cup	60
Brussels sprouts, cooked	½ cup	70
Cabbage	½ cup	20
Greens, cooked		
Collards	½ cup	70
Kale	½ cup	50
Mustard greens	½ cup	35
Spinach	½ cup	25
Turnip greens	½ cup	50
Parsley, raw	1 small bunch	20
Potatoes	2 tablespoons	34
Tomato	1 medium	25
Tomato juice	¾ cup	30

The remaining vitamins are fat-soluble. This means they can be stored in our bodies and do not have to be provided each and every day through the foods we eat. Provitamin A and beta carotene, the food source from which the body can produce vitamin A, are both essential to our health. Each has been credited with playing a possible role in preventing disease and is also important in vision and in the health of the skin and other body tissues. Fruits and vegetables provide more than half of your vitamin A. The second major source is meat, fish, poultry, and eggs. Spinach, carrots, sweet potatoes, asparagus, tomatoes, kale, broccoli, apricots, papaya, watermelon, and peaches are all good sources. Once again, however, the best source of all is our old friend liver. The table below shows some good sources of vitamin A and beta-carotene (provitamin A).

Table 11. Provitamin A Content of Selected Foods

Food	Serving Size	Vitamin A (Units)
Fruits		
Apricots, fresh	½ cup	2,250
Cantaloupe	½ cup	2,750
Orange	1 medium	300
Papaya, raw	½ cup	1,400
Peaches	½ cup	1,100
Vegetables		
Asparagus, cooked	½ cup	900
Broccoli, cooked	½ cup	2,400
Carrots, raw	½ cup	9,000
Greens		
Collard	½ cup	5,400
Kale	½ cup	4,600
Mustard	½ cup	5,800
Spinach	½ cup	7,300
Turnip	½ cup	4,800
Squash, winter	½ cup	4,300
Sweet potatoes	½ cup	7,800
Tomatoes, raw	1 small	900
Meat		
Liver		
Beef	3 oz	45,000
Calf	3 oz	19,000
Chicken	3 oz	27,000

Vitamin E is another vitamin that has been touted for its potential in reducing the risk of cancer. In animals, it plays a role in preventing sterility. Other benefits have been attributed to this vitamin, such as enhancing sexual performance, slowing aging, enhancing athletic abilities, and reducing damage from air pollutants, as well as reducing the risks of cancer and heart disease. But a recent study was disappointing—Vitamin E did not lower the risk of heart disease and may actually have increased the risk. The major sources of vitamin E are oils and fats in the diet. Most oils, with the exception of coconut oil and olive oil, have high quantities of vitamin E. The table below shows some good sources of vitamin E.

Table 12. Vitamin E Content of Selected Food

Food	Vitamin E in mg per 100 g
Mayonnaise	50
Margarine (corn oil)	46.7
Cornmeal, yellow	3.4
Bread, whole wheat	2.2
Spinach	2.0
Liver, beef, broiled	1.6
Egg	1.4
Broccoli	1.3
Haddock, fillet broiled	1.2
Butter	1.0
Tomatoes, fresh	0.85
Green peas, frozen	0.65
Ground beef	0.63
Pork chops, pan-fried	0.60
Chicken breast	0.58
Corn flakes	0.43
Banana	0.42
White bread	0.23
Carrots	0.21
Orange juice, fresh	0.20
Potato, baked	0.055

Vitamins D and K are vitamins we do not have to obtain from the foods we eat. Vitamin D is often called the sunshine vitamin because it is produced by the body when the skin is exposed to sunlight. It plays an important role in bone formation and kidney function and controls calcium absorption in the body. In children, a lack of vitamin D can lead to rickets. But this disease is now rare because vitamin D is added to milk and various other foods. Deficiency of vitamin D is found in people who have limited exposure to sunlight, for example, in Muslim women whose outdoor garments completely cover them, or during the winter season in people who live in more polar latitudes. Sunscreen may also limit the amount of vitamin D that is made by the skin.

Vitamin K is produced by microorganisms in the intestine. This vitamin is essential for controlling clotting of the blood, but dietary intake is not necessary in healthy people.

The bottom line on vitamins is that most of us can obtain adequate levels of vitamins through our diet with little special effort. There may be a possible benefit, however, to taking a vitamin supplement. I do not recommend taking "mega-doses" of individual vitamins, but a daily multiple vitamin, with Vitamin C, Vitamin E, and beta-carotene, along with B-complex, will certainly do no harm.

Minerals
Several minerals are key to our survival. Calcium is one of those vital minerals. Without it, our bones would collapse. With aging, the skeleton loses calcium, which can lead to hip and spine fractures. By age thirty, we have achieved maximum body calcium levels. After that, calcium is gradually lost from the skeleton.

Consequently, getting calcium early in life is essential. More than 75% of our calcium comes from milk and milk products. Other food groups provide smaller amounts. People who cannot drink milk or eat milk products must rely on other sources. Yogurt may help, since the making of yogurt breaks up the lactose sugar that presents digestive problems to some people. Sardines, almonds, sesame seeds, cabbage, and turnip greens are other good sources of calcium. Orange juice enriched with calcium is also a good source. Since achieving satisfactory amount of calcium can be a challenge from foods, and since higher levels of calcium intake may reduce body weight and certainly do not cause weight gain, I recommend extra calcium.

Magnesium is another important mineral and is used by the body in the nervous system and in producing energy. The great thing about magnesium is that all the groups in MyPyramid contribute to our magnesium supply. Rich sources include cocoa, nuts, soybeans, whole grains, molasses, and spices. Clams, spinach, and cornmeal are also good sources. Most meats, milk, eggs, and most fruits and vegetables are poor sources of magnesium.

Potassium is another mineral that is available in a wide range of foods. Among the rich sources of potassium are avocados, dried apricots, cantaloupe, and lima beans. Good sources include bananas, liver, chicken, salmon, milk, broccoli, and potatoes. Many other fruits, vegetables, and meats have modest amounts of potassium. Only a few items, such as breads, cereals, cheese, and eggs, have low levels of potassium. The DASH diet (discussed earlier) containing fruits and vegetables that have high levels of potassium and magnesium, along with low-fat dairy products as a source of calcium, lowered blood pressure significantly in men and women with normal-range blood pressure.[15,16]

Sodium is one component of table salt. It is important to monitor the sodium in our foods because blood pressure in some people is sensitive to sodium. More than half of the sodium we receive comes from prepared foods. Less than half is added by using the salt shaker. Moderate amounts of sodium are found in milk, chicken, eggs, celery, canned tomato juice and other vegetable juices, and cottage cheese. High amounts are present in many canned products, cured ham, sauerkraut, bacon, green olives, processed cheese, and many cereals. Fresh fruits and vegetables have very little sodium.

The LowFructose Approach to Weight Control

While salt is not a problem for most of us, I still recommend that you refrain from reaching for the salt shaker when cooking or eating. Another major source of sodium is from processed foods. The message again is to eat fresh fruits and vegetables that are naturally nutrient rich. The following table compares the sodium and potassium content of some fresh and prepared foods.

Table 13. Sodium and Potassium Content of Selected Foods

Food	Portion Size	Sodium (mg)	Potassium (mg)
Asparagus	4 spears	trace	73
Beans, frozen cooked	½ cup	trace	105
Beans, kidney, cooked	½ cup	3	315
Banana	1 medium	1	500
Chicken, white meat, cooked	1 piece	20	110
Egg	1	60	65
Beef, round, cooked	3 oz	65	300
Milk	1 cup	120	350
Bread, white	1 slice	140	29
Shrimp raw, fried	3 oz	140	29
Cheese, cheddar	1 oz	200	200
Flounder, cooked	3 oz	200	500
Beef, broth	1 cup	1600	Trace

Iron is essential for producing blood, which carries oxygen from the lungs to our body tissues. For women, the monthly menstrual flow is a major source of iron loss. We once got plenty of iron by cooking in iron pots. A lack of iron can lead to anemia if the iron is not adequately replaced. Liver leads the list as a source of iron. Other meats and dried fruits are good sources of iron, as are oysters, lima beans, spinach, and cooked mustard greens.

Finally, there is much recent research supporting the importance of antioxidants in preventing disease and helping the body heal itself. Antioxidants are naturally occurring substances that can be found in many fresh fruits and berries, which underscores yet again the importance of these naturally fat-free foods for good nutrition as well as for maintaining a healthy weight. Table 14 shows the antioxidant scores for some fresh fruits, berries, and nuts.

Table 14. Antioxidant Scorecard

Food	Serving Amount	Score
Blueberries	1 cup	9,019
Cranberries	1 cup	8,983
Blackberries	1 cup	7,701

Raspberries	1 cup	6,058
Strawberries	1 cup	5,938
Red Delicious apple	1	5,900
Red kidney beans, cooked	½ cup	5,569
Pecans	1 oz	5,095
Pinto beans, cooked	½ cup	4,983
Sweet cherries	1 cup	4,873
Black plum	1	4,844
Walnuts	1 oz	3,846
Green pear	1	3,172
Hazelnuts	1 oz	2,739
Orange, navel	1	2,540
Red cabbage, cooked	½ cup	2,359
Potato, russet, cooked	6 oz	2,325
Pistachios	1 oz	2,267
Green tea	1 cup	2,231

Source: Prevention Feb 2006

Appendix. Fiber Content and Energy Density of Selected Foods

Food Item	Portion Size	Fiber (g)	Energy Density Calories/ 100 grams
Cereal (100% bran)	1 cup	19.9	132
Apricots, dried	½ cup	15.6	169
Prunes, dried	5	8.2	130
Apple	1 medium	7.9	80
Broccoli, cooked	1 medium	7.4	47
Coconut	2" × 2" piece	6.1	156
Spinach, cooked	½ cup	5.7	21
Blackberries	½ cup	5.3	42
Almonds	¼ cup	5.1	212
Pinto beans (raw)	¼ cup	4.8	166
Red raspberries	½ cup	4.6	35
Shredded wheat	1 cup	4.3	124
Peas, cooked	½ cup	4.2	57
Banana	1 medium	4.0	101
Dates, dried	¼ cup	3.9	122
Potato, baked	1 medium	3.9	145
Pear	1 medium	3.8	100
Lentils, cooked	½ cup	3.7	106
Corn, cooked	1 ear	3.6	70

Lima beans, cooked	½ cup	3.5	126
Sweet potato, cooked	1 medium	3.5	172
Apple pie	⅛ pie	3.1	302
Blackberry pie	⅛ pie	3.1	287
Peanuts	¼ cup	2.9	210
Brown rice, raw	¼ cup	2.8	180
Corn flakes	1 cup	2.8	97
Oats, rolled	½ cup	2.8	156
Orange	1 medium	2.6	64
Raisins	¼ cup	2.5	105
Brussels sprouts, cooked	4	2.4	30
Navy beans, raw	¼ cup	2.4	174
Peanut butter	1 tablespoon	2.4	188
Bread, whole wheat	1 slice	2.4	61
Apricots, fresh	3 medium	2.3	55
Carrot, raw	1 medium	2.3	30
Beets, cooked	½ cup	2.1	27
Peach	1 medium	2.1	58
Kale greens, cooked	½ cup	2.0	22
Summer squash, raw	½ cup	2.0	13
Zucchini, raw	½ cup	2.0	11
Parsnips, cooked	½ cup	1.9	51
Beans, snap, raw	½ cup	1.9	18
Tomato, raw	1 medium	1.8	27
Turnips, cooked	½ cup	1.7	18
Barley, raw	⅛ cup	1.6	87
Okra, raw	½ cup	1.6	18
Strawberries	½ cup	1.6	28
Tangerine	1 medium	1.6	39
Walnuts	¼ cup	1.6	196
Chili con carne, canned	1 cup	1.5	169
Green pepper, raw	1 large	1.5	36
Black bean soup, canned,	1 cup	1.3	116
Fruit salad, canned	½ cup	1.3	43
Wheat bran	1 tablespoon	1.3	6
Cherries, sweet	10	1.1	47
Endive	1 cup	1.1	36
Cauliflower, raw	½ cup	1.0	14
Pineapple	¾" slice	1.0	44
White rice, raw	¼ cup	1.0	177
Asparagus, cooked	4 medium	0.9	12
Cabbage, raw	½ cup	0.9	9
Mushrooms, raw	½ cup	0.9	0

Popcorn, popped	1 cup	0.9	23
Sprouts	¼ cup	0.8	12
White bread	1 slice	0.8	76
Big Mac	1	0.7	541
Celery, raw	1 stalk	0.7	7
Cream of asparagus soup, canned	1 cup	0.7	87
Pea soup, canned prepared in water	1 cup	0.7	164
Grapefruit	½ medium	0.6	40
Onions, raw	¼ cup	0.6	16
Plums	3 medium	0.6	20
Grapes, seedless	10	0.5	34
Minestrone soup, canned, water prep	1 cup	0.4	79
Cucumber	½ cup	0.2	8
Cayenne	⅛ teaspoon	0.1	0.8
Chili powder	⅛ teaspoon	0.1	1

CHAPTER SIX

The Roadmap to Good Nutrition Three:

Beverages and Your Weight

Beverages provide our major source of water, and they may also provide energy, and in some cases such as milk or soups, they may have protein, fat, and carbohydrates. Prior to the Industrial Revolution three hundred years ago, milk, water, juice from crushed fruits, tea, coffee, and alcoholic beverages were the standard.[1] It wasn't until the nineteenth century that carbonated, sweetened beverages appeared.

The number and kind of beverages we drink has changed steadily. Between 1977 and 2001, the amount of energy we got from calorically sweetened soft drinks and fruit drinks containing "bad fructose" increased threefold. In 1977 these beverages with "bad fructose" accounted for 2.8% (50 cal/day) to 7.0% (144 cal/day) of our energy needs. With this rising tide of "bad fructose" from soft drinks, there was a decrease in milk intake.[2] As recently as 1999–2000, our daily beverages gave those of us older than two years of age more than 20% of our calories each day. Unfortunately, much of this beverage intake is nutritionally poor, calorie-rich beverages sweetened with one of the forms of "bad fructose." They are displacing other important foods we should be eating. We are thus getting lesser amounts of Vitamin E, magnesium, potassium, and fiber than we need. No wonder beverages deserve a special chapter.

To help you and me select the type and amount of beverages we drink, I am providing a table on guidance for beverage choices, prepared by some of the leading nutritionists in America.[3]

Table 1. Guidance for Beverage Intake[3]

Category	Maximum Number of Servings/Day (*)	
	Men	**Women**
Total Daily Intake[§]	13	9
Water	13	9
Coffee-unsweetened = 0 Cal	4	4
Tea-unsweetened = 0 Cal	8	8
Skim/Low-Fat milk	2	2
Diet soft drinks or tea and coffee with artificial sweetener	4	4
100% fruit juice/whole milk or sports drinks	1	1
Soft drinks/juice drinks	≤ 1	≤ 1

*A serving is considered to be 8 ounces (240 ml)

§ Total daily intake can be entirely water, which explains why these two are the same. The other numbers are recommended upper limits.

Water: How Much Do We Need?

The human body is nearly 70% water.[4] Each day we need about 1 to 2 quarts (or liters, four to eight 8-ounce glasses) of water from varying sources just to replenish our water losses. More than half of this water comes from the beverages we drink. The remainder is provided when food is burned in the body, which produces water as one end product. This is because the percentage of water in most of the foods we eat is higher than the 60–70% water that exists in the human body. Lettuce and asparagus, for example, are more than 90% water. The fresh or frozen meat we buy has about 50–70% water before cooking. On down the water list is cheese, with less than 40% water, and bread, with about 30% water. Dried and pickled foods contain hardly any water.

The National Research Council Recommended Dietary Intakes[5] describe our nutrient needs in terms of an "adequate intake." An adequate intake of water for young men is about 3½ quarts (3 liters) per day and for women about 2½ quarts (2 liters). Beverages provide well over half of this, so select your beverages carefully.

One of the nice things about water is that it contains absolutely no calories. One of the ways in which foods are made to contain fewer calories is to increase the amount of water they have. Helping yourself to more water and less fat is an important concept in managing your weight. Drinking water at each meal can provide an important part of your daily water need, can substitute for other beverages that might contain calories, and can slow your eating. In hot weather and when you are exercising, your body needs even more water. So don't forget to take water with you to drink when you go for a walk or to the gym.

When your body burns up food to produce the energy you need each day, it also makes water (and carbon dioxide). Water must then leave the body through the kidneys, the lungs, or the skin. But your kidneys do the bulk of the work. For that reason, our kidneys are essential to eliminating the water we drink and the water we produce from eating and digesting food. If this process trips up and doesn't work right away, as it does from time to time, our body weight may go up simply because we do not get rid of the water we drink and the water we make each day from digesting and metabolizing food. In fact, for every pound of fat we burn, we metabolically produce slightly more than a pound of water. This is one of the causes for the day-to-day variation in body weight we all experience. There is more than one way to reduce the energy (calories) in your diet. Selection of the correct mix of beverages is a good step in that direction. One study showed that people who consume a larger amount of water on average weigh less.[6] Thus get lots of "cool, clear water."

Coffee

Many people prefer drinking coffee over drinking plain water. Some health benefits have been claimed for filtered coffee, including lowering the risk of Type II diabetes.[7] Coffee is a good source of caffeine, and drinking it in the morning is a "waker-upper" for many people (including me). Too much coffee can produce jitters because of the caffeine, and stopping coffee consumption if you drink a lot can result in headaches. When cream or sugar is added to coffee, it adds calories. For this reason, I prefer non-caloric sweeteners.

The caffeine in coffee and tea is a mild stimulant that increases alertness.[8] The stimulant effect of added caffeine in some soft drinks may be one of the reasons why people consume so many of them—to get a caffeine fix. You could also get your "caffeine fix" from the caffeine-containing diet beverages.

Tea

When you tire of just drinking water, you can select green tea, black tea, or herbal teas. These have been popular drinks for many, many years. If you don't add milk or sugar, they have no calories—just like water. But tea does provide small amounts of flavonoids, which may have some health benefits. Some green teas also have small amount of a substance that slightly increases metabolism. Called epigallocatechin gallate (EGCG), this substance stimulates energy expenditure slightly. Some tea can provide caffeine, and if this is a problem for you, you can drink decaffeinated tea. Adding table sugar (sucrose - 1 teaspoon = around 16 cal) to tea adds to your daily caloric intake, so I recommend you sweeten it, if you desire, with artificial sweeteners, like I do.[9]

Skim Milk and Low-fat Milk

Milk is the first beverage we get, preferably from our mothers' breasts as infants. Breast milk provides very good nutrition and also protection from some diseases through the antibodies it provides. Breast milk is free of bacteria and doesn't need to be heated or pasteurized to sterilize it.

As we grow up, some people can no longer tolerate milk—it produces gastrointestinal problems. For these people, other sources of calcium are needed. For the rest of us, milk remains a great drink. It provides calcium and vitamin D. Pediatricians recommend whole milk for children after age 1 year and until age 2 years because of its mix of fatty acids that are so important to the cells of your body.

From school age on, milk remains a good drink, but it is healthier without the fat. One-percent milk and skim milk, including yogurt drinks, can be part of a healthy diet. Whole or full-fat milk is rich in saturated fat as well as extra calories. An 8-ounce glass of whole milk has 150 calories, compared to 90 calories in the same size glass of skim milk—a nearly 50% difference.

Fortified soy milk can replace cow's milk and related products and can be found in low-fat, as well as higher-fat, versions. Large amounts of "bad fructose" (sugar (sucrose) or HFCS)), however, are often added to soymilk and must be limited for the soymilk to be a healthy beverage option. The preparation of yogurt beverages reduces the milk sugar (lactose) that some people cannot digest. Like milk, yogurt is an important source of calcium, protein, and other essential nutrients. Unfortunately, many yogurt manufacturers add "bad fructose" (sugar (sucrose) or HFCS) to make it sweeter. The presence of HFCS or sugar (sucrose) on a label is a sign of a highly purified product. I try to find ones without these additives, which is often plain yogurt or ones sweetened with artificial sweeteners.

In the United States, milk is fortified with vitamin D. Rickets, once a common bone disease, has almost disappeared after the addition of vitamin D to milk.

Diet Drinks and Artificial Sweeteners

The next category is diet drinks. These are separated from the other soft drinks because they do not contain energy—they are almost entirely water with some flavor. They are sweetened with one of several "artificial" chemicals that give them the sweet taste.[10] Aspartame is a combination of two amino acids—the building blocks of protein. It is 200 times sweeter than sugar (sucrose) and was first approved for use to sweeten foods in 1981. When aspartame is eaten, the two amino acids that are connected in aspartame are split into their separate parts—methanol, aspartic acid, and phenylalanine. Phenylalanine is a problem for people with a specific genetic disease (phenylketonuria or PKU), and for them this sweetener should be avoided. To date no studies have shown adverse health effects from aspartame, except for those with phenylketonuria. This warning appears in the foods and drinks that are sweetened with aspartame (marketed as Equal).

Saccharin has a long history, being discovered in the nineteenth century (1879). It is 200 to 700 times sweeter than sugar (sucrose) and was widely used to sweeten foods. For a short time, it carried a warning label because of concerns that it might cause cancer, but these concerns have not been supported and the warning label was removed in 2000.

Acesulfame K (potassium) is a more recent addition to the list of sweeteners, being approved in 1988. It is about 200 times sweeter than sugar (sucrose) and has "no calories." A large number of studies show this compound is safe to consume.

Sucralose is made from sugar (sucrose), but it can't be digested in the intestine. Following a thorough review, this product which is 600 times sweeter than sugar (sucrose), was approved by the U.S. Food and Drug Administration in 1998.

Neotame is similar to aspartame but is 7,000 to 13,000 times sweeter than sugar (sucrose). Although it contains phenylalanine, the amount released is so small that there is no warning for people with phenylketonuria. Like the other sweeteners, there are a large number of clinical and animal studies that show its safety.

100% Fruit Juice
Beverages consisting of 100% fruit juices are different from "juice drinks." Please shop carefully to avoid being confused! I often pick up the wrong bottle or container, until I read the label and it says "high-fructose corn syrup." This is a sign of "bad fructose" and that the product is highly purified and manmade. Return to the 100% juice shelf. Another phrase to watch out for is "made from concentrate." "Concentrate" is another word for "sugar." The juice from the fruit is squeezed out and then treated to remove the water and other "volatile" parts. This leaves behind primarily the sugar. It can then be used as a "sweetener" for fruit juice, resulting in more sugar and "bad fructose." Just as with high-fructose corn syrup, I try to avoid those juices made from "concentrate," since I know it is largely "sugar" (bad fructose) and not much else.

Having selected 100% juice, you will have a naturally nutrient-rich food, but you will usually miss the fiber of whole fruit and get a relatively high energy (calorie) intake. I recommend you select the fruit over the fruit juice because it is closer to nature's own. It was increasing the fruits and vegetables in a dietary plan that lowered blood pressure in a study of dietary patterns and blood pressure that we discussed earlier.[11,12] When you use 100% juices, limit your total intake to 4–8 ounces per day. To show the amount of fruit needed to get fruit juice, I have compiled a short table.

Table 2. The number of pieces of fruit required to produce an 8-ounce glass from four different fruits

Fruit	Amount of Fruit needed to make 8-ounce glass of juice
Apple	12 medium
Grapes	¾ pound
Orange	2-3
Grapefruit	1 medium

Whole Milk

Whole milk—just as it comes from the cow and after Pasteurization to make it safe to drink—is a separate category from skim and low-fat milk because of the higher fat content of whole milk. Pediatricians recommend whole milk for children between ages 1 and 2 years, but thereafter lower-fat milks provide all of the calcium and vitamin D without the saturated fat. I prefer 1% or skim milk and would encourage you to make this shift for you and your family—a way to help you help yourself and those around you.

Sports Drinks

These are a separate category of beverages because they contain minerals—usually potassium—that are lost during vigorous exercise.[13] For athletes who are riding bicycles or running, these beverages are useful since they provide water, glucose, and minerals to replace what is being lost with exercise. For the ordinary individual who is not exercising, sports drinks are another source of "bad fructose," and you would be well advised to save them for the times when you are being much more active. Sports drinks may contain as much as 70% of the calories of soft drinks. Nonetheless, we should limit intake of sports drinks just as we do other calorically sweetened soft drinks. A well-balanced, nutritious diet provides the same ingredients as sports drinks. The carbohydrate, water, and sodium in sports drinks can, however, be an advantage during high levels of physical activity (more than 60 minutes), since they provide sodium, potassium, and fluid along with HFCS.

Soft Drinks and Bad Fructose

Soft drinks—cola, ginger ale, and others—are very popular. They are aggressively advertised. In the United States, soft drinks with calories are almost all sweetened with "bad fructose" (high-fructose corn syrup or sugar (sucrose)). In other countries, sugar (sucrose) is the major caloric sweetener and source of "bad fructose." Some people, including me, think we consume too much HFCS. Earlier I told you how HFCS is made from U.S. government-subsidized corn. It is thus cheap and sweet. One of my colleagues once wrote a book in which he described sugar as "pure, white and deadly."[14] The same thing might be said about HFCS. It is the fructose molecule that, in my opinion, is the bad actor in both sugar (sucrose) and HFCS. It is present in both table sugar (sucrose) and HFCS.

I am often asked whether there are any differences between high-fructose corn syrup and sugar (sucrose) once they are digested. Yes, there are several, and the differences start even before digestion. To describe these differences, let me use an analogy in which fructose and glucose in HFCS can be thought of as balloons. We will color the fructose balloon red and the glucose one green. In HFCS, these balloons are free to float around independently in their container. Either color of balloon can hit any wall without necessarily interfering with the other-color balloon. Sugar (sucrose) can also be viewed in this analogy as made of green and red balloons, but in this case the balloons are "connected" to each other at a fixed distance. When the green one moves one direction, the red one has to follow. If the red one hits a wall, the green one has to be close by, but not necessarily on the wall. Thus the balloons in the sugar solution move together; those in the HFCS solution move independently. This difference makes HFCS a very good product to use in preparing foods that will be frozen because the separation of the molecules of glucose and fructose prevents freezer burn better than with the same quantity of sugar (sucrose). There are other cooking advantages to HFCS as well, particularly in making soft, calorically rich cookies and pastries. Beware!

The difference in the number of separate particles in a 10% solution of HFCS and a 10% solution of sugar (sucrose) (the concentration found in soft drinks) gives the fructose and glucose in HFCS competitive access to the taste receptors on the tongue. If the fructose in sugar (sucrose) gets to the sweet receptor, the glucose attached to it cannot because of the "bond" that separates them. This probably accounts for the slight differences in sweetness between HFCS and sugar (sucrose).

When a 10% HFCS or a 10% sugar (sucrose) solution is swallowed, there is also a difference in the amount of water that enters the stomach to produce a solution that can pass into the intestine. HFCS has more particles and thus requires somewhat more water. Once the right concentration is reached in the stomach, the HFCS and sugar (sucrose) solutions enter the intestine. Once in the intestine, the fructose and glucose in HFCS can start to be absorbed immediately, since they are already separated. Before the fructose and glucose in dietary sugar (sucrose) can be absorbed, the sugar (sucrose) must be split into two parts to make glucose and fructose. The liver has the primary metabolic machinery in the body for dealing with fructose. When fructose from any source enters the liver, it uses an important energy source (ATP), whose concentration drops as fructose is used. Fructose in the liver can be turned into the backbone of fat, which is why an increase in blood fats is seen in some studies when people are given fructose in their diet.[15] It can also be turned into glucose. Although there are subtle differences in the ways "bad fructose" in sugar (sucrose) and in high-fructose corn syrup are handled by the body, the key point for us is that "bad fructose" is still "bad fructose," whether from dietary sugar (sucrose) or from high-fructose corn syrup. These differences are not important compared to the effects of bad fructose on the body.

Regardless of whether they contain HFCS or sugar (sucrose), calorically sweetened beverages should be replaced when possible with calorie-free beverages by anyone attempting to manage his or her weight, simply because the noncaloric beverages (water, diet sodas, tea, coffee, and other "diet" drinks) don't have calories. *Tip:* Reach for water first or one of the diet drinks or flavored-water drinks without calories.

One additional problem with soft drinks or fruit drinks containing either HFCS or sugar (sucrose) is that the body fails to recognize their calories as easily as it does the calories in milk or soup.[16] Why is this? One explanation is that the HFCS or sugar (sucrose) produces strong positive tastes on the tongue that make you want more. A second element may be that sweet mixtures of water and sugar (sucrose) or HFCS rapidly leave the stomach for the intestine, leaving the stomach feeling "hungry." Whatever the explanation, the calories in the HFCS (or sugar (sucrose))-sweetened soft drinks or fruit drinks do not suppress your appetite well enough.

Alcohol

Americans, on average, get 2–3% of their energy from alcoholic beverages. Alcohol contains about 7 calories per gram of energy. An ounce of beer has 12.5 calories per ounce, or 150 calories in the 12-ounce can. Wine has about 25 calories per ounce, and 80-proof liquor has about 70 calories per ounce. In beer, about 60% of the calories come from alcohol and the remainder mainly from carbohydrate. In wine, 80% of the calories come from alcohol and the remainder from carbohydrate. In hard liquor, all of the calories come from alcohol.

Alcoholic beverages can have some health benefits for adults, but they need to be consumed in moderation. A moderate intake for women is one drink daily and for men two drinks daily. By definition, one drink is 12 ounces of beer, 5 ounces of wine, or 1½ ounces of hard liquor (distilled beverages). Yes, alcohol provides calories to the body and depending on how much you drink, this can be important.

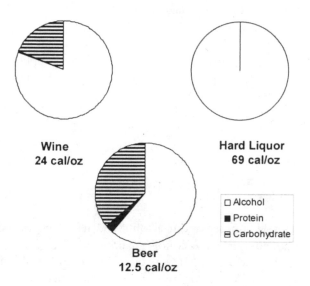

Figure 1. Alcohol Content of Various Types of Alcoholic Beverages

Excessive alcohol may cause a number of serious health and social problems. There is a relation between alcohol consumption and early death; light to moderate consumption is associated with lower rates of death—mostly from lower risks of cardiovascular diseases—than avoiding alcohol, while at the other end of the spectrum, heavy alcohol intake is associated with increased risk of early death. These effects are mainly from the alcohol and not from the other things in these beverages. Intake of alcoholic beverages, even moderate intake, is linked to higher risk of birth defects, and pregnant women should not consume alcoholic beverages. Intake of alcoholic beverages is also related to the risk of breast cancer. Heavier alcohol use is linked with some other cancers.

Table 2 is the amount of calories in various kinds of alcoholic beverages, and Table 3 shows the amount of time you have to spend in various activities to balance the alcohol intake in the beverages shown in the table.

Table 2. Calorie content in various types of alcoholic beverages

Item	Serving Size	Calories
Beer (Regular can)	12 fluid oz	150
Wine, dry	5 fluid oz	115
Liquor	1½ fluid oz	105

Table 3. Exercise needed to burn alcoholic beverage calories

FOOD	Weight 1 oz (30 g)	Calories	Walking	Bicycling	Swimming	Jogging
			Minutes of Activity			
Beer 8 oz	240	115	22	18	14	12
Gin, dry 1½ oz	43	108	20	16	12	11
Manhattan cocktail 3½ oz	100	165	32	25	19	17
Martini cocktail 3½ oz	100	140	27	22	16	14
Rum 1½ oz	45	105	20	16	12	11
Scotch 1½ oz	45	105	20	16	12	11
Sherry 2-oz glass	60	85	16	13	10	9
Vermouth 3½ oz glass	100	105	20	16	12	11

1½ oz of liquor = 1 jigger

There is a lot of concern about alcohol and its effects on people who drive or use other equipment. Alcohol impairs mental functions to variable degrees. We have all learned that you don't drink and drive. *Tip:* Don't drink and diet, either. A glass or two of wine, a few beers, or a couple of mixed drinks can take the edge off. But part of the edge they take off is your ability to help yourself to control your food selection. My advice is "don't drink and diet."

There is another face to alcoholic beverages. A drink or so a day is claimed to improve the "good cholesterol" (HDL-cholesterol), which can lower your risk of heart attacks. If you accept this reasoning, the best time to have the drink might be after dinner, once you have already made the rest of your nutritional choices. To have it before dinner, unless it is well before, runs the risk of lowering your ability to make good nutritional choices. The choice is yours.

Caffeine

For many of us, coffee tastes good. Others prefer tea or chocolate. All of these drinks contain stimulants. Caffeine is the best known of these. Caffeine makes us more alert; it is a good picker-upper. It can also increase our metabolism. I have shown a list of caffeinated drinks below. Caffeine does not cause any diseases, but it can keep you awake. In moderation, caffeine and its relatives can be part of a healthy lifestyle.

Table 4. Caffeine content of beverages and medications

Item	Caffeine Content (mg/unit)
Coffee (6 oz - 1 cup)	
Brewed: Percolator	90-120
Dripolator	120-150
Instant (freeze-dried)	50-80
Decaffeinated	2-5
Tea (6 oz = 1 cup)	
Brewed (5 min)	
Black	50-80
Green	35-50
Mint or herb	0
Soft drinks (12 oz)	
Coca Cola	65
Diet Coca Cola – caffeine free	0
Dr. Pepper	60
Pepsi Cola	43
Diet Pepsi – caffeine free	0
Royal Crown (RC) Cola	36
Medications:	
Nodoz	100
Excedrin	64.8
Anacin	32.5
Bromo-seltzer	35.5
Emprin Compound	32.2
Pre-Mens-forte	100

What Are You Drinking?

Now its time to find out what you are drinking and how much of it contains "bad fructose," which can come from high-fructose corn syrup (HFCS), sugar (sucrose), or concentrate it contains. To do this I will introduce the system we use throughout this book. It is based on writing down what you use on a 3x5 card or some other convenient and small piece of paper or cardboard you can carry with you. A PDA (Personal Digitial Assistant) could also be used. On the form or your PDA, record each beverage you drink during the day and then note next to it the sources of calories in that beverage. We will have a longer discussion of calories and how to record them in Chapter 10.

Bray Plan Monitor **MONITOR FOR BEVERAGES**						
Day Beverage Consumed	Amt Oz	From Conc	HFCS	Sugar	Art Sweet	Alc

Amt Oz = amount in ounces; From Conc = beverage made from concentrate (a form of "bad fructose"); HFCS = high-fructose corn syrup (a form of "bad fructose"); sugar (a form of "bad fructose"); Art Sweet = artificial sweeteners including saccharin (Sweet'N Low®, Sweet Twin®, Necta Sweet®), aspartame (NutraSweet® and Equal®), sucralose (Splenda®), Acesulfame-K (Sunett® and Sweet One®); Alc = alcohol.

Do this for a period of seven days, which will cover the usual times during the work or school week and the weekend where beverages are used differently. Be honest. You have only yourself to benefit. Write down every time you drink something, including a glass of water. Writing it down helps make you conscious of helping yourself record things and knowing what you have taken into your body. After all, it is your body, and the more you know about it, the easier it is to help yourself keep it healthy.

Now let's summarize what you have done for the past week. Below is a recording form where you can enter the number of times during the week when you drank beverages with different things.

| Bray Plan Monitor ANALYSIS OF BEVERAGES | | | | | | | | | | | | | | | | |
Sweetener	1	2	3	4	5	6	7	8	9	10	11	12	13	14	Add'l	Total
From Conc																
HFCS																
Sugar																
Art Sweet																
Alcohol																

From Conc = From Concentrate (a form of "bad fructose"); HFCS = high-fructose corn syrup (a form of "bad fructose"); sugar (a form of "bad fructose"); Art Sweet = artificial sweeteners that include saccharin (Sweet'N Low®, Sweet Twin®, Necta Sweet®), aspartame (NutraSweet® and Equal®), sucralose (Splenda®), Acesulfame-K (Sunett® and Sweet One®); Alc = alcohol.

From your first day, put a check mark or blacken a box for each time the beverage you had contained one of the sweeteners or alcohol. If you have more than fourteen beverages that contained "bad fructose" in any of the categories, just note these in the additional ("add'l") category. Now go to the next day and so on until you have listed all of the beverages you consumed during the week. With this in mind, you can now repeat the recording by focusing of reducing the amount of "bad fructose" you are getting from your beverages. Increase water, decrease the checks in the HFCS, from concentrate and sugar categories, and increase the artificial sweeteners category. Good luck!

CHAPTER SEVEN

Become More Active

Are You Ready?
This chapter is about helping you help yourself BECOME MORE ACTIVE. This is a vital element in your successful weight-loss plan. We know this because successful people, those who have lost and maintained their weight loss, tell us that one essential strategy for keeping the weight off is to become more active.[1] You need to build this into your plan for managing your weight, too.

The flip side of being more active is to be less inactive. Here television is a big culprit. Most children and adults spend many hours watching television each week, often with food nearby. The more television people watch, the more likely they are to be overweight.[2] When children were provided with rewards for being less inactive OR for being more active, the rewards for being less inactive produced more weight loss than those for being more active. *Tip:* Reduce the time in your day when you are inactive.

Your body weight is a balance between what you eat and what you burn up through exercise and metabolism. Reducing the number of calories you get from the foods you eat by avoiding fructose and fat affects one end of the balance of fat stores. Increasing the number of calories you burn by being more active works on the other end in reducing energy balance, like spending money reduces the balance in your bank account. But most Americans are not enamored with the idea of physical activity. Working up a sweat and improving endurance are hard work for many people. Help yourself by thinking small when starting an exercise program.

Figure 1 shows this idea of a balance. On the right is a column the height of the food you eat. The left-hand column is divided up roughly into the amounts you spend in each form of "energy expenditure." Roughly two-thirds (2/3) of the amount of food energy you eat is used by your body for the daily tasks of keeping your body warm, digesting food, keeping your blood circulating, and so on. The remaining one-third (1/3) is devoted to the activity that moves your muscles. For some people with very physically demanding jobs, this can be much higher, but for people with a weight problem, the proportions shown on this figure are about right.

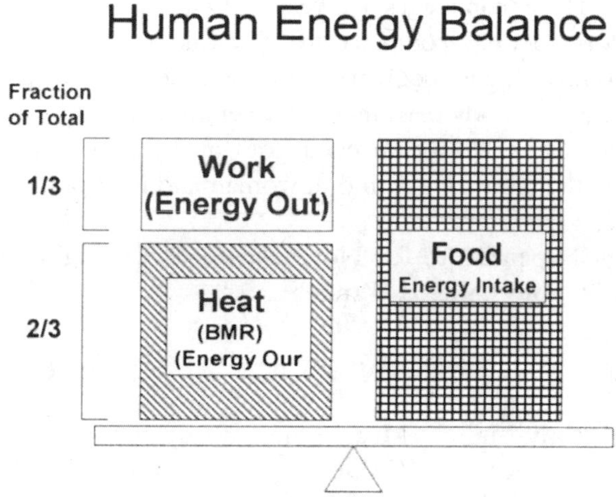

Human Energy Balance

Figure 1. Energy Balance Diagram. This illustration shows the relation between food intake and exercise, which is one basic principle of weight loss.

How do we know how high these bars are? We have already talked about food intake and how difficult that is to measure well. We do have a lot of information about it, however, and can provide reasonably good ideas about how much food people need. The energy expenditure bars on the left can also be measured. One technique that has been particularly useful was developed only within the last twenty-five years. It is called doubly labeled water, or DLW for short. When your energy account is in balance, it means the money going in equals what is coming out—just like a bank account. When you are in energy balance, ALL that comes out is carbon dioxide and water. Remember the carbon dioxide cycle? Plants take carbon dioxide from the air and make it into plant food. Human beings and other animals burn this food to produce carbon dioxide and water. If we know how much carbon dioxide and water you are producing, we can estimate how much food you had to eat to do that. With the doubly labeled water technique, we do just that by giving you markers for the water and carbon dioxide you produce and then collecting these markers. From this information, we can calculate how much energy your body uses.

Using this DLW technique, the energy needs for Americans have been estimated for various ages and both sexes by the National Research Council.[4] These numbers can help you know what your energy levels are. Using the now familiar body mass index (described in Chapter 1) and the method of measuring energy expenditure that we just described, we can see that people who are overweight burn *more* calories and thus must eat more calories to *maintain* their weight. The children ages 3–8 years with a body mass index of 15.4 needed 1441 calories per day, compared to 1728 calories per day for children the same age who had a higher body mass index averaging 19.8—chubby children, indeed. When the body mass index is several units higher, as shown in this table, the number of calories needed goes up by 200 to 700 per day, depending on whether you are a man or a woman and how old you are.

Table 1. Energy Expenditure for Normal and Overweight Males and Females Using Doubly Labeled Water

Age Group, Years	Normal Weight		Overweight	
	Body Mass Index	Mean Total Energy Expenditure (kcal/d)	Body Mass Index	Mean Total Energy Expenditure (kcal/d)
Males				
3-8	15.4	1,441	19.8	1,728
9-13	17.2	2,079	25.4	2,451
14-18	20.4	3,116	—	—
19-30	22.0	3,081	29.6	3,599
31-50	22.6	3,021	30.8	3,598
51-70	23.0	2,469	29.6	2,946
>70	22.8	2,238	27.8	2,510
Females				
3-8	15.6	1,487	20.3	1,669
9-13	17.4	1,907	24.7	2,346
14-18	20.4	2,302	27.6	2,798
19-30	21.4	2,436	29.8	2,677
31-50	21.6	2,404	31.9	2,895
51-70	22.2	2,066	30.4	2,176
>70	21.8	1,564	27.6	1,763

Adapted from Dietary Reference Intakes for Energy, Carbohydrate, Fiber, Fat, Fatty Acids, Cholesterol, Protein, and Amino Acids. Washington, D.C.: The National Academies Press, 2002–2005[5]

Using these numbers, the people at the U.S. Department of Agriculture and the U.S. Department of Health and Human Services, who prepare our dietary guidelines, have estimated energy needs for various age groups at three different levels of activity (Table 2). As you begin to manage your weight, keep in mind that you are balancing calories expended in activity with those obtained in food. The more active you are, the more food calories you can eat and still keep your weight in line.

Table 2. Estimated energy requirements in calories per day in relation to age and gender at three levels of physical activity

Gender	Age, years	Activity Level		
		Sedentary	Moderately Active	Active
Boys & Girls	2-3	1,000	1,000-1,400	1,000-1,400
Female	4-8	1,200	1,400-1,600	1,400-1,800
	9-13	1,600	1,600-2,000	1,800-2,200
	14-18	1,800	2,000	2,400
	19-30	2,000	2,000-2,200	2,400
	31-50	1,800	2,000	2,200
	>50	1,600	1,800	2,000-2,200
Male	4-8	1,400	1,400-1,600	1,600-2,000
	9-13	1,800	1,800-2,200	2,000-2,600
	14-18	2,200	2,400-2,800	2,800-3,200
	19-30	2,400	2,600-2,800	3,000
	31-50	2,200	2,400-2,600	2,800-3,000
	>51	2,000	2,200-2,400	2,400-2,800

Adapted from the Dietary Guidelines 2005[3]

The quickest way to lose your enthusiasm for being more active is to try to do too much too fast. As Covert Bailey,[6] author of *Fit or Fat*, puts it, start so slowly that "people will make fun of you." But before suggesting an activity program, here are a few basic pointers about energy and activity.

First, let's make sure being more active is for you. If you answer "no" to either of the two following questions, you need to consult your doctor before trying to become more active. (1) Can you walk half a mile without stopping or without pain? (2) Are you able to climb one flight of stairs without becoming winded? If you answered "yes" to both of these questions, then ask yourself the following questions. Do you have a convenient place for your activity? Remember, you need to be able to be active in all kinds of weather. Do you have someone to join you in being more active? A buddy who wants to walk with you makes it more fun. Beware of picking someone who is highly trained if you are not up to that level. This can both tax you physically and take away the fun and rewards.

Can you make a commitment of time? Being more active requires time. You need to budget the time into your schedule. Do you believe that being active will make you feel better or feel less tired? If so, and if you have tried exercising before and liked the feeling, sometimes called an "endorphin" high because of those pesky pleasurable peptides produced in your brain, then you are on the right path.

The amount of energy you burn every day of your life is roughly equivalent to the amount of heat generated over a twenty-four-hour period by a 60-watt lightbulb. As you increase your level of activity, you may increase this. But even if you are very active, you will still rarely produce much more heat or energy than a 100-watt lightbulb when it is turned on.

The lightbulb lights up your room because an electric power plant somewhere is producing electricity that is sent to your house. In turn, the electric power plant is burning fuel to produce the electrical energy. Your food is the fuel that is burned by your power plant. The power plant can only produce energy as long as there is fuel available for it to burn. If the electric power plant runs out of coal, gas, or whatever other fuel it uses, it cannot supply electricity to your house to light your light bulb. The fat stored on your body is like the coal or gas stored by the power plant. It is the reserve fuel stored to power your body's generator. In weight management, we are trying to reduce the extra stores of this energy in fat by burning it up.

Think of the fat on your body as the gasoline in your car's fuel tank. When the gas in your tank runs out, your engine stops. That is why we keep fuel in our tank. It is a source of energy available whenever we need it to drive our car. The fuel you store on your body is composed largely of fat—protein contributes a bit and glucose very little. If you compared the energy you have available in your body to the amount of gasoline in a car's fuel tank, it would be comparable to an oil tanker being pulled by a compact car. The energy stored in fat is enormous when compared to the energy stored as gasoline in the fuel tank of your car.

So each day we are burning about the same amount of fuel that would be required to light a 60-watt lightbulb. We replenish that energy by eating food. We can talk about the amount of energy in the foods we eat in terms of calories. While sitting quietly in a chair, most of us use a little less than one calorie per minute, depending on our age, size, and sex. Bigger people will use more energy than smaller people. Just sitting around all day requires approximately 1500 calories to keep our human engine running at idle.

An 8-oz (240 ml) glass of skim milk has about 100 calories (so does 8 oz of soda, but with "bad fructose" and without the other nutrients in milk). To burn off those 100 calories, you would have to walk about a mile. Now consider that a pound of fat contains about 3,500 calories. That means we would have to walk about 35 miles to burn up a pound of fat.

Table 3 is a short list of foods and the number of minutes that are required to talk them off at a rate of 3 miles per hour for individuals of 3 different weights. Table 5 (at the end of the chapter) is a longer list of foods and the minutes needed to use the calories for different kinds of exercise. You can look at Table 3 in two different ways. First, you may say, why bother? Walking makes such a little difference that it isn't worth it. But remember, you're taking the positive approach to helping yourself (Chapter 3). You can walk a mile a day, every day for 35 days, and burn off one pound. But that's 10 pounds a year or 50 pounds in five years. The glass is emptying. Exercise is obviously important. It's just that exercise alone is not a good way to lose a lot of weight in a short time.

Table 3. Minutes of Walking to Burn the Calories in Various Foods

Foods	Calories in Food	Minutes to Burn Calories Walking at 3 miles per hour Body Weight (lb)		
		120	160	200
Apple (2¼-in diameter)	75	21	17	14
Apple Pie (1/6 of 9-inch pie)	410	115	93	78
Beer (12 oz)	170	47	38	31
Blueberries (1 fresh cup)	87	23	19	16
Beef steak (4 oz)	300	83	68	57
Bologna (1 slice)	88	23	22	19
Biscuit (2-inch diameter)	130	36	30	24
Bread (1 slice)	65	18	15	12
Broccoli (1 cup)	50	14	12	10
Cola drink (8 oz - 250 ml)	100	28	23	19
Cereal (1 cup cooked)	165	46	38	31
Cheese (1 oz)	100	28	23	19
Chocolate Cake (1 slice 2×3×2" with no icing)	165	46	38	31
Egg (1 medium)	78	22	18	15
Flounder (4 oz raw)	78	22	18	15
Frankfurter	124	34	28	23
Hamburger & bun (3 oz High-fat meat)	400	111	91	76
Milk (8 oz whole milk)	166	46	38	31
Orange (large 3-3/8 inch)	115	32	27	23
Potato (1 baked no skin 2½-inch diameter)	100	28	23	19
Salmon (3½ oz canned)	200	56	46	38
Strawberries (1 cup)	54	15	12	10

But helping yourself to a regular activity program makes a statement about your commitment to a new lifestyle. It means making a commitment to success and improved health. It's also very important in maintaining your weight after you have reached your goal, which we will discuss in greater detail in a later chapter.

You can help yourself by following through with your activity plan. Here's an example from a research study: Two groups of policemen volunteered to find out whether being physically active after losing weight made any difference in their long-term weight control.[7] The policemen ate one of four different diets. Half of the officers in each group exercised, under supervision, for 90 minutes three times per week, while the others did not.

Exercising while dieting added very little extra weight loss for these police-men during the initial 8 weeks (Figure 2). But the picture at both 8 months and 18 months later tells a very different story. The solid lines during the follow-up period in the graph below show what happened to the men who continued their activity and the dashed lines what happened to the men who stopped being active.

Effect of Exercise on Initial Rate of Weight Loss and on Subsequent Weight Status

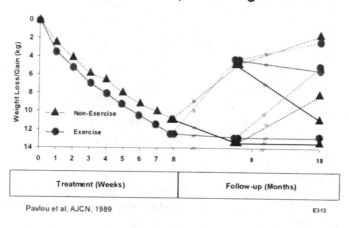

Pavlou et al, AJCN, 1989   E313

Figure 2. Weight loss and regain over 18 months. The policemen lost weight by diet, but exercise added only a little bit more weight loss in this first 8 weeks. After the end of the first 8 weeks, whether men stayed lighter or regained their weight was predicted best by whether they continued to exercise (solid line) or not (dashed lines).[7]

By 8 months, the men who were physically active, whether or not they were initially in this group, maintained their twenty-five-pound weight loss. Between 8 and 18 months, some policemen continued to be more active (solid lines) and others did not. Those who continued their active lifestyle kept their weight down, those who did not regained weight. The bottom line is simple: Being physically active helps you help yourself keep your weight down or prevents it from rising.

Exercise for Health and Fun

Let's face it, though. Being more active can be a real chore for some people. That's not surprising, once you consider activity (work) itself. Work, a way of measuring the amount of energy you produce, is composed of two parts. The first is the distance you cover. The second is the weight you move over

119

that distance. If you are twice as heavy as your buddy, you will need to use twice as much energy to move the same distance. In short, this means an overweight person spends more energy moving his or her body than does a person of normal weight. That's why overweight people get hot, sweaty, and uncomfortable very quickly when increasing their activity.

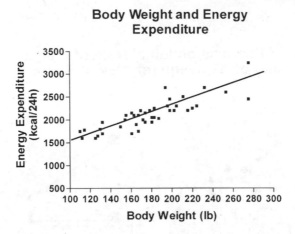

Body Weight and Energy Expenditure

Figure 3. Energy expenditure and body weight. This figure shows the energy that individuals of various weights used when moving the wheels on a bicycle. The heavier they were, the more energy it took simply to move their legs.[8]

Make no mistake about it, being active requires energy and hard work. But you don't have to run a mile right out of the starting gate. One activity you already do every day is walking. Increasing the amount of walking you do is within the grasp of nearly everyone and is the best way you can help yourself. You already walk around your living room and your kitchen. Now help yourself to walk an additional amount every day. Figure 3 shows the results of women of different weights pedaling on a bicycle. Heavier people have heavier legs, and this figure shows that moving heavier legs (the rest of the body was sitting on a bicycle seat) increased as body weight increased. Thus moving heavier legs in a heavier person takes more effort.

If you are more than 20 pounds overweight, increase your activity slowly, say, by only five minutes each day or so. But make activity a regular, routine part of your life. It is the commitment you make to incorporating movement and activity into your everyday lifestyle that is important. Also try to introduce as much walking into your day as possible. Park farther away from the supermarket door, the shopping center entrance, or your office door. Take the stairs instead of an elevator. Every little bit helps you help yourself.

Counting your steps is a useful way to find out how you are doing. Small step counters (pedometers) that you can put on your waist record the steps you take. These little devices are good for giving you feedback on how you are doing and for helping you set new goals. Each 2,000 steps you walk add up to about 1 mile and require some 300 kcal, depending on your weight. Get yourself a step counter at the sports store and begin to wear it every day for a week, then record how many steps you take by using the Step Counting Form.

Bray Plan Monitor	
MONITOR FOR STEP COUNTER	
Day of the Week	Number of Steps
Monday	
Tuesday	
Wednesday	
Thursday	
Friday	
Saturday	
Sunday	

Add up how many steps you walked and divide by 7 to get your average daily walking distance. For the next week, try to add 500 or 1000 steps per day. If you increase slowly over a few weeks, you can get your number of steps up to 5,000 steps per day or more. The longer-term goal is to reach 10,000 steps per day or about 5 miles. Using step counters is one part of the national movement called "America on the Move." There is an Internet website for those interested in advice about using the step counter (*www.americaonthemove.org*).

The next step will help you in your long-term weight-loss program. As you start your weight-loss program, you will lose weight. As your weight decreases, two things will happen: First, your daily activities will require less energy, that is, fewer calories, because there will be less of you to move around, so to speak. In order to maintain your *current* body weight, you need to eat about 10 calories per pound. For example, a middle-aged man or woman who weighs 240 pounds will maintain that weight when consuming approximately 2,400 calories or more per day. But if this same person loses 80 pounds (so that the new weight is 160 pounds), the requirement drops to roughly 1,600 calories or more per day—*a decrease of 800 calories per day*. This change in the amount of energy required is like replacing a 100-watt lightbulb with a 60-watt lightbulb. Less heat and light are generated. The second result is that you will feel cooler. And it is not unusual; many of my patients have complained about being cold after losing weight.

It is important to note that you require fewer calories per day to *maintain* your new body weight after you lose weight. If you now weigh 160 lbs, you will only need about 1,600 calories or more to maintain that weight. This is where that mile of walking can play an important role. The 100 calories per day or more that you burn through increased activity will help narrow that margin when combined with your new nutritional lifestyle.

I am often asked whether I recommend aerobic exercise, such as jogging or running. Aerobic exercise is activity that increases oxygen consumption by your entire body and improves the efficiency of your heart and lungs. Sure, aerobic exercise is great if you like it and are in shape to do it. But it is more important for you to make a commitment to yourself to get regular movement into your life, even if you only begin with 5 to 10 minutes a day. Start out with walking. Walking is the easiest and safest exercise. If you are later motivated to take up more vigorous aerobic exercise, such as jogging, swimming, bicycling, or climbing stairs, then that's wonderful. But the most important step is to simply begin moving. Any type of extra movement will help you on the way to a more active lifestyle.

Aerobic Exercise

Aerobic exercise refers to the increased oxygen delivery required for vigorous muscular activity. The benefits of an aerobic exercise program include a healthier, stronger heart and a more efficient respiratory system. You can only work so hard. There is a maximum amount of work that you can sustain, which we call your maximum aerobic capacity. This is the highest rate at which your cardiovascular system can deliver oxygen to your body. This rate is related to your *maximum heart rate*. Since your maximum heart rate declines with age, so does your maximum aerobic capacity, or your body's ability to do maximal work. As a guideline, your maximal heart rate is 220 beats per minute minus your age in years. Now let's stop and figure out your maximum heart rate.

Table 4. Relationship between heart rate and age for various percentages of maximal output

Age (years)	Heart Rate (beats/min) to Achieve % of Maximum			
	55% Max	60% Max	90% Max	Maximum
20	110	120	180	200
25	107	117	177	195
30	104	114	173	190
35	102	111	168	185
40	99	108	163	180
45	96	105	159	175
50	93	102	153	170

55	91	99	149	165
60	88	96	143	160
65	85	93	140	155
70	82	90	135	150
75	80	87	132	145
80	77	84	129	140

This table is only an approximation for any individual's response and will not apply when certain rate-altering medications are being taken, such as beta-blockers and some calcium antagonists.

55% of maximum is the minimum heart rate for health benefit designated by the American College of Sports Medicine; 60% is the minimum rate for fitness designated by the ACSM; Maximum exercise heart rate designated by the ACSM
Adapted from the American College of Sports Medicine[9]

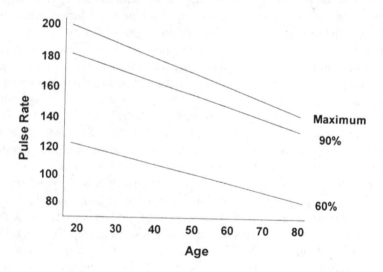

Figure 4. Relation of heart rate to age for different levels of percentage maximal heart rate. The maximal rate is your age subtracted from 220 as shown in Table 4. The 90% and 60% numbers are 90% and 60% of this maximal value.

Maximum heart rate = 220 minus Your Age (years)=_____.

To know whether you are doing enough aerobic exercise, you must determine your pulse rate and raise it to the appropriate level. As a guide, your maximum obtainable pulse rate is 220 minus your age in years. If you are 40 years old, this means your maximum obtainable pulse rate is approximately 180 beats per minute. For aerobic exercise, you should raise your pulse rate to approximately 60 to 75% of this maximum for at least 10 to 20 minutes per day. So for our forty-year-old, this means a pulse rate of about 108 to 135 beats per minute. This elevated heart rate should be obtained during exercise or very shortly after it is stopped. Measuring your heart rate requires a watch with a second hand. I recommend counting the pulse for 6 seconds at the wrist, if it is easy to feel, or in the neck. The number of heartbeats in 6 seconds, multiplied by 10, results in the pulse rate of beats per minute.

Dr. Peter Lindner identifies several steps for increasing activity levels in his book *From Fatness to Fitness.*[8] The first step is to help yourself think positively about being more active. If you think about being more active and commit yourself to it, you will have many more opportunities to be active than if your mind is on something else.

The second step is to loosen up. This is a good idea before beginning any type of activity. As soon as you wake up in the morning, stretch your arms, legs, hands, and feet. Stretching is a good form of activity and a great way to stretch the tendons and warm up the muscles before beginning any more vigorous activity. Also try stretching your neck by lifting your chin high. Stretch the muscles in your back, abdomen, and sides by twisting your body to the right and left several times. Stretch your back muscles by bending over and pulling your shoulders toward your knees as far as they will go. Some of the most effective meetings I've attended had the attendees participate in stretch breaks, rather than a morning coffee break. Five minutes were set aside for participants to stretch by standing, bending, and moving.

The third step is to spend more time on your feet. Standing increases the amount of energy you burn by 10%. Obviously, the more time you spend on your feet, the more energy you will burn. Stand while talking on your cell phone. Do your ironing, do your hair, put on makeup, do your emails, and prepare a shopping list while standing, if you can. In my opinion, television remote controls are one of the scourges of modern society. Lock that remote control in a drawer. This means you'll have to get up to change the channel or the volume. Studies have shown that even fidgeting in a chair can be an effective way to keep your muscles moving and burning energy. Move your foot up and down, even if there isn't any music.

Many modern conveniences have reduced the amount of energy we burn. Even switching from the typewriter to the omnipresent computer to prepare documents conserves about 17.5 calories per hour. That may seem trivial, but look at it this way: If you save 17.5 calories per hour, in a forty-hour week you will have saved about 700 calories. Since a pound of fat contains 3,500 calories, you could put on 1 pound over 5 weeks—10 pounds of fat in 50 weeks just by switching from an electric typewriter to a word processor. Other labor-saving devices such as electric mixers, electric toothbrushes, and automatic dishwashers have deprived us of ways to burn energy. The moral of the story is that it is sometimes better to do things the old-fashioned way and at the same time help yourself to increase your activity.

Tips to Help You Be More Active

Here are a number of tips you can use to help yourself get moving:

1. Take your pet for a walk. If you don't have a dog, take the neighbor's dog for a walk. Maybe you could adopt a shelter dog.
2. Take the baby or grandchild for a walk.
3. Play catch or throw a Frisbee with a family member, friend, or neighbor.
4. When you go shopping, park your car at the far end of the parking lot.
5. At work, park as far away from the door as practical. This gets you to walk further.
6. Do shopping and other errands more frequently.
7. Mow your lawn or garden more often.
8. Join a walking or hiking club.
9. Visit outdoor historical sites, where you need to walk to see the exhibits.
10. Take a walk with your spouse or a good friend.
11. Get up from the chair or sofa for a walk during the television commercials.
12. Do volunteer work that keeps you up and active.
13. If you ride a bicycle or swim, do it regularly.
14. Take dancing lessons or join a dance club.
15. Take up an active hobby that will keep you moving.
16. Use a step counter.
17. Set up a home gym and use it instead of watching television.
18. For birthdays and other holidays, give gifts that encourage activity.
19. To see how active you are, take the president's challenge as a family. See *www.presidentschallenge.org.*
20. Have an activity party—bowling or skating, for example.

Walking can do all this for you. I hope it is clear that I believe walking is the best activity you can incorporate into your daily lifestyle. You must do it regularly. You must decide where you are going to walk and then get some estimate of the distance you are planning to walk. A one-mile walk or 2000 steps is a reasonable place to start. Measure a walking course by driving it in your car or find an already marked course. Don't dawdle during your walk. Keep yourself moving. Try using your iPOD or other source of music during your walk. A good pace for a mile is about 20 minutes for a mile. If you are over 240 pounds, I recommend a slightly slower pace, maybe a mile in 25 minutes. At this pace, you will burn off about 10 pounds of fat in a year if you help yourself by not eating more. Remember, begin your walking with a 5- to 10-minute warm-up period. After your walk, begin a cool-down routine by walking at a gradually slower pace.

Covert Bailey[6] offers what I think is a great piece of advice about activity: "If you can't do it right, do it often." He says that even if you can't move as rapidly or effectively as you might like, it isn't an excuse for not moving at all. With that in mind, Bailey says never exercise with a fit friend. It's the quickest way to become discouraged. There are no excuses for missing one of your activity sessions. Bailey sums it up by saying: "I am not burning a lot of calories when I am exercising, but my body is changing into a better fat-burning machine." The purpose of increased activity is to help you help yourself change your fat-burning chemistry. I think this is excellent advice. Recall the earlier discussion on activity and fat.

What can you do if your joints hurt when you become more active? This is certainly a problem for some people. In some of our programs where we want to get people moving more, we have them do water aerobics. Doing your bending and other activities while standing in the shallow end of a swimming pool is a good approach. You can also use the pool as an opportunity to swim.

Table 5. Time Required to Use Calories in Various Foods with Different Types of Activity

Food	Weight 1 oz-30g	Calories	Walking	Bicycling	Swimming	Jogging
				Minutes of Activity		
Bread						
Bread + butter						
1 slice + 5 g (1 tsp)	28	96	18	16	11	10
Biscuit 2" diam	35	130	25	20	15	13
Muffin 4" diam	40	120	23	18	14	12
Roll, hard	36	109	21	16	13	11
Tortilla, 6" diam	30	65	13	10	8	7
Pancake 4" diam	45	105	20	16	12	11
Waffle, plain						
5½" diameter	75	210	40	32	25	21
Cereal and Pasta						
Bran flakes ¾ cup,						
milk ½ cup + sugar 5 g (1 tsp)	153	212	41	32	15	21
Oatmeal 1 cup cooked,						
+ milk ¼ cup,						
+ sugar 1 tsp (5 g) sugar	301	260	50	39	31	26
Macaroni or pasta, cooked 1 cup	140	205	39	31	24	21

Vegetables

Brussels sprouts					
2/3 cup	100	36	7	5	4	4
Carrots, cooked, drained 2/3 cup	100	31	6	5	4	3
Celery 2 small stalks 5"	40	6	1	1	1	1
Corn, sweet 1 ear	140	70	14	10	8	7
Eggplant, cooked ½ cup	100	19	4	3	2	2
Lettuce, romaine 3½ oz	100	18	3	3	2	2
Mushrooms, fresh raw,						
10 small or 4 large	100	28	5	4	4	3
Onions, cooked ½ cup	105	30	6	4	4	3
Peas, green cooked ½ cup	80	58	11	9	7	6
Potato, baked, 1 medium	99	90	17	14	11	9
Potato, baked 1 medium						
+ 2 pats butter	110	160	31	24	19	16
Potato chips 10 pieces (2" diam)	20	115	22	17	14	12
Potatoes, French fried						
20 pieces (½"× ½" × 2")	100	274	53	41	33	27
Spinach, cooked ½ cup	90	20	4	3	2	2
Squash, summer cooked ½ cup	105	14	3	2	2	1
Tomato, cooked ½ cup	100	26	5	4	3	3
Turnip greens, cooked ½ cup	145	30	6	4	4	3

Fruits

Apple, raw, 1 medium						
(2½" diameter)	150	87	17	13	10	9
Applesauce 1/3 cup	100	90	17	14	11	9
Apricots, raw 3 medium	100	50	10	8	6	6
Avocado, raw ½ pitted	100	167	32	25	20	17
Banana, 1 medium	150	127	24	19	15	13
Blackberries, raw 1 cup	144	84	16	13	10	8
Blueberries, raw 5/8 cup	100	62	12	10	7	6
Boysenberries, frozen						
without sugar 4/5 cup	100	48	9	7	6	5
Cantaloupe, raw ¼ melon						
5" large	100	30	6	4	4	3
Cherries, sweet, raw 24 small,						
15 large	100	70	14	10	8	7
Grapefruit, raw ½ medium	100	40	8	6	5	4
Honeydew, raw ¼ small						
(5" diameter)	100	33	6	5	4	4
Nectarine, raw 1 medium	50	32	6	4	4	3
Olives, green, packed, 4 medium	26	9	6	4	4	3

Olives, ripe 4 large	40	74	14	11	9	7
Orange, raw 1 medium (3" diameter)	150	73	14	11	9	7
Peaches, raw 1 medium	100	38	7	6	4	4
Pears, raw 1 medium	200	122	24	18	14	12
Pineapple, raw 1 slice (3½ × ¾")	84	44	9	7	5	4
Pineapple, canned, heavy syrup 1 large slice	100	74	14	11	9	7
Plums, raw 2 medium	100	66	13	10	8	7
Raisins, dried 1 teaspoon	10	30	6	4	4	3
Raspberries, raw, black 2/3 cup	100	75	14	11	9	8
Strawberries, raw, 10 large	100	37	7	6	4	4
Strawberries, frozen, with sugar ½ cup	126	140	27	22	17	14
Tangerine, raw 1 large	100	46	9	7	6	5

100% Fruit Juices

Apple juice, fresh 8 oz	240	120	24	18	14	12
Grapefruit juice, 8 oz	240	94	18	14	12	10
Orange juice, 8 oz	240	108	20	16	12	10
Punch, Hawaiian 8 oz	240	216	42	34	26	22
Tomato juice 8 oz	240	46	8	6	3	4
Vegetable juice, canned 8 oz	240	42	8	6	6	4

Milk, Yogurt, and Cheese

Cheese, blue 1 oz	30	103	20	15	12	10
Cheese, American 1 slice (1 oz)	30	112	22	17	13	11
Cheese, Parmesan 1 oz	30	130	25	20	16	13
Cottage cheese 1 round tablespoon	30	30	6	4	4	3
Ice cream 1/6 quart = 5 round tablespoons	90	186	36	28	22	19
Ice cream sundae, 2 dips	75	326	63	49	39	33
Ice milk 1/6 quart = 5 round tablespoons	90	137	26	21	16	14
Milk, buttermilk 8 oz	240	88	17	13	10	9
Milk, skim 8 oz	240	88	17	13	10	9
Milk, 2%, 8 oz	240	126	24	19	15	13
Milk, whole, 8 oz	240	160	36	24	19	16
Yogurt, from skim milk, 1 cup	240	122	24	18	14	12

Fish, Poultry, Meat, Dry Beans, Eggs, and Nuts
Fish

Food						
Bass, baked 1 serving (3" × 3"× ½")	115	287	55	43	34	29
Carp, fried, 3½ oz in 1 tablespoon oil	100	280	53	42	34	28
Catfish, fried 3½ oz in 1 tablespoon oil	100	270	51	40	32	27
Clams, 5 large or 10 small	100	80	15	12	10	8
Flounder or sole, baked 1 serving	100	202	38	31	24	20
Haddock, fried 1 fillet (3"× 3"× ½")	100	165	31	25	20	17
Halibut, broiled, 4 oz	120	214	41	32	26	21
Lobster, boiled with butter 1 and 2 tablespoons butter	334	308	59	46	37	31
Mackerel, broiled 1 fillet (4½ oz)	130	300	58	45	36	30
Perch, fried 1 serving	65	108	21	16	13	11
Salmon, baked 3½ oz	100	182	35	27	22	18
Trout,brook, raw 3½ oz	100	100	19	15	12	10
Tuna, canned in oil, drained 3 oz	90	170	32	26	20	17
Tuna, canned in water, ½ cup	100	127	24	20	15	13

Poultry

Food						
Chicken, breast, broiled ½ breast	72	105	20	16	13	11
Chicken, breast, fried, ½ breast	76	155	29	23	19	16
Chicken, leg, broiled 1 medium	35	52	10	8	6	5
Chicken, leg, fried 1 medium	38	90	17	14	11	9
Chicken, roasted 2 slices (3"× 3"× ¼")	80	158	30	24	19	16
Duck roasted 2 slices (3½"× 2½" × ¼")	70	218	42	33	26	22
Turkey, roasted 2 slices (3" × 3" × ¼")	80	160	31	24	19	16
Turkey, roasted with gravy 2 slices; 2 tablespoons gravy	115	240	46	36	29	24

Meat
Beef

Food						
Club steak, broiled 3 oz	90	175	33	26	21	16
Hamburger, cooked 1 patty (3" diameter × 1" thick)	85	224	43	34	27	22
Porterhouse, broiled 3oz	90	175	33	26	21	18

Rib roast 2 slices					
(4" × 2½" × ½")	105	240	46	36	29	24
Round, broiled 1 slice					
(4" × 3" × 1")	120	218	41	33	26	22
Rump roast 2 slices					
(4" × 1¼" × ½")	90	165	31	25	20	17
Short ribs, broiled					
1 serving (3 oz)	90	220	42	33	26	22
Frankfurter 1 (2 oz)	56	170	32	26	20	17
Ham, fresh, cooked 2 slices (3 oz)	90	254	49	38	30	25
Lamb chop 2 chops (3 oz)	90	205	39	31	25	21
Liver, beef or pork 2 slices					
(3" × 2¼" × 3/8")	75	170	33	26	20	17
Meat loaf, beef 1 slice					
(4" × 3" × 3/8")	70	140	27	22	17	14
Pork chops, lean 2 chops (3 oz)	90	260	49	39	31	25
Pork roast 3 slices					
(2½" × 1" × ½")	70	160	31	24	19	16

Sausages

Bologna 1 slice (4½" diameter)	30	66	13	10	8	7
Frankfurter 1 (2 oz)	56	170	32	26	20	17
Luncheon meat 1 slice					
(4½" diameter × ¼")	30	80	15	12	10	8
Pork sausage 1 patty					
(2" diameter)	22	100	19	15	12	10

Nuts

Almonds, dried, salted 12-15 nuts	15	93	18	14	11	9
Cashew nuts, roasted 6-8 nuts	15	84	16	13	10	8
Coconut, shredded,					
dried 2 tablespoons	15	83	16	12	10	8
Mixed nuts 8-12 nuts	15	94	18	14	11	9
Peanuts, dry roasted 8-10 nuts	16	80	15	12	10	8

Fats, Oils, and Sweets

Butter 1 pat (1" × 1" × 1/3")	5	35	7	5	4	4
Margarine 1 teaspoon	5	36	7	5	4	4

Desserts
Cakes

Angel food 1 piece					
(1½" × 1" × 1/3")	53	135	26	20	16	14

Chocolate with icing 1 piece					
(2½" diameter)	55	205	39	31	24	21
Cupcake with icing 1					
(2½" diameter)	36	130	25	20	16	13
Plain cake with icing 1 slice					
(1/12 of 9" cake)	50	186	36	28	22	19
Cheesecake 1 slice					
(1/12 of 9" cake)	5	160	30	25	19	16
Doughnut 1 average	32	125	24	19	15	13

Pies (1/6 of 9" pie)

Fruit pies	160	400	77	60	47	40
Pecan	160	670	129	100	78	67
Pumpkin	150	320	62	48	38	32

PART TWO
THE STEPS TO SUCCESS

CHAPTER EIGHT

The Roadway to Success

Different Strokes for Different Folks

K now Yourself
We can all learn to read a road map or electronic map from our global positioning device and follow it to where we want to go. Sometimes one way is the easiest, and sometimes another way. With modern global positioning technology, finding where you want to go is much easier. We don't yet have the global weight-loss system that can unfailingly guide us to where we want go. Thus we need to work with what we have and keep testing new highways and byways to find the best way for us. In this chapter, I am going to describe several ways you can manage your weight using today's technology. I have called them roadways to emphasize they are like a map. More than one road will often get you where you want to go. That is certainly true in the field of weight management. Whichever road you take, beware that "bad fructose" and fat are the potholes on that road, the ones you want to avoid.

When I first began helping people manage their weight, I had a lot to learn, too. I knew saturated fat in a high-fat diet was bad for heart health, but I didn't know the best way to help people lower their fat intake. I knew excess fat combined with "bad fructose" (the deadly duo) meant a positive caloric balance, but I didn't know how to help people reduce these foods easily in order to reduce their calories. I tried counting calories and found it hard. I also didn't know how to cook or how to plan meals—typical of men of my generation. I needed to learn how to help my patients focus on the important nutritional values of the foods they were eating. Increased activity was not a part of my daily life, although I was getting older. In learning about each of these roadways, I have driven into many potholes along on the way. In the process, however, I have learned to help countless people with their weight-management problem. This chapter and the following chapters are intended to do that for you.

We have already talked about the arithmetic of being overweight. You have consumed over months to years about 50–200 calories more per day than you needed to gain your extra weight. Now we need to address the imbalance. You have "saved" too much—now we need to spend this excess fat energy to make you thinner for life. The fat in your diet, the "bad fructose"-based but sweet-tasting refined carbohydrates (HFCS and sucrose), the size of servings you eat, and eating away from home are all part of the problem. Reducing fructose and fat are two ways to help you get control of your "fat account" and to spend it down. Remember that a 12-oz soft drink or 12-oz glass of fruit drink has about 140 kcal. Reducing your intake by one 12-oz soft drink each day will bring you into a new balance—neither gain nor loss, providing you don't change other parts your lifestyle.

So first, let me give you an overview of the roadways that are available for you to choose from in this journey we will take together. The system I developed slowly evolved as I treated more and more patients, and it is still evolving. Several truths became apparent to me. First, each patient is different. You are a unique individual. There is no one else exactly like you in the entire world. Your needs are unique. And you need special attention to satisfy those needs. Furthermore, what works for you may not work for someone else. Additionally, what works for you now may not work for you later.

Thus the old adage "know thyself" is very important. In previous chapters, we have provided a general background on dealing with positive thinking, nutrition, activity, and the basics of managing your weight. Whether you want to lose weight now, later, or never, you now know how to deal effectively with your nutritional and activity needs. This chapter, therefore, will focus on you and your eating habits.

While you are unique, there are still similarities between you and large groups of other people. For example, while hair color varies broadly among individuals, we can still group hair colors into blond, brunette, black, redhead, and gray. The same holds true with eating and menu planning. Your eating habits and preferences can be organized into several categories we will use to identify the best approach to help you manage your weight. There are people who like to eat large quantities of food, with little regard for the kind of food. Others seek sweets and chocolates. Binge eaters eat a great deal of food in a very short period of time.

How Do You Eat?

The central message of my approach is to switch from foods that contain "bad fructose" and fat to those that do not. This will reduce your intake of calorie-sweetened soft drinks and fruit drinks, which have "bad fructose," and provide more fruits and vegetables, which have "good fructose." It will reduce your consumption of pastries, cakes, muffins, brownies, cookies, doughnuts, etc., but will increase your meat and protein intake. Now that you are on the low fructose-low fat path to weight control, let's examine some other features of eating.

What kind of eater are you? Do you eat quickly? Do you eat often or infrequently? Is there a specific time of the day you eat? Do you eat everything you can lay your hands on? Does your weight fluctuate during the year? Are chocolates, cookies, and candy the only things that will satisfy your cravings? Is your idea of a satisfying meal a huge steak and a couple of baked potatoes? Determining what kind of eater you are is a vital first step in designing a weight-loss program that addresses your individual needs.

It is clear that many people who are overweight are binge eaters. These people eat very large meals at a single sitting. Binge eaters have comprised as many as 30% or more of the patients I have seen. For binge eaters, a low-fructose and low-carbohydrate/high-protein diet may be the answer. Medications have also been helpful for many people with binge-eating disorder. A high-carbohydrate diet composed of fruits and vegetables is also a high-fiber diet, which tends to increase the feelings of fullness—another option to try.

The increase in weight that occurs as we hit our middle years is well documented. Women, particularly, may consciously restrain their eating in order to avoid weight gain. For those restrained eaters, the key to maintaining this control is to avoid events that lead you to loosen your control over eating. For such individuals, alcohol can be a major trigger for loss of control. *Tip*: Drink soda water with a twist of lemon at cocktail parties and leave the alcohol for others. Situations that produce frustration can also lead to loss of control. The techniques discussed in Chapter 3 on positive thinking are particularly useful to folks who fall into this category.

Some people overeat because they constantly feel hungry. For these individuals, the roadway to successful weight management needs to include frequent stops for food; therefore, we will outline a procedure to increase the frequency of eating. A number of different food items will be made available to allow for frequent low-calorie snacking. This will allow the "always-hungry" eater to control hunger with a minimum of excess calories.

A final type of eating behavior includes folks who are fond of sweet, high-fat foods. For these individuals, the use of a low-fat, higher-fiber diet is useful. We will describe a low-fat procedure as one of the options for dealing with weight problems.

You've Got to Move

The foods you eat provide the energy you need. If your weight is stable, you are in "energy balance." This means your "checkbook" of energy is in balance—you are burning up as much energy as you are taking in. Of the food energy we eat every day, about two-thirds are devoted to running the day-to-day needs of your body. This so-called "resting" level of metabolism is the energy you require during sleep or even if you don't bother to get out of the bed in the morning (Chapter 5). The remaining one-third of your food energy is used to power your muscles and move you about.

The more you weigh, the more energy is needed by your body to perform basic activities (Chapter 7). An overweight person expends more energy when walking around the block or getting dressed than does a person of average weight. This is because it requires more work to move a heavier body. Being more active causes overweight people to perspire more readily, and they frequently find even moderate activity levels downright uncomfortable. From sleeping to scrubbing floors, energy expenditure may go up as much as five times. Activity is important. People who succeed in losing weight need to be more active. We know that overweight people tend to sit an average of 2½ hours per day more than leaner people.[2] *Tip*: Stand up when you talk or make phone calls from your cell phone. Remember, cell phones are portable. Walk and talk at the same time in this multi-tasking world. As your nutritional program takes hold, you can be even more active. For me, more activity means first and foremost walking more. We can all walk more, and you need to develop that in your activity plan. My plan for increasing your activity is in Chapter 7.

You do not live by bread alone. You do not lose weight by diet or by exercise alone. You will maintain your weight loss longer if you also change your eating habits.

Eating habits include a lot of things: where you eat, when you eat, what you eat, how hungry you are, who you are with, and so on. Changing your behavior is a key component of successful weight management. Behavior change (behavior modification) to help with weight loss came into its own thirty years ago.[3] Today there are manuals and more manuals on how to do it.[4,5] *Monitoring* is a key part. It means watching yourself by writing down what you do. This will help you keep your eye on the goals—less fructose and fat, smaller portions, and a more active lifestyle.

In college, I took a psychology course and learned about "conditioning." One kind of conditioning gives you rewards for doing things right,[6] the other kind punishes you for doing them wrong.[7] The rewarding kind works better. But to know when to reward yourself, you have to keep records—monitors, I call them. Recording your weight is one kind of monitor.

It is a direct measure of how your energy balance (your fat store) is doing. If done at the same time of day, every day, with the same clothing, it can help you plot your progress and pick up any backsliding easily. Recent studies show that people who regularly weigh themselves tend to lose more weight. An important study focused on people who are "relapsing," that is, regaining weight they have lost. When the most helpful things to prevent weight regain were identified, weighing oneself regularly was one of the most important. *Tip*: Weigh yourself regularly—same time of day.

Self Monitoring

In order to help *you* learn how to monitor your behavior, I had to learn first. The first type of monitor I tried was one that is still widely used. It was a sheet of paper on which I wrote down the time I started and stopped a meal, the place where I ate it, my physical position (such as standing or sitting), whether I ate the meal alone or with others, whether there were other activities going on at the same time, and finally the amount of food and its calorie value. Table 1 shows such a one-page form. Some of you may like this, and if it works for you, use it.

When I started carrying around a large piece of paper, I found that I was either losing it, forgetting it, or messing it up. To get around this problem, I broke the monitor page up into simple single steps. One of these for recording the food you eat is shown below.

Since the large sheets of paper didn't work well for me, I tried using only parts of the sheet of paper. After a number of trials and a lot of errors, I finally decided the best forms for me were 3×5-inch cards that can be carried in a pocket or purse. I call these Bray Plan Monitors. You will be using these monitors throughout the rest of this book. They can be a real asset. These monitors are your continuing reminder that you are succeeding. We know that people who are successful at weight management continue to monitor their eating and other behaviors. Because there are several to choose from, you can use them to monitor the behaviors that are your biggest challenge. Like choosing a nutritional plan for success, the monitor or monitors you decide to use should fit into your plan for success. You have many choices. There are monitors for exercise, monitors for counting fat grams, monitors for calorie counting, and even behavioral monitors to track where and when you eat. Try a few, or try them all, and find out which works best for you. The choice of monitors is up to you. But not to choose is like not being active. You reduce your chances of long-term success.

Table 1. Long Form for Monitoring Eating and Related Activities

	Name		Date
Antecedent	What Eaten	Time Eaten	What Happened Next

Bray Plan Monitor		
MONITOR FOR PLACES OF EATING		
Day		
Food Eaten		Place

The Road Signs for Success with Food

By this time, you are ready. You have made up your mind that you really want to make some lifestyle changes that will help you lower and control your weight. You may also have decided that you want these changes to last a long time. There are a number of tips and strategies you can use in dealing with foods. I have tried to pull together some of the more important ones here.

First: "Bad fructose" (HFCS and sucrose) is a marker for "highly refined" foods. When "bad fructose" is coupled with fat, this "deadly duo" is the key to fattening. Choose foods that do not have fructose (HFCS or sucrose), that are less refined, and that have lower fat.

Second: Eat a lower-fat diet. We will focus on the low-fat diet in detail in Chapter 9. Lower-fat, particularly lower-saturated-fat sources, are healthful and have important metabolic effects that help you control your weight.

Third: Protein: Be generous with the protein in your diet.

Fourth: To be repetitive—get moving and keep moving. Not only will it help you stay away from food, it will help you keep your weight down once you have lost your weight.

Fifth: Monitor your activity, monitor your fat intake, monitor your life. Whichever strategy you choose to help you lose weight and keep it off, monitoring is critical. I have given you models from my experience, but you may have a better way. If so, use it. The success will be yours! And if you do have a better way, I would like to hear about it so I can share it with others. I am always learning from my patients, and I want to learn from you.

Sixth: Weigh yourself regularly.

Seventh: Plan ahead of time when you are eating away from home. More and more, we eat meals away from home. These situations can complicate controlling your weight. The social situation can be filled with cues and urges to eat. Think positively. Think assertively. You have the right to say no. You have the right to choose. So choose wise nutrition based on what you like and what you have learned from the road maps for good nutrition.

141

The Gatekeeper

Eating at home is usually, though not always, an easier way to control what you eat than eating away from home. We tend to be creatures of habit. At home, you are the gatekeeper. Or your spouse is the gatekeeper. Or you may both be gatekeepers. If you are living with someone else, it is essential to have their support. Ms. G. was a married woman who came to see me because she had just tipped the scale at 300 pounds. She was fed up. She wanted to lose weight. The huffing and puffing as she moved around had become too much. She was tired of feeling hot and sweaty after just a little bit of exertion. She wanted to lose weight in the worst way. We talked for a while, and I gave her some ideas about what she would need to do and asked her to talk with her husband. She went home for that talk and came back a week later almost in tears. Her husband said if she were successful in losing weight, he would divorce her! She had given serious thought to her predicament and decided to proceed. Even without support at home, she was successful in losing nearly 100 pounds. Her husband did as he promised and divorced her, only to marry another 300-pound woman some months later.

When you are the gatekeeper of the home, the problem is easier than when you have to rely on someone else. If your mate wants you to be the way you are, s/he can sabotage you in many ways. Fortunately, most mates and significant others are eager to have you lose weight and are highly supportive. The role of the gatekeeper is particularly important for overweight children. Younger children get their food from home, at a friend's house, or from school. They are highly dependent on adults, unlike "independent" teenagers, who believe they know everything and can do everything. The best time to set good nutritional standards is in the early years. That is when children are most likely to learn and continue good eating habits. Helping yourself manage your weight may help others, too—remember, excess weight may be "contagious."[8]

Tips for Following the Road Signs

As gatekeeper, you begin your management at home and in the grocery store and continue when you eat out, as Americans do more and more each year.[9] The food you eat at home mostly comes from the grocery store. Decide ahead of time what you are going to buy. Read labels to identify "bad fructose" (HFCS and sucrose) as an indicator of highly processed foods. Use the ideas we have provided so far and the more detailed ones to come. Always shop from a list. Do not shop when you are hungry. Do not take the children. Their eyes light up every time they see one of the advertised "goodies" from television or tempting treats conveniently placed at their eye level. When they are along on shopping trips with you, it can be difficult for you to say no. So don't take them shopping!

Shop more often rather than less often. In preparing your shopping lists and meals, remember that you want to make eating enjoyable and healthful. Know which foods cause trouble—usually the ones that "melt in your mouth"—the high-fat sweets with tasty "bad fructose" (HFCS or sucrose). If you buy them, you may have difficulty not eating them. If they're not in the house, you can't as easily be tempted by them.

Remember, the food you eat may be the food you keep. You digest and then absorb it into your body. If it is fat, the fat you eat goes to your fat cells. And all too often, that is where it stays. So buy less fat and eat less fat and particularly the combination of "bad fructose" and fat—the deadly duo. Your body will thank you. Keep a clear mental picture of the smooth, "melt-in-your-mouth" foods. They are often "high mark-up" foods for the grocer and are heavily advertised by food manufacturers.

Drink more water and avoid beverages that have "bad fructose" (HFCS or sucrose) as sweeteners. The body has a harder time detecting these liquid calories than calories in solid foods.[10] By drinking water, you are getting the essential element of any beverage but without the caloric waste, which may end up on your waist. Eat more foods with high water content. Fresh fruits and vegetables are good examples. Dehydrated foods, such as pretzels, potato chips, and dried fruits, are not good choices. Remember, 20% of your daily water comes from the food you eat. Fresh fruits and vegetables, for example, have a lot of water in them. Some have over 90% water. Water has no calories. Since we are nearly three-quarters water, we need 6–8 glasses (1.5–2 liters) of water every day. Water also helps cleanse your body through the actions of the kidneys. Choose the fruits and vegetables with more water—tomatoes, lettuce, and cabbage (see Chapter 5).

Alcohol as a "social drink" can be a big problem when you want to manage your weight. Beware of alcoholic drinks. Even small amounts can cloud your mind, change your positive thinking, and dull your willpower. I advise my friends and patients not to consume alcoholic beverages while they are trying to manage their weight. Try carbonated water with a twist of lemon instead. Savor it and you can savor your success.

Choose crunchy foods. As a rule, if food seems to melt in your mouth, it is sliding its way from your lips to your hips. Soft, smooth foods tend to have fat in them. But you can't always tell how much fat is in a particular food, although reading the food labels will help (see Chapter 5 and the Appendix). That delicious-looking pastry may be teeming with fat and "bad fructose" just itching to become part of your body. Eat only the fat you want to keep.

Crunchiness in foods often signifies they are rich in fiber. Most of us get too little fiber in our diet. We need more. Fiber comes in crunchy forms, like bran, but also in the vegetables we call legumes. We have provided you with a lot of information about fiber in Chapter 5. But remember, foods with higher fiber content fill the stomach more completely, digest more slowly, and tend to have more nourishment.

Watch less television, or preferably do something that can replace watching television.[11] Advertisers know they can sell you on buying things with television. That is why a minute of television advertising time can be worth millions of dollars. Food ads are a big part of television. You are bombarded by television ads, by Internet ads, by newspaper ads, by billboard ads, and by radio ads. If you are going to win at weight loss, you need a clear strategy to see fewer ads, particularly those with food in them. Use the mute. Do errands during ads. TiVo your favorite programs to fast-forward past the food ads. Be imaginative—it's in your best interest.

Avoid being distracted while eating. Watching television takes very little energy. It floods you with ads for food. It distracts you from other things. Normally, when we eat, we gradually slow down the pace of our eating and finally stop.[12] After the first few bites, the next few come more slowly. When we are distracted, like when we are watching television, this natural slowdown can be lost. My motto is, if you watch television, do not eat at the same time.

Watch out for sauces and dressings. Mayonnaise, vegetable oils, most gravies, butter, and margarine are all high in fat. Putting dressing on your salad can put on more calories than what are in the salad itself! At a restaurant, ask the waiter to put the dressing on the side. Lemon juice, balsamic vinegar, and pepper provide a way of adding flavor to a salad with few, if any, calories. Other spices can also substitute for dressings and gravies to give foods a good taste. If you still feel you need dressings, try the "low-calorie" dressings. When we talk about the NUTRITION FACTS on the nutrition label again (Chapters 8 and 9), you will learn more about how to make the nutrition label your friend.

Fats in dressings, margarines, and butter are easy to take care of when you plan ahead. It is equally easy to cut the fat off of the cuts of meat you buy. Cattlemen are now sending leaner animals to market. But you still need to trim off fat when it is visible. Ground beef can be particularly high in fat unless you have it ground for you from a lean piece of meat.

Monitoring is one key. Monitor yourself by writing down what you eat. This will focus your attention on fat and dressings.

Proper preparation of foods is also important. For meats, broil, bake, or grill them. Fried foods have the fat they came with plus the fat from the frying skillet. When I was a youngster, my mother served bacon. But before she served it, it was well cooked to remove as much fat as possible and then blotted between paper towels to remove more of the fat. Extra fat can be removed from ground beef by browning it, draining the fat, putting it in a dish, covering it with water, and then placing it in the refrigerator. The residual fat will rise to the top and solidify, making it easy to remove. The ground beef is then a very low-fat ground beef.

Food manufacturers are becoming more imaginative. Turkey can be used to prepare "turkey sausages" and "turkey hot dogs," which are much lower in fat than regular sausage or hot dogs. You might give them a try.

In the chapters that follow, I will give you more specific ideas about how to choose a way to lose weight that will satisfy you today and tomorrow.

Restrained Eating: Women and the Cult of Thinness

Most of my patients are women, and this is true in all weight-loss programs. Yet just as many men have health-related weight problems as women. Why are more women interested in losing weight? Women are more concerned about their appearance, particularly since more skin is usually visible.

This concern for appearance is reflected in art as well as society.[13] One of my friends likes to visit art museums. While there, he has been measuring the women who are painted in the pictures. He makes two measurements. The first is the distance from the top of the head to the pubic bone. The second is the length of the lower segment, which is the distance from the pubic bone to the floor. In you and me, these two distances are almost exactly the same: It is the same distance from the top of your head to your pubic bone as it is from your pubic bone to the floor. Beginning nearly four hundred years ago, the way artists drew women's bodies began to change. The artists began to draw them with longer legs than in real life. This has been a gradual change but a real and continuing one.

You can also see this trend in the advertisements in your local newspaper. Look at the drawings of women who model clothes. They are much "leggier" than the models who are photographed. To accent the longer, leggier look, photographers often take the picture from the floor looking up. In either case, it shows women as unnaturally thin and long-legged. High heels and platform shoes are other ways of accentuating height.

The gradual change toward "thinness" is also seen in the Miss America Pageant winners.[14] Over the years from the end of World War II until the late 1980s, contestants became progressively leaner. One of my patients was a former Miss State Champion, who was in the Miss America contest from her state. She told me of the severe diets she went on to reach her contest weight. When I saw her at nearly forty years of age, this thinness had disappeared and she was desperately battling "the bulge." The lean-model appearance was long gone.

So we have a cultural bias toward thinness. This has been a concern to some women, particularly in this age where women's rights are a national priority. Are women being victimized by this bias toward thinness? Some think so. Others think not. Thinness seems to be more common in women who are married to highly paid executives and professionals than in women who are struggling to put food on the table. This important social difference among women has been emphasized over and over again. It is true in the United States and around most of the world.

Are the women who are married to executives and professionals genetically different? Certainly not. What, then, do they do differently? Many of them appear to be "restrained eaters." A restrained eater is someone who is holding their eating in check. This is the strategy many women use to control their weight. The concept was introduced by Drs. Herman and Polivy[1] and is solidly based on their research.

Eating Restraint

Restrained eating is very common. At the Pennington Center, we wanted to study a group of restrained and unrestrained eaters to see if there were any differences in their metabolism. To find women over forty years of age who were of normal weight and who were not restrained eaters proved difficult. We had to test more than four hundred women to find the twenty we wanted. Restrained eating is common. Indeed, I now believe that most women over age forty who are at or near normal weight are restrained eaters.

What is a restrained eater? To understand this, let me take you on a brief trip through two terms: "hunger" and "satiety." Hunger is obvious. We know it when our stomach growls. We know it when we have not eaten for more than twenty-four hours. It is a tension. It can produce headaches. It can sap our energy. It can drive us to eat. Most of our eating, however, is not done for hunger. In Chapter 18, I will tell you how to focus more on your own hunger signals. Identifying what makes you hungry and satisfying that before it becomes ravenous can be important in taking control of your eating and keeping a lid on it.

Satiety or satiation is the feeling you have when you are full. At Thanksgiving and other holidays, we frequently eat "more than we should" and feel "stuffed." This is an exaggeration of satiety. Normally you eat most rapidly at the beginning of a meal and then slow down until you finally stop. The early food you eat may in fact stimulate you to eat more. As time passes during your meal, you will eat less and less and then stop. If you are controlling your weight automatically, you will satisfy your hunger and your body needs at the same time. If your weight is slowly creeping up, your hunger and satiety are not correctly matched to your energy needs. Restraint is a way of matching them.

Restraint is using your self-control to replace the hunger-satiety controls, which do not do their job correctly. It is a form of willpower. It is applying many of the lessons we have already talked about before weight becomes a problem. One of my friends illustrated this clearly. For her, exercise on a daily basis was essential to control her weight. For her, restraint was regular exercise.

Movement, physical activity, and exercise are important. It is one of the themes of this book. It is one of the keys of restraint. It is also one of the keys to success.

A second key to restrained eating is to plan ahead. In Chapter 18 on Success at Behavioral Control, you will learn about planning ahead. You will also learn strategies for avoiding "food traps." Your background in nutrition from Chapters 4, 5, and 6 will be used every day. So will your skills at thinking positively. Assertiveness is a key tool for the restrained eater. Knowing what you want to eat will allow you to assert yourself and only eat what you want.

The third key is a low-fat, low-fructose diet. As you learn more and more about the fat you eat, you will create your own mental list of the low-fat foods you like and you will avoid the sources of "bad fructose." This applies particularly to snacks and main courses as well. Use this list to help you be an effective restrained eater with fat as well as "bad fructose" (HFCS and sucrose).

The fourth key is knowing when to make substitutions: sparkling water with lemon instead of a gin and tonic, a diet soda instead of one containing "bad fructose," healthy fats instead of saturated and *trans* fats.

CHAPTER NINE

Eating for Success

Low-fat Diet and Counting Fat Grams

Fats in Foods

Low-fat diets, high-fat diets, no-fat diets—what difference does it make, anyway? A lot. Give animals high-fat diets to eat, and they almost always become fat. Look at the dogs and cats that eat the "leftovers" many pet owners provide from their own high-fat diets. Obesity is now a major problem for our pets[1]—and for us, too. Fat pets usually have fat owners. The similarity of body size between pets and their owners[2] shows us again that it is what we choose to eat, not our genes, that is primarily responsible for the current overweight epidemic.

For most people, eating a high-fat diet is a sure way to increase your weight. Fat packs more than twice the energy (9 calories per gram) as does the same amount of carbohydrate or protein (4 calories per gram). To provide the same number of calories for the stomach means you have to eat twice as much carbohydrate-containing or protein-containing foods as fat-rich foods.

One of my major research interests has been to understand why high-fat diets produce an increase in body weight.[3] As I said above, if animals are given high-fat diets to eat, almost all of them become fat. A few "resistant" animals do not, probably because they are genetically different. The same is true of you and me. When we eat the typical American diet (which contains more than 35% fat), it is easy to become fat, particularly when that fat is sweetened with "bad fructose" (sucrose or HFCS). Those who do not become fat use one of several strategies.

Some of you are genetically resistant to becoming overweight even when eating the high-fat, high-fructose American diet. Some people eat

148

low-fat diets. For others, dietary "restraint" is their strategy. Increased movement, physical activity, or exercise is another strategy. We showed this at the Pennington Center by asking men who volunteered to eat a high-fat diet with little or no exercise and then to eat the same diet again with exercise.[4,5] The first day they ate a 35%-fat diet, similar to what most Americans eat. For the next four days, they ate a 50%-fat diet while we measured their metabolism. We found their bodies were slow to adjust to the high-fat diet. After four days living a sedentary lifestyle, only two of the six men had made the complete adjustments in their metabolism to allow them to burn this extra fat. We then exercised the subjects with the same diet. With exercise, all six men adjusted their metabolism more quickly, and they were able to burn the extra fat in the high-fat diet. Thus physical activity or extra movement is important for you to be able to adjust your body to burn dietary fat effectively. There is more about success by being more active in Chapter 7. In this chapter, we will talk about controlling the fat you eat and counting fat grams.

It is very uncommon for a vegetarian to be overweight. Vegetarians eat much less fat than do people who eat the typical American diet. Most of us, however, aren't going to become vegetarians. But we can all benefit from reducing our fat intake, and this chapter will give you a way to count the grams of fat in your diet and lower fat intake as much as you can in order to reduce your body weight.

What is fat? We talked about this some in Chapter 5. Briefly, the fat in our diet comes from two sources, animals or plants, although some of it may be disguised. From animals, we get fat in whole milk, cheese, and butter fat; we also get the visible fat on meats and the invisible fat in the meat that is part of the meat itself. Lard is pig fat; tallow is beef fat. In poultry, the fat is located primarily under the skin and to a small extent as part of the meat. In fish—salmon, for example—it is part of the flesh. Fish caught in cold waters are a particularly rich source of so-called "fish oils," which have omega-3 fatty acids—"good" fats. Fish oils contain particular fats that can help us lower our risk of heart disease[6] (see Chapter 5). Saturated fat and cholesterol in our diet comes from animal sources but is particularly high in the yolks of eggs, in liver and organ meats, and in some shellfish.

Plants are the second source of fat in our diet. Most plant seeds have fats or oils in them. Corn oil, peanut oil, sunflower oil, coconut oil, palm oil, and palm kernel oil are all examples of dietary fats and oils from plants or seeds. One major difference among these plant oils is the amount of saturated fat they contain. Saturated fatty acids increase the risk of heart disease. Palm oil, coconut oil, and palm kernel oil fall into the saturated fat category. But they are very cheap and hence widely used. *Tip*: Select monounsaturated fats, such as olive oil or canola oil, over saturated fats. Vegetable oils with predominantly mono-unsaturated fatty acids do not increase the risk of heart disease.

You have already heard of polyunsaturated fats. These fats can come from plants, animals, or fish. Small amounts are essential for life. Whether large amounts of these fats are good or bad for you is not yet settled. In this case I follow the rule of Aristotle, the famous Greek philosopher: "Moderation in all things." Moderate your intake of saturated fats and replace them with monounsaturated fats and polyunsaturated fats.

Fats can be hidden from view. Baked foods contain fat and "bad fructose"—the deadly duo. Fried foods are cooked in fat. The soft taste of chocolate and the smoothness of rich ice cream are due to the fat they contain. We Americans eat more fat now than at the beginning of the twentieth century. We also eat less carbohydrate. Hidden fat is often the most difficult to deal with. Fat is an important part of many recipes. It is these "hidden" fats you must learn to detect. How can you do this? First, we will show you how to estimate your fat grams in relation to your total energy needs. Then we will show you the kinds of foods that are likely to contain fats. You will also learn about fat content from food labels. Food labels tell you a lot about fat. Food companies must provide you with information about total fat, saturated fat, and *trans* fat in all packaged foods. This will make it even easier to count your fat calories. *Tip*: If the food melts in your mouth, it is probably high in fat. Along with watching out for "bad fructose," watching out for hidden fat can help you avoid extra "fat calories." Remember, it is the combination of "bad fructose" and high fat (the deadly duo) that underlies many of the ills that currently afflict people eating westernized diets.

Why am I spending so much time on fat? Because the amount of fat you eat now and how much you eat after losing weight tells you how successful you will be. How do I know? By monitoring patients and determining who succeeds in losing weight and what they do to help themselves keep weight off. This question is important to you, to me, and to all of us who work with overweight people. There is growing evidence that successful dieters change their diet to eat less fat.[7] They also exercise more.[7] These are the three principles: Lower the fat in your diet, avoid "bad fructose," and become more active.

Did you know the more French fries, dairy products, sweets, and meats you eat, the more likely you are to increase your body weight? Losing weight is harder if you eat cheese, butter, snack foods, fast foods, fried foods, and desserts. When you eat in a fast-food restaurant, you eat differently.[8] On days when people eat in a fast-food restaurant as compared to days when they do not, people consume more soft drinks and less milk and more French-fried potatoes but fewer vegetables. If you switch to a low-fat diet, you are more likely to lose weight.[3,9,10] Certainly part of the reason is the difference in energy (calories) between fat and other foods. Fats are more than twice as high in calories per ounce (or gram) as either carbohydrate or protein.

One recent study evaluated more than one hundred people. Fat intake, as well as the intake of other food items, was measured. The people who changed the amount of energy or calories they got from fat lost the most weight. Reducing fat predicted success better than reducing calories for most people. When we measured food intake in a group of dietitians, we found the more fat they ate, the more energy they ate.[11]

The low-fat message was a popular one during the 1990s. When the population kept gaining weight, some nutrition experts concluded that a message to eat less fat was the wrong message.[12] But it is clear that the number of overweight people in various countries increases as their average fat intake rises.[3] In developing countries, we are watching an epidemic of obesity as fat and fructose intakes rise. A recent large-scale trial in the U.S. showed that women assigned to a low-fat diet not only lost weight in the first year but didn't gain as much weight over the several years of the trial as those who ate a higher-fat diet.[9] It is particularly important that the less fat a woman eats, the more fat she loses. We and others have shown that over six months, the weight loss when eating a low-fat diet is about what is predicted from the change in fat intake. But diets don't cure your weight problem; they just help you control it against a sea of outside advertising. From my perspective, the low-fat message is a valuable one, particularly for people who have lost weight and want to keep it off.

Fat slips into your fat cells easily. Carbohydrate and protein can be turned into fat, but the body does not do it easily. Your metabolism goes up after eating. When fat is spread on bread and then eaten, your metabolism does not rise any more than if you had eaten the bread alone.[13] For some people this extra fat "slips through the cracks," so to speak, and ends up around the belly or on your thighs. Remember, the fat you eat is the fat you get. In a recent study at the Pennington Center, we fed normal people all they wanted on one day when the choices had a lot of fat and on another day when the choices were instead high carbohydrate with very little fat. When the choices were high-fat foods, they ate nearly 50% more than when the choices were low in fat. The amount of carbohydrate they ate on both days was very similar. If we weighed the food, they ate the same weight of high- or low-fat food, but they got many more calories from the high-fat foods. This and other studies suggest that we preferentially eat for either the "weight" of food or for carbohydrate, rather than the amount of calories the food contains.[14]

The amount of fat we eat each day is equivalent to much less than 1% of the fat we have stored in our bodies (Chapter 5). In contrast, our daily consumption of protein is nearly 1% of the amount of protein we have stored. At the other extreme, the carbohydrate we eat daily is nearly equal to the amount of carbohydrate stored in our body. This means each day your body burns virtually all of the carbohydrate you eat. This is why eating carbohydrate is important for your metabolism. The finding that healthy people eat as much carbohydrate during a day when they have choices of high-fat foods as when they have choices of low-fat foods says that our bodies can estimate our carbohydrate needs. It also explains why eating a high-fat diet can lead to weight gain. Since high-fat foods tend to be low in carbohydrate, we must eat more of a high-fat diet than a low-fat diet to get the same amount of carbohydrate for our bodily need. You now have a reason to eat more foods that are rich in carbohydrate (but not "bad fructose") and eat less food that is high in fat. But avoid the "bad fructose"!

How much fat do you need? The current American diet is typically 35% or more fat. The U.S. Government, as well as many other governments, recommends that we eat less than 20–35% fat. Vegetarian diets can be in the range of 10% fat. For most people, however, these levels include too few of the foods they want to eat.

Can you eat less fat? Certainly, you can. I do. When I finished medical school, I used to love sausage, hot dogs, fried foods, and beef. I ate hot dogs more than once a week. When I began to learn more about nutrition and the relationship between fat and the risks for heart disease, high blood pressure, overweight, and some forms of cancer, my diet changed. I gave up whole milk in favor of skim milk or milk with 1% fat. Hot dogs and sausages are no longer on my shopping list. When I buy meat, it is lean cuts, and I only seldom eat fried foods.

Our tastes are partly acquired and partly inborn. Some cultures like hot spicy foods; others do not. Vegetarians for religious and other reasons avoid meat. That is one reason weight problems are less common among vegetarians.

Calculating Your Fat Grams
You can easily calculate how much fat you can eat. Most overweight adults who are physically inactive need about 10 calories for each pound they weigh. Some active people and young individuals may need up to 15 calories or more for each pound, but we'll use 10 calories for this calculation since that applies to most overweight people. To begin, multiply your weight in pounds by 10.

Actual Weight _____ × 10 = _____ = Rough Estimate of Calories Needed per Day

Now multiply this number by the percentage of fat calories you want in your diet. Let's say you have selected 30% as your target.

Calories (from above)_____ × 0.30 = _____ = Fat Calories

Fat has just over 9 calories per gram (270 calories per ounce). For simplicity, we will use the number of 10 calories per gram for fat to make calculation easier.

_____Fat Calories ÷ 10 = _____ = Grams of Fat You Should Eat

This can be made easier. Get out your calculator. Now simply multiply your weight in pounds by 0.3 if you want 30% of your calories from fat, 0.25 if you want 25% of your calories from fat, or 0.2 if you want 20% of your calories from fat. This will give you an estimate of the number of fat grams you can eat.

Another counter for fat grams comes from the U.S. Government, and their advice for how to reduce your risk of getting diabetes is printed below. You can copy it to take with you if you want. A category for your weight is on the left. Select the category where you fit. With a calorie goal like the one shown in the fourth column, your fat-gram intake shown in the second column will provide about 25% of your total calories.

Weight (Pounds)	Fat Goal (grams)	Calories from Fat (9 × grams)	Calorie Goal	Percent Calories from Fat
120-174	33	297	1,200	24.75%
175-219	42	378	1,500	25.2%
220-249	50	450	1,800	25.0%
250+	55	495	2,000	24.75%

From: Small Steps-Big Rewards. Your Game Plan for Preventing Type 2 Diabetes 2007.[15]

Fat Gram Self Monitor

As a way of keeping track of fat, I have developed a monitor to help you count your fat grams. It is shown below. It is the size of a 3×5-inch card. To do your own fat-gram counting, you will need to buy a package of 3×5-inch cards with lines on them.

The lines make it easier to keep things in columns. As an exercise, I want you to write down each item of food you eat. Opposite the food put serving size, calories, and then the grams of fat it contains. In many cases, you can get the grams of food from the food label.

Bray Plan Monitor					
MONITOR FOR FAT GRAMS					
Day					
Food Eaten	Serving Size	Calories	Grams of Fat	Sat'd Fat	*trans* Fat

Figure 1. Bray Plan Fat Monitor. This 3×5-inch form can be duplicated onto 3×5-inch cards to allow you to record the foods you eat along with their fat contents.

The important point is to estimate the *amount* of food you ate because the amount of fat varies with the size of the portion. Put check marks under saturated or *trans* fats if they are listed on the label. Keep a running total each day for the next week. I have provided you with a table of the fat grams in many foods (Appendix). Keep in mind that products may change. Always check nutrition labels for food lists with update information. You might also look up restaurant menus on the website to find out calorie values of meals. When you look at other fat-counting systems, you will note they usually include the percentage of fat and often the cholesterol and saturated fat as well. From what you have already read here, you have a good feeling about where saturated fat comes from. You get saturated fat from animal products (red meats, milk fat, lard, etc.) and from some tropical oils. You have already learned about tropical oils and that when possible you need to substitute these with monounsaturated fats (olive oil or canola oil).

The Nutrition Facts Label now lists *trans* fatty acids. *Trans* fats are naturally part of many animal products in low quantities. More importantly, they are produced when vegetable oils are partially hydrogenated to make them more "solid." Foods must now be labeled with the amounts of *trans* fats. I use the Nutrition Facts Label to avoid *trans* fats just like I use it to reduce my intake of "bad fructose." When I buy peanut butter, for example, I select from among those with zero *trans* fats. Using good-quality margarines is a better idea, since these usually have little or no *trans* fats.

Fat Grams in Food

Take a minute to look at the Fat Counter Table. I have let the MyPyramid be my guide. I have arranged the foods according to the Food Groups used to build MyPyramid. First comes the bread, cereal, rice, and pasta group, which is one side of the pyramid. As a rule, foods in this group have very little fat. In contrast, baked foods are often laden with fat. Whether they have cholesterol or not depends on whether they were made with vegetable shortening or contain animal products (eggs, whole milk, or meat). By looking at the percentage of fat in the food, you can tell whether it is a high-fat food. Pastries are particularly high in fat, as are things like doughnuts. Fruits as a group are very low in fat. Only when cream or other items with fat are added do they become high in fat. Vegetables are likewise low in fat, unless they are prepared and served in a sauce that has fat. *Tip*: Beware of the sauce—it can be loaded with fat.

The meat, fish, poultry, dry beans, eggs, and nuts group is the most variable in fat and types of fat and will take the most work on your part. Topping the list are prepared meats, sausages, etc. In general, fish and skinless poultry are lower in fat. Fast food can be a problem. I have prepared a separate list of fast-food items, since many of them are high in fat. Like sauces, beware of fast foods if you want to keep your fat intake low.

Like the meat group, the milk, yogurt, and cheese group is also variable in the amount of fat these foods contain. Yogurt and milk both come in full-fat and low-fat versions and now in fat-free versions. The butterfat and cream from milk are very high in fat and in saturated fat.

Some items in the miscellaneous group of MyPyramid are almost entirely fat, such as the margarines and butter and many dressings, but some have no fat at all but do have "bad fructose (HFCS or sugar/sucrose) such as syrups or alcoholic beverages.

To keep your fat intake where you want it:
- Eat fresh fruits and vegetables.
- Choose fish and remove skin from chicken.
- Choose bread or bagels over rolls or muffins.
- Choose whole-grain products.
- Trim the visible fat from meat.
- Choose skim or ½% milk and low-fat yogurt.
- Eat less cheese.
- Eat fast food sparingly, and when you do, choose the chicken or salad items.
- Use butter and margarine sparingly.

I have chosen to use fat grams and percentage of fat in the foods for my table. Looking at the percentage tells you immediately whether the food is high in fat. There is one limitation to the use of percentages. One gram of margarine could be 100% fat, but it is only 1 gram. When you have figured out how much fat you want, it is in terms of grams. So we will work in grams. If you want more detailed information about saturated fat, polyunsaturated fat, and cholesterol in the foods you are recording, I would suggest you buy the book *A Consumer's Guide to Fats*,[16] or another comprehensive book containing this information. For our purpose, however, the use of fat grams from food labels and a knowledge of the types of fats in various foods will serve you perfectly well.

Now you are ready to review your fat-intake record. Use the form below.

Bray Plan Monitor **ANALYSIS OF FAT GRAMS EATEN**										
Number of Grams of Fat at Each Eating Event										
Day	1	2	3	4	5	6	7	Add'l	Total
1									
2									
3									
4									
5									
6									
7									

Figure 2. Bray Plan Fat Gram Analysis Form. This form gives you a way of recording your daily fat gram intake over several days. By the time you have completed this, you will have a good picture of your fat gram intake.

This form provides a line for each day of the week and a column for fat at each eating event. Make a 3×5-inch card like this, and write down the amount of fat you ate each day. There will be differences from day to day. Now add up the week's total. Divide by 7 to get your average fat grams each day. How does this compare with the fat gram level you chose earlier? If you are close and you chose 30% fat or less as your goal, give yourself extra credit. If the fat grams were well above your goal, review the daily cards and identify the foods that were high in fat. Now for the next week, you should repeat the exercise. As you count the fat grams in your food week after week, you will get a clearer picture of the high-fat foods you prefer AND a picture of the foods you like that are lower in fat. Make a list of the two groups of foods like the one shown below. As the list gets longer from week to week, you will get a better and better idea of how to choose low-fat foods you like that have less fat.

Foods I Like

High-fat	Low-fat
_____	_____
_____	_____
_____	_____
_____	_____
_____	_____
_____	_____
_____	_____
_____	_____
_____	_____
_____	_____
_____	_____
_____	_____
_____	_____
_____	_____
_____	_____
_____	_____
_____	_____
_____	_____
_____	_____
_____	_____

Table of Calories and Fat Grams in Some Foods

Food/Portion Size	Calories	Total Fat Grams	Fat as Percent of Calories
Bread, Cereal, Rice, and Pasta			
Biscuits			
Baking powder, home recipe, 1 biscuit	100	5	45
Bread			
Boston brown, canned, 3¼×½-inch slice	95	1	9
Cracked wheat, 1 slice	65	1	14
French, enriched, 5×2½ × 1-inch slice	100	1	9
Frozen bread dough, Honey Wheat, Rhodes,			
1 slice, approx 28 g (1 oz)	69	1	13
Frozen bread dough, Texas Whole Wheat, Rhodes, 2 oz	129	1	7
Italian, enriched, 4½×3¼×¾-inch slice	85	Tr	n/a
Oat, Hearty Slices Crunchy Oat Bread,			
Pepperidge Farm, 1 slice	95	2	19
Oat, Oat Bran Bread, Roman Meal, 1 slice	70	Tr	<1
Pita, enriched, white, 6-inch diameter, 1 pita	165	1	5
Pumpernickel, 2/3 rye, 1/3 wheat, 1 slice	80	1	11
Raisin, enriched, 1 slice	65	1	14
Rye, 2/3 wheat, 1/3 rye, 4¾×3¾×7/16-inch slice	65	1	14
Vienna, enriched, 4¾×4×½-inch slice	70	1	13
Wheat, Soft, Brownberry, 1 slice	70	1	13
Wheat, Stoneground 100% wheat, Wonder, 1 slice	70	1	13
White, Country White Hearty Slices, Pepperidge			
Farm, 2 slices	190	2	9
White, Home Pride Buttertop, 1 slice	70	1	13
White, Wonder, 1 slice	70	1	13
Cake			
Angel Food Cake mix, Duncan Hines, 1/12 of cake	140	0	0
Chocolate Loaf, Fat & Cholesterol Free,			
Entenmann's, 1-oz slice	15	0	0
Cupcakes Lights, Hostess, 1 cupcake, 1½ oz	130	2	14
Devil's Food Cake Mix, Moist Deluxe, Duncan Hines			
1/12 of cake, regular recipe	280	15	48
Gingerbreaad Cake & Cookie Mix, Betty Crocker,			
1/9 of cake (1.6 oz), regular recipe	220	7	29
Orange Supreme Cake Mix, Duncan Hines,			
1/12 of cake, regular recipe	260	11	38
Pound Cake, All Butter, Sara Lee, 1 oz	130	7	48

Pound Cake, Free & Light, Sara Lee, 1 oz	70	0	0
Twinkies Lights, Hostess, 1 cake, 1½ oz	130	2	14
White Cake Mix, Lovin' Lites, Pillsbury (using egg whites), 1/12 of cake	170	2	11
White Cake Mix, Moist Deluxe, Duncan Hines, regular recipe, 1/12 of cake	270	12	40
Yellow Cake Mix, Moist Deluxe Duncan Hines, regular recipe, 1/12 of cake	260	11	38

Cookies

Chocolate Chip, Chips Ahoy, Nabisco, 1 cookie	50	2	36
Chocolate chip, refrigerated dough, 1 cookie	56	3	48
Fig Newtons, Nabisco, 1 cookie	60	1	15
Oreos, Nabisco, 1 cookie	50	2	36
Shortbread, commercial, 1 small cookie	39	2	46
Sugar, refrigerated dough, 1 cookie	59	3	46
Wafers, vanilla, 5 cookies	93	4	39

Pastry

Coffee cake, Easy mix, Aunt Jemima, 1/8 of cake	170	5	26
Danish, fruit, 4¼-inch round pastry	235	13	50
Danish, plain, 1 oz	110	6	49
Danish, plain, 4¼-inch round, 1 pastry	220	12	49
Toaster, 1 pastry	210	6	26

Pie (all pies include crust made with enriched flour and vegetable shortening)

Apple, 1/6 of 9-inch pie	405	18	40
Blueberry, 1/6 of 9-inch pie	380	17	40
Cherry, 1/6 of 9-inch pie	410	18	40
Custard, 1/6 of 9-inch pie	330	17	46
Lemon meringue, 1/6 of 9-inch pie	355	14	35
Peach, 1/6 of 9-inch pie	405	17	38
Pecan, 1/6 of 9-inch pie	575	32	50
Pumpkin, 1/6 of 9-inch pie	320	17	48

Miscellaneous

Brownies, Fudge Brownie Mix, Duncan Hines, 1 brownie	130	5	35
Doughnuts, cake, plain, 1 doughnut	210	12	51
Doughnuts, yeast, glazed, 1 doughnut	192	13	61

Cereals, Cold

40% Bran Flakes, Post, 1 oz (2/3 cup)	90	Tr	<1

100% Bran Cereal, 1 oz (1/3 cup)	70	1	8
100% Natural, Oats & Honey, Quaker, 1 oz (¼ cup)	130	6	40
Alpha-Bits, Post, 1 oz	110	1	8
Apple Jacks, Kellogg's, 1 oz	110	0	0
Bran Flakes, 1 oz	90	0	0
Bran Flakes, Kellogg's, 1 oz (¾ cup)	90	0	0
Cap'n Crunch, Quaker, 1 oz (¾ cup)	120	3	23
Cheerios, 1 oz (1¼ cups)	110	2	16
Cocoa Puffs, 1 oz	110	1	8
Common Sense Oat Bran, Kellogg's, 1 oz	100	1	9
Corn Chex, Ralston, 1 oz	110	0	0
Corn Flakes	100	0	0
Corn Flakes, Total, 1 oz (1 cup)	110	1	8
Cracklin' Oat Bran, 1 oz	110	4	33
Crispy Wheats & Raisins, 1 oz	110	1	8
Froot Loops, 1 oz (1 cup)	110	1	8
Frosted Mini-Wheats, 1 oz	100	0	0
Fruit & Fibre	90	1	10
Fruity Pebbles, 1 oz	113	1	8
Golden Grahams, 1 oz (¾ cup)	110	1	8
Granola, 1 oz (1/3 cup)	125	5	36
Grape Nuts, Post, 1 oz	110	0	0
Honeycomb, Post, 1 oz	110	0	0
Just Right with Fiber Nuggets, Kellogg's, 1 oz	100	1	9
Kix, 1 oz	110	0	0
Life, 1 oz	111	2	16
Lucky Charms, 1 oz (1 cup)	110	1	8
Mueslix Five Grain, 1 oz	96	1	9
Nutri Grain Biscuits, 1 oz	90	0	0
Oat Bran, Quaker, 1 oz	110	2	16
Product 19, 1 oz (¾ cup)	110	Tr	<1
Puffed Rice, Quaker Oats, ½ oz	54	Tr	<1
Puffed Wheat, Quaker Oats, ½ oz	54	Tr	<1
Raisin Bran, 1 oz (¾ cup)	120	1	8
Rice Chex, Ralston, 1 oz	110	1	11
Rice Krispies, 1 oz (1 cup)	110	0	0
Shredded Wheat, Nabisco, 1 biscuit, 5/6 oz	80	<1	n/a
Shredded Wheat, Spoon Size, Nabisco, 1 oz	90	<1	n/a
Smurf-Berry Crunch, 1 oz	110	Tr	<1
Special K, 1 oz (1-1/3 cups)	110	Tr	<1
Super Golden Crisp, 1 oz	110	0	0
Trix, 1 oz (1 cup)	110	1	8
Wheat Chex, 1 oz	100	0	0

Wheat Germ, Honey Crunch, Kretschmer, 1 oz	105	3	26
Wheaties, 1 oz (1 cup)	100	Tr	<1

Cereals, Hot

Corn grits, regular/quick, enriched, 1 cup	145	Tr	n/a
Cream of Wheat, regular/quick/instant, 1 cup	149	Tr	<1
Malt-O-Meal, Chocolate, 1 oz	100	0	0
Oat Bran, Quaker Oats, 1 oz	92	2	20
Oats, Instant, Apple Cinnamon, Quaker Oats, 1¼ oz	134	2	13
Oats, Instant, Maple & Brown Sugar, Quaker Oats, 1½ oz	163	2	11
Oats, Instant, Regular, Quaker Oats, dry, 1 oz	109	2	17
Oats, Quick or Old Fashioned, Quaker Oats, dry, 1 oz	100	2	17
Wheateena, 1 oz	100	1	9
Whole Wheat Hot Natural, Quaker Oats, 1 oz	92	1	10

Crackers

Cheese, plain, 1-inch square, 10 crackers	50	3	54
Graham, plain, 2½-inch square, 2 crackers	60	1	15
Oat Bran, Sunshine, 8 crackers	80	4	45
Ritz, Nabisco, 4 crackers	70	4	51
Rye wafers, whole grain, 2 wafers	55	1	16
RyKrisp (Natural) 1 cracker	80	0	0
Saltines, 4 crackers	50	1	18
Snack-type, standard, 1 round cracker	15	1	60
Town House, Low Sodium, Keebler, 4 crackers	70	4	51
Wheat, thin, 4 crackers	35	1	26

Muffins

Apple Streusel, Breakfast, Hostess, 1 muffin	100	1	9
Banana Nut, Frozen, Healthy Choice, 1 muffin	180	6	30
Blueberry, Bakery Style, Muffin Mix, Duncan Hines, 1 muffin	180	5	25
Blueberry, Frozen, Healthy Choice, 1 muffin	190	4	19
Blueberry, mix, 1 muffin	140	5	32
Bran, mix, 1 muffin	140	4	26
Brain, with Raisins, Pepperidge Farm, 1 muffin (2 oz)	170	6	32
English, plain, enriched, 1 muffin	140	1	6
English, Thomas', 1 muffin, 57 g (2 oz)	130	1	7

Rolls

Dinner, enriched commercial, 1 roll	85	2	21
Frankfurter/hamburger, enriched, commercial, 1 roll	115	2	16

Hard, enriched commercial, 1 roll	155	2	12
Hoagie/submarine, enriched commercial, 1 roll	400	8	18

Miscellaneous

Bagel, plain/water enriched, 1 bagel	200	2	9
Breadsticks, Pillsbury, 1 stick	100	2	18
Croissant, with enriched flour, 1 croissant	235	12	46
Melba toast, plain, 1 piece	20	Tr	n/a
Pancakes and Waffle Mix, 3 to 4 pancakes	190	6	28
Stuffing, Herb Seasoned, Pepperidge Farm, 1 oz	110	1	8
Stuffing Mix, Croutettes, Kellogg's, Approx. ¾ oz	70	2	26
Stuffing mix, moist, prepared from mix, 1 cup	420	26	56
Taco Shell, Ortega, 1 shell	70	3	39
Tortilla, corn, 1 tortilla	65	1	14

Pasta

Egg Noodles, Creamette, 2 oz	210	3	13
Egg Noodles Substitute, Cholesterol Free, No Yolks, 2 oz, dry	200	1	5
Linguine, Fresh, Di Giorno, Cholesterol Free, 3 oz	250	3	11
Macaroni, enriched, cooked, firm, hot, 1 cup	190	1	5
Macaroni, enriched, cooked, tender, cold, 1 cup	115	Tr	n/a
Macaroni, enriched, cooked, tender, hot, 1 cup	155	1	6
Noodle Roni Parmesano, prepared with margarine and 2% milk, ½ cup	250	14	50
Noodle Roni Romanoff, prepared with margarine and 2% milk, ½ cup	213	8	34
Noodle Roni Stroganoff, prepared with margarine and 2% milk, ½ cup	290	11	34
Noodles, chow mein, canned, 1 cup	220	11	45
Noodles, Creamette, all types except egg, 2 oz	210	1	4
Noodles, egg, enriched, cooked, 1 cup	200	2	9
Spaghetti, enriched, cooked, firm, hot, 1 cup	190	1	5
Spaghetti, enriched, cooked, tender, hot, 1 cup	155	1	6

Rice

Beef Flavor, Rice-A-Roni, prepared with margarine, ½ cup	170	5	26
Brown, cooked, hot, 1 cup	230	1	4
Brown & Wild, Mushroom Recipe, Uncle Ben's, ½ cup	130	1	7
Chicken Flavor, Rice-A-Roni, prepared with margarine, ½ cup	171	5	26

Chicken Vegetable, Rice-A-Roni, prepared			
with margarine, ½ cup	139	3	19
Extra-Long-Grain, Riceland, ½ cup	100	0	0
Herb Rice Au Gratin, Country Inn, Uncle Ben's			
prepared with margarine, ½ cup	170	5	26
Instant, ready-to-serve, hot, 1 cup	180	0	0
Long Grain, Natural, Converted, Uncle Ben's, 2/3 cup	120	0	0
Long Grain & Wild, Original Recipe,			
Uncle Ben's 28 g (about ½ cup cooked)	100	<1	<9
Long Grain & Wild, Rice-A-Roni, prepared			
with margarine, ½ cup	137	3	20
Minute Rice, w/o salt or butter, 2/3 cup	120	0	0
Parboiled, cooked, hot, 1 cup	185	Tr	n/a
Parboiled, raw, 1 cup	685	1	1
Savory Broccoli Au Gratin, Rice-A-Roni, prepared			
with margarine, ½ cup	178	10	51
Savory Rice Pilaf, Rice-A-Roni, prepared			
with margarine, ½ cup	186	5	24
White, enriched, cooked, hot, 1 cup	225	Tr	n/a

Fruit

Apples, raw, unpeeled, 3¼-inch diameter, 1 apple	125	1	7
Applesauce, canned, Regular or Chunky, Mott's, 1 cup	114	0	0
Applesauce, canned, sweetened, 1 cup	195	Tr	n/a
Applesauce, canned, unsweetened, 1 cup	105	Tr	n/a
Apricots, canned, heavy syrup pack, 3 halves	70	Tr	n/a
Apricots, canned, juice pack, 3 halves	40	Tr	n/a
Apricots, dried, cooked, unsweetened, 1 cup	210	Tr	n/a
Apricots, dried, uncooked, 1 cup	310	1	3
Apricots, raw, 3 apricots	50	Tr	n/a
Avocados, raw, ½ avocado	160	14	
Bananas, raw, 1 banana	105	1	9
Blackberries, raw, 1 cup	75	1	12
Blueberries, frozen, sweetened, 10 oz	230	Tr	n/a
Blueberries, raw, 1 cup	80	1	11
Cantaloupe, raw, ½ melon	95	1	9
Cherries, sweet, raw, 10 cherries	50	1	18
Cranberry sauce, sweetened, canned, strained, 1 cup	420	Tr	
Dates, chopped, ½ cup	245	<1	2
Dates, whole, w/o pits, 1 date	23	Tr	
Figs, dried, 1 fig	48	Tr	4
Fruit, Mixed, in Syrup, Birds Eye Quick Thaw Pouch,			
5 oz	120	0	0

Fruit Cocktail, Del Monte, ½ cup	80	0	0
Grapefruit, canned, w/ syrup, 1 cup	150	Tr	n/a
Grapefruit, raw, ½ grapefruit	40	Tr	n/a
Grapes, Thompson seedless, 10 grapes	35	Tr	n/a
Honeydew melon, raw, 1/10 melon	45	Tr	n/a
Kiwifruit, raw, w/o skin, 1 kiwifruit	45	Tr	n/a
Lemons, raw, 1 lemon	15	Tr	n/a
Mangos, raw, 1 mango	135	1	7
Nectarines, raw, 1 nectarine	65	1	14
Olives, canned, green, 4 medium or 3 extra large	15	2	100
Olives, ripe, mission, pitted, 3 small or 2 large	15	2	100
Oranges, raw, whole, w/o peel and seeds, 1 orange	60	Tr	n/a
Papayas, raw, ½-inch cubes, 1 cup	65	Tr	n/a
Peaches, canned, heavy syrup, 1 cup	190	Tr	n/a
Peaches, canned, juice pack, 1 cup	110	Tr	n/a
Peaches, dried, uncooked, 1 cup	380	1	2
Peaches, frozen, sliced, sweetened, 1 cup	235	Tr	n/a
Peaches, raw, whole, 2½-inch diameter, 1 peach	35	Tr	n/a
Pears, Bartlett, raw, w/skin, 1 pear	100	1	9
Pears, canned, heavy syrup, 1 cup	190	Tr	n/a
Pears, canned, juice pack, 1 cup	125	Tr	n/a
Pears, Halves, Lite, Libby's, ½ cup	60	0	0
Pineapple, Canned, Heavy Syrup (all cuts), Dole, ½ cup	91	0	0
Pineapple, Canned, Juice Pack (all cuts), Dole, ½ cup	70	0	0
Pineapple, canned, juice pack slices, 1 slice	35	Tr	n/a
Pineapple, raw, diced, ½ cup	38	Tr	n/a
Plums, canned, purple, juice pack, 3 plums	55	Tr	n/a
Plums, raw, 1½-inch diameter, 1 plum	15	Tr	n/a
Prunes, dried, cooked, unsweetened, 1 cup	225	Tr	n/a
Prunes, dried, uncooked, 4 extra large or 5 large	115	Tr	n/a
Raisins, seedless, ½ cup	220	Tr	
Raspberries, frozen, sweetened, 1 cup	255	Tr	n/a
Raspberries, in Lite Syrup, Birds Eye Quick Thaw Pouch, 5 oz	100	1	9
Raspberries, raw, 1 cup	60	1	15
Rhubarb, cooked, added sugar, 1 cup	280	Tr	n/a
Strawberries, frozen, sweetened, sliced, 1 cup	245	Tr	<1
Strawberries, halved, in Lite Syrup, Birds Eye Quick Thaw Pouch, 5 oz	90	0	0
Strawberries, raw, whole, 1 cup	45	1	20
Tangerines, raw, 2-3/8-inch diameter, 1 tangerine	35	Tr	n/a
Watermelon, raw, 4×8-inch wedge, 1 piece	155	2	12
Watermelon, raw, diced, 1 cup	50	1	18

Vegetables

Alfalfa Seeds, sprouted, raw, 1 cup	10	Tr	n/a
Artichokes			
Globe or French, cooked, drained, 1 artichoke	53	Tr	n/a
Jerusalem, red, sliced, 1 cup	14	Tr	n/a
Asparagus			
Cuts & tips, cooked, drained, from raw, 1 cup	45	1	20
Spears, cooked, drained, from raw, 4 spears	15	Tr	n/a
Bamboo shoots			
Canned, drained, 1 cup	25	1	36
Beans			
Baby Lima, Birds Eye, Regular Vegetables, approx 3-1/3 oz	98	0	0
Fordhook Lima, Birds Eye Regular Vegetables, approx 3-1/3 oz	94	0	0
Green, Whole, Birds Eye Deluxe Vegetables, 3 oz	25	0	0
Sprouts, (mung), cooked, drained, 1 cup	25	Tr	n/a
Beets			
Cooked, drained, diced or sliced, 1 cup	55	Tr	n/a
Greens, leaves and stems, cooked, drained, 1 cup	40	Tr	n/a
Broccoli			
Cooked, drained, from frozen, 1 piece (4½—5 inches long)	10	Tr	Tr
Cooked, drained, from frozen, chopped, 1 cup	50	Tr	Tr
Brussels Sprouts			
Cooked, drained, from raw, 1 cup	60	1	15
Cabbage			
Common varieties, cooked, drained, 1 cup	30	Tr	n/a
Carrots			
Cooked, Sliced, drained, from raw, 1 cup	70	Tr	n/a
Cauliflower			
Cooked, drained, from raw (florets), 1 cup	30	Tr	n/a
Celery			
Pascal type, raw, pieces, diced, 1 cup	20	Tr	n/a
Collards			
Cooked, drained, from raw (leaves without stems), 1 cup	25	Tr	<1
Corn			
Sweet, canned, cream style, 1 cup	185	1	5
Sweet, cooked, drained, from frozen, 1 ear (3½ inch)	60	Tr	n/a
Sweet, cooked, drained, kernels, 1 cup	135	Tr	n/a
Cucumber			
Peeled slices, 1/8 inch thick (large 2-1/8 inch diameter,			

small 1¾-inch diameter), 6 large or 8 small	5	Tr	n/a
Eggplant			
Cooked, steamed, 1 cup	25	Tr	n/a
Endive			
Curly (including escarole), raw, small pieces, 1 cup	10	Tr	n/a
Greens			
Dandelion, cooked, drained, 1 cup	34	1	26
Mustard, cooked, drained, 1 cup	20	Tr	n/a
Turnip, cooked, 1 cup	50	1	19
Turnip, cooked, drained, from raw (leaves and stems), 1 cup	30	Tr	n/a
Kale			
Cooked, drained, from raw, chopped, 1 cup	40	1	21
Kohlrabi			
Thickened bulblike stem, cooked, drained, diced, 1 cup	50	Tr	n/a
Lettuce			
Crisphead, as iceberg, raw, ¼ of head, 1 wedge	20	Tr	n/a
Crisphead, as iceberg, raw, pieces, chopped, shredded, 1 cup	5	Tr	n/a
Looseleaf (bunching varieies including romaine or cos), chopped or shredded, 1 cup	10	Tr	n/a
Mixed vegetables			
Baby Carrots, Peas, Pearl Onions, Birds Eye Deluxe Vegetables, 1-1/3 oz	50	0	0
Broccoli, Baby Carrots, Water Chestnuts, Birds Eye Farm Fresh Mix, 3-1/5 oz	28	0	0
Broccoli, Cauliflower, Carrots, Birds Eye Farm Fresh Mix, 3-1/5 oz	20	0	0
Broccoli, Corn, Red Pepper, Birds Eye Farm Fresh mix, 3-1/5 oz	40	0	0
Broccoli, Green Beans, Pearl Onions, Red Peppers, Birds Eye Farm Fresh Mix, 3-1/5 oz	20	0	0
Broccoli, Red Peppers, Bamboo Shoots, and Straw Mushrooms, Birds Eye Farm Fresh Mix, 3-1/5 oz	20	0	0
Brussels Sprouts, Cauliflower, Carrots, Birds Eye Farm Fresh Mix, 3-1/5 oz	24	0	0
Cauliflower, Baby Carrots, Snow Pea Pods, Birds Eye Farm Fresh Mix, 3-1/5 oz	24	0	0
Chinese Style, Birds Eye international Recipe, 3-1/3 oz	79	5	57
Chinese Style, Birds Eye Stir-Fry Vegetables, prepared with soybean oil, 3-1/3 oz	107	8	67
Chow Mein Style, Birds Eye International Recipe, 3-1/3 oz	89	3	30

Corn, Green Beans, Pasta, Birds Eye Combination			
Vegetables, 3-1/3 oz	109	5	41
Mushrooms			
Canned, drained, solids, 1 cup	35	Tr	n/a
Cooked, drained, 1 cup	40	1	23
Raw, sliced, or chopped, 1 cup	20	Tr	n/a
Okra			
Pods, 3×5/8 inch, cooked, 8 pods	27	Tr	n/a
Onions			
Cooked, whole or sliced, drained, 1 cup	60	Tr	n/a
Rings, breaded, pan-fried, frozen prepared, 2 rings	80	5	56
Parsley			
Raw, 10 sprigs	5	Tr	n/a
Parsnips			
Cooked, diced or 2-inch lengths, drained, 1 cup	125	Tr	n/a
Peas			
Black-eyed, immature seeds, cooked, drained, from raw,			
1 cup	180	1	5
Green, frozen, cooked, drained, 1 cup	125	Tr	n/a
Peppers			
Sweet, 1 pepper	20	Tr	n/a
Pickles			
Bread and Butter Sticks, Vlasic, 2 sticks	18	0	0
Cucumber, dill, medium whole, 1 pickle (3¾ inch long,			
1¼ inch diameter)	5	Tr	n/a
Cucumber, fresh-pack slices, 2 slices (1½ inch diameter,			
¼ inch thick)	10	Tr	n/a
Cucumber, sweet gherkin, small, pickle (whole, about			
2½ inches long, ¾ inch diameter)	20	Tr	n/a
Potatoes			
Baked (about 2 per lb, raw, with skin) 1 potato	220	Tr	n/a
Boiled (about 3 per raw), peeled after boiling,			
1 potato	120	Tr	n/a
French fried strip (2 to 3½ inches long), oven heated,			
10 strips	110	4	33
Sweet, canned, solid packed, mashed, 1 cup	260	1	3
Sweet, cooked (baked in skin), 1 potato	115	Tr	n/a
Pumpkin			
Cooked, from raw, mashed, 1 cup	50	Tr	n/a
Radishes			
Raw, stem ends and rootlets off, 4 radishes	5	Tr	n/a
Spinach			
Cooked, drained, from raw, 1 cup	40	Tr	n/a

Squash

Summer (all varieties) cooked, sliced, drained, 1 cup	35	1	26

Tomatoes

Juice, canned, 1 cup	40	Tr	n/a
Raw, 2-3/5-inch diameter (3 per 12 oz pkg), 1 tomato	25	Tr	n/a
Vegetable Juice, V-8, 6 fl oz	35	0	0

Meat, Fish, Poultry, Dry Beans, Eggs, and Nuts
Meat
Beef

Chipped, dried, 2½ oz	118	3	23
Chuck blade, lean only, braised/simmered/pot roasted, approx 2¼ oz	168	9	48
Corned, canned, 3 oz	213	16	68
Corned, lean, Carl Buddig, 1 oz	40	2	45
Ground, patty, broiled, regular, 3 oz	245	18	66
Ground patty, lean, broiled, 3 oz	230	16	63
Heart, lean, braised, 3 oz	150	5	30
Liver, fried, 3 oz	185	7	34
Roast, eye of round, lean only, oven cooked, approx 2½ oz	135	5	33
Roast, rib, lean only, oven cooked, approx 2¼ oz	150	9	54
Round, bottom, lean only, braised/simmered/ pot roasted, 2-4/5 oz	175	8	41
Steak, sirloin, lean only, broiled, 2½ oz	150	6	36

Franks and Sausage

Frankfurter, Chicken, Healthy Valley, 1 frank	145	12	74
Franks, Beef, Oscar Mayer, 1 link	144	14	88
Franks, Eckrich, 1 frank	190	17	81
Franks, Healthy Choice, 1 frank	50	1	18
Franks, Jumbo Beef, Eckrich, 1 frank	190	17	81
Franks, Lite, Eckrich, 1 frank	120	10	75
Sausage, beef and pork, frankfurters, cooked, 1 frank	120	10	75
Sausage, pork, brown and serve, browned, 1 link	50	5	90
Sausage, pork, links, 1 link (1 oz)	50	4	72
Sausage, pork, Regular, Jimmy Dean, 1 patty (1-1/5 oz)	140	13	84
Turkey, Breakfast Sausage, Louis Rich, 1 oz	54	4	67
Wieners, Oscar Mayer, 1 link	144	13	81

Game

Buffalo, roasted, 3 oz	111	2	16
Venison, roasted, 3 oz	134	3	20

Lamb

Chops, shoulder, lean only, braised, approx 1¾ oz	135	7	47
Leg, lean only, roasted, approx 2-2/3 oz	140	6	39
Loin, chop, lean only, broiled, approx 2-1/3 oz	182	10	49
Rib, lean only, roasted, 2 oz	130	7	48

Luncheon Meats

Bologna, Beef, Oscar Mayer, 28 g (1 oz)	90	8	80
Bologna, Lite, Oscar Mayer, 28 g (1 oz)	70	6	77
Bologna, Oscar Mayer, 15 g (1 oz)	100	8	72
Braunschweiger sausage, 1 oz	102	9	79
Chicken, roll, light, 1 oz	45	2	40
Ham, chopped, 8-slice (6-oz) pack, 1 slice	49	4	64
Ham, cooked, Eckrich Lite, 1 oz	25	1	36
Ham, extra lean, cooked, 2 slices (1 oz)	38	1	36
Ham, regular, cooked, 2 slices (2 oz)	105	6	51
Pork, canned lunch meat, spiced/unspiced, 2 slices, 42 g (1½ oz)	140	13	84
Salami sausage, cooked, 2 oz	141	11	70
Salami sausage, dry, 12-slice (4 oz) pack, 2 slices	84	6	64
Sandwich spread, pork/beef, 1 tbsp	35	3	77
Turkey, Breast, Light, Eckrich, 1 oz	30	1	30
Turkey, breast meat, loaf, 8-slice (6 oz) pack, 2 slices	45	1	20
Turkey, Oscar Mayer, ¾ oz	22	1	41
Turkey, thigh meat, ham cured, 2 oz	75	3	36
Turkey Bologna, Louis Rich Turkey Cold Cuts, 28 g (1 oz)	61	5	74
Turkey Breast, Healthy Choice, 2 oz	60	1	15
Turkey Breast, Oven Roasted, Eckrich Lite, 1 oz	30	1	31
Turkey Ham, Louis Rich Turkey Cold Cuts, 21 g (¾ oz)	25	1	36
Turkey Ham, Smoked, Louis Rich Turkey Cold Cuts, 28 g (1 oz)	34	1	26
Turkey Pastrami, Louis Rich Turkey Cold Cuts, 23 g (4/5 oz)	24	1	38
Vienna sausage, 7 per 4-oz can, 1 sausage, 16 g (approx ½ oz)	45	4	80

Pork

Bacon, Canadian, cured, cooked, 2 slices	86	4	42
Bacon, low salt, Armour, 1 slice	38	4	85
Bacon, regular, cured, cooked, 3 medium slices	108	9	75
Chop, loin, fresh, lean only, broiled, 2½ oz	163	7	39

169

Chop, loin, fresh, lean only, pan fried, approx 2½ oz	181	10	50
Ham, Boiled, Oscar Mayer, 21 g (¾ oz)	26	1	35
Ham, Breakfast Slice, Oscar Mayer, 1 slice	50	2	36
Ham, canned, roasted, 3 oz	140	7	45
Ham, leg, fresh, lean only, roasted, 2½ oz	156	8	46
Ham, light cure, lean only, roasted, approx 2½ oz	107	4	34
Ham, Lower Salt, Light Eckrich, 1 oz	25	1	36
Ham, Low Salt, Armour, 1 oz	40	3	68
Rib, fresh, lean only, braised, 2½ oz	173	8	42
Shoulder cut, fresh, lean only, braised, 2-2/5 oz	169	8	43
Tenderloin, roasted, lean, 3 oz	139	4	26
Turkey Bacon, Louis Rich, 1 slice	32	2	56

Veal

Cubed, lean only, braised, 3½ oz	188	4	19
Cutlet, leg, lean only, braised, 3½ oz	203	6	27
Rib, lean only, roasted, 3½ oz	177	7	36

Fish and Shellfish

Catfish, breaded, fried, 3 oz	194	11	52
Catfish, skinless, baked w/o fat, 3 oz	120	5	38
Clams, canned, liquid and solids, Doxsee, ½ cup	59	Tr	Na
Clams, raw, meat only, 3 oz	65	1	14
Cod, fillets (frozen), Booth, 4 oz	90	1	10
Cod, skinless, broiled w/o fat, 3 oz	90	1	10
Crabmeat, canned, 1 cup	135	3	20
Fish sticks (frozen), reheated, 4×½-inch stick	70	3	39
Flounder, baked, with lemon juice, w/o added fat, 3 oz	80	1	11
Haddock, breaded, fried, 3 oz	175	9	46
Haddock, skinless, baked w/o fat, 3 oz	90	1	10
Halibut, broiled, with butter and lemon juice, 3 oz	140	6	39
Herring, pickled, 3 oz	190	13	62
Lobster, boiled, 3 oz	100	1	9
Mackerel, skinless, broiled w/o fat, 3 oz	190	12	57
Orange roughy, broiled, 3 oz	130	7	48
Oysters, breaded, fried, 1 oyster	90	5	50
Oysters, raw, meat only, 1 cup	160	4	23
Perch, ocean, breaded, fried, 1 fillet	185	11	54
Perch, Ocean, Natural Fillets (frozen) Taste O' Sea, 4 oz	100	3	27
Pollock, skinless, broiled w/o fat, 3 oz	100	1	9
Salmon, Pink, Bumble Bee, 3½ oz	138	6	39
Salmon, Pink (in spring water), Chicken of the Sea, 2 oz	60	2	30
Salmon, red, baked, 3 oz	140	5	32

Salmon, smoked, 3 oz	150	8	48
Sardines, canned in oil, drained, 3 oz	175	11	57
Sardines (in olive oil), King Oscar, 3¾ oz	460	16	31
Scallops, breaded (frozen), reheated, 6 scallops	195	10	46
Scallops, broiled, 3 oz (5–7 large or 14 small)	150	1	6
Shrimp, boiled, 3 oz	110	2	16
Shrimp, canned, drained solids, 3 oz	103	1	9
Shrimp, French fried, 3 oz (7 medium)	189	9	43
Snapper, cooked by dry heat, 3 oz	109	2	17
Sole, baked, with lemon juice, w/o added fat, 3 oz	90	1	10
Surimi seafood, crab flavored, chunk style, ½ cup	84	Tr	n/a
Trout, Rainbow, skinless, broiled w/o fat, 3 oz	130	4	28
Tuna, Albacore (in water), Bumble Bee, 2 oz	70	1	13
Tuna, Chunk Light (in spring water), StarKist, ½ cup	77	1	12
Tuna, Chunk Light (in vegetable oil), Bumble Bee, 2 oz	160	12	68
Tuna, Chunk Light (in water), Bumble Bee, 2 oz	70	1	13

Poultry

Chicken, boneless, canned, 5 oz	235	11	42
Chicken, breast, flesh only, roasted, 5 oz	140	3	19
Chicken, broiler-fryer, breast, w/o skin, roasted, 3½ oz	165	4	22
Chicken, drumstick, roasted, approx. 1.6 oz	75	2	24
Chicken, light and dark meat, flesh only, stewed, 1 cup	332	17	46
Chicken, liver, cooked, 1 liver	30	1	30
Chicken, white and dark meat, w/o skin, roasted, 3½ oz	190	7	33
Cold cuts, chicken or turkey, see Luncheon Meats in Meat section			
Duck, flesh only, roasted, ½ duck, approx 7¾ oz	445	24	49
Frankfurters, chicken or turkey, see Franks and Sausages in Meat section			
Turkey, dark meat only, w/o skin, roasted, 3½ oz	187	7	34
Turkey, flesh only, 1 light and 2 dark slices, 85 g (3 oz)	145	4	25
Turkey, flesh only, light and dark meat, chopped or diced, roasted, 1 cup (140 g; 5 oz)	240	7	26
Turkey, flesh only, light meat, roasted, 2 pieces, 85 g (3 oz)	135	3	20
Turkey, frozen, boneless, light and dark meat, seasoned, chunked, roasted, 3 oz	130	5	35
Turkey, Ground, Lean, Louis Rich, cooked, 1 oz	52	2	35
Turkey, Ground, Louis Rich, cooked, 1 oz	60	4	60
Turkey, patties, breaded, battered, fried, 1 patty	180	12	60
Turkey, white meat only, w/o skin, roasted, 3½ oz	157	3	17
Turkey and gravy, frozen, 5-oz pkg	95	3	28

Eggs

Egg Beaters, Fleischmann's ¼ cup (2 oz)	25	0	0
Egg Substitute, Scramblers, 4 oz	120	6	45
Large, fried in butter, 1 egg	83	7	76
Large, hard cooked, 1 egg	80	6	68
Large, poached, 1 egg	80	6	68
Large, raw, white only, 1 white	15	0	0
Large, raw, whole, 1 egg	80	6	68
Large, raw, yolk only, 1 yolk	65	6	83
Scrambled, with milk, cooked in margarine, 1 egg	100	7	63

Legumes and Nuts
Beans

Black, dry, cooked, drained, 1 cup	225	1	4
Chick peas, dry, cooked, drained, 1 cup	270	4	13
Lentils, dry, cooked, 1 cup	215	1	4
Lima, dry, cooked, drained, 1 cup	216	1	4
Peas (Navy), dry, cooked, drained, 1 cup	258	1	3
Pinto, dry, cooked, drained, 1 cup	234	1	4
Pork and Beans, Van Camp's, 1 cup	226	1	5
Red kidney, canned, 1 cup	216	1	4
Refried, canned, 1 cup	268	3	10
Snap, canned, drained, solids (cut), 1 cup	25	Tr	n/a
Snap, cooked, drained, from frozen (cut), 1 cup	35	Tr	n/a
Snap, cooked, drained, from raw (cut and French style), 1 cup	45	Tr	n/a
Sprouts (mung), raw, 1 cup	30	Tr	n/a

Nuts

Almonds, shelled, whole, 1 oz	165	15	82
Almonds, sliced, 1 oz	170	13	69
Brazil, shelled, 1 oz	185	19	92
Cashew, salted, roasted in oil, 1 oz	108	8	69
Chestnuts, European, roasted, shelled, 1 oz	44	1	8
Coconut, raw, piece, 45 g (1 oz)	100	10	84
Filberts (hazelnuts), chopped, 1 oz	119	10	79
Macadamia, salted, roasted in oil, 1 oz	136	13	85
Mixed, with peanuts, salted, dry roasted, 1 oz	170	13	69
Mixed, with peanuts, salted, roasted in oil, 1 oz	175	14	72
Peanut Butter, 1 tbsp	95	8	76
Peanuts, Dry Roasted, Planter's, 1 oz	160	14	79
Pecans, halves, 1 oz	94	8	81
Pistachios, dried, shelled, 1 oz	165	13	71

Walnuts, black, chopped, 1 oz	94	8	73
Peas			
Black-eyed, dry, cooked, 1 cup	190	1	5
Split, dry, cooked, 1 cup	230	1	4
Seeds			
Pumpkin/squash kernels, dry, hulled, 1 oz	155	13	75
Sunflower, dry, hulled, 1 oz	160	14	79
Soy Products			
Miso, 1 cup	568	14	22
Soybeans, dry, cooked, drained, 1 cup	298	13	39
Tofu, firm, 1 cup	328	5	55

Yogurt and Cheese

Yogurt

Blueberry, Dannon, 8 oz	259	3	10
Blueberry, Dannon Fresh Flavors, 8 oz	216	4	17
Blueberry, Dannon Light, 8 oz	100	0	0
Blueberry, Lite n' Lively, 5 oz	150	1	6

Cheese

American, Pasteurized Process Cheese Slices, Deluxe, Kraft, 1 oz	110	9	74
American Flavored, Singles, Pasteurized Process Cheese Product, Light n' Lively, 1 oz	70	4	51
American Flavor Process Cheese, Low Sodium, Weight Watchers, 1 slice	35	1	26
Blue, 1 oz	100	8	72
Camembert, 1 wedge (1/3 of 4-oz container)	115	9	70
Cheddar, Natural, Kraft, 1 oz	110	9	74
Cheddar, Free n' Lean, Alpine Lace, 1 oz	35	0	0
Cheddar, Sharp, Process Cheese, Borden Lite-Line, 1 oz	50	2	36
Cheese Spread, Pasteurized Process, Velveeta, 1 oz	80	6	68
Cheese Spread, Slices, Pasteurized Process, Velveeta, 1 oz	90	6	60
Cheez Whiz, Pasteurized Process Cheese Spread, 1 oz	80	6	68
Cottage, creamed, large curd, 1 cup	235	10	38
Cottage, creamed, small curd, 1 cup	215	9	35
Cottage, Lite n' Lively, 4 oz	80	1	11
Cottage, Lowfat, Lite-Line, or Viva, Borden, ½ cup	90	1	10
Cottage, low-fat (2%), 1 cup	205	4	18
Cottage, uncreamed, dry curd, 1 cup	125	1	7
Cream Cheese, Philadelphia Brand, 1 oz	100	10	90
Edam, Natural, Kraft, 1 oz	90	7	70
Feta, 1 oz	75	6	72

Gouda, Natural, Kraft, 1 oz	110	9	74
Jalapeno Singles, Pasteurized Process Cheese Food, Kraft, 1 oz	90	7	70
Limberger, Natural, Little Gem Size, Mohawk Valley, 1 oz	90	8	80
Monterey Jack Singles, Pasteurized Process Cheese Food, Kraft, 1oz	90	7	70
Mozzarella, Low Moisture, Casino, 1 oz	90	7	70
Mozzarella, made with part-skim milk, 1 oz	72	5	63
Mozzarella, Truly Lite, Frigo, 1 oz	60	2	30
Muenster, 1 oz	104	8	69
Munster, Lo-Chol Cheese Alternative, Dorman's, 1 pz	100	7	63
Parmesan, grated, 1 tbsp	25	2	72
Parmesan, Natural, Kraft, 1 oz	100	7	63
Provolone, 1 oz	100	8	72
Ricotta, Natural Nonfat, Polly-O-Free, 1 oz	25	0	0
Ricotta, Reduced Fat, Polly-O-Lite, 1 oz	35	2	51
Romano, Grated, Kraft, 1 oz	130	9	62
Romano, Natural, Casino, 1 oz	100	7	63
Sandwich Slices with Vegetable Oil, Lunch Wagon, 1 oz	90	7	70
Swiss, 1 oz	105	8	69
Swiss Pasteurized, Process Cheese Slices, Deluxe, 1 oz	90	7	70
Swiss Singles Pasteurized Process Cheese Food, Kraft, 1 oz	90	7	70

Miscellaneous
Candy

Almond Joy, 1 bar (1.76 oz)	250	14	50
Baby Ruth, 1 bar (2.1 oz)	290	14	43
Butterfinger Bar, 1 bar (2.1 oz)	280	12	39
Butter Mints, Kraft, 1 mint	8	0	0
Caramels, Kraft, 1 caramel	30	1	30
Chocolate, sweet, dark, 1 oz	152	10	59
Chocolate Fudgies, Kraft, 1 fudgie	35	1	26
Crunch, Nestle, 1.4 oz	200	10	45
Fudge, chocolate, plain, 1 oz	117	3	23
Gum drops, 1 oz	100	Tr	n/a
Hard candy, 1 oz	110	0	0
Jelly beans, 1 oz	105	Tr	n/a
Jet-Puffed Marshmallows, Kraft, 1 marshmallow	25	0	0
Kisses, Hershey's, 9 pieces	220	13	53
Kit Kat, 1-3/5 oz	172	9	47
M&Ms Peanut Chocolate Candies, 1 oz	150	7	42

M&Ms Plain Chocolate Candies, 1 oz	140	6	39
Marshmallows, 1 oz	91	0	0
Milk chocolate, plain, 1 oz	147	9	55
Milk chocolate, with almonds, 1 oz	152	9	53
Milk chocolate, with peanuts, 1 oz	154	10	58
Milk chocolate, with rice cereal, 1 oz	140	7	45
Milk Chocolate Bar, Hershey's, 1 bar	250	12	43
Milky Way Bar, 1 bar (2.15 oz)	280	11	35
Miniature Marshmallows, Kraft, 10 marshmallows	18	0	0
Mr. Goodbar, Hershey's, 1.65 oz	240	15	56
Party Mints, Kraft, 1 mint	8	0	0
Peanut Brittle, Kraft, 1 oz	130	5	35
Peanut Butter Cups, Reese's, 2 cups	280	17	55
Snickers, 1 bar	280	13	42
Special Dark, Hershey's 1 bar	220	12	49

Creams and Creamers

Coffee Rich, ½ oz	20	2	90
Cool Whip Extra Creamy Dairy Recipe Whipped Topping, Birds Eye, 1 tbsp	14	1	64
Cool Whip Non-Dairy Whipped Topping, Birds Eye, 1 tbsp	12	1	75
Cream Sour 1 tbsp	25	3	100
Cream, Sour, Land O' Lakes, 1 tbsp	20	1	45
Cream, Sour, Light n' Lively Free, Kraft, 1 tbsp	10	0	0
Cream, Sour Half and Half, Breakstone's Light Choice, 1 tbsp	20	2	90
Cream, sweet, half-and-half, 1 tbsp	30	3	90
Cream, sweet, light/coffee/table, 1 tbsp			
Cream, sweet, whipping, unwhipped, heavy, 1 tbsp	52	6	100
Cream, sweet, whipping, unwhipped, light, 1 tbsp	44	5	100
Cream, whipped topping, pressurized, 1 tbsp	10	1	90
Creamer, sweet, imitation, liquid, 1 tbsp	20	1	45
Creamer, sweet, powdered, Cremora Lite, 1 tsp	8	Tr	n/a
Cream, Topping, Real, Kraft, ¼ cup	35	3	77
Whipped topping, sweet, imitation, frozen, 1 tbsp	15	1	60
Whipped topping, sweet, imitations, pressurized, 1 tbsp	10	1	90
Whipped topping, sweet, powdered, prepared with whole milk, 1 tbsp	10	1	90
Whipped Topping Mix, Dream Whip, prepared with water, 2 tbsp	10	0	0
Whipped Topping Mix, Reduced Calorie, D-Zerta, prepared, 1 tbsp	8	1	100

Fast Foods

Arby's

Light Roast Beef Deluxe Sandwich	294	10	31
Light Roast Chicken Deluxe Sandwich	263	6	21
Light Roast Turkey Deluxe Sandwich	260	5	17
Salad, Chef	205	10	44
Salad, Garden	109	5	41
Salad, Roast Chicken	184	7	34
Salad, Side	25	Tr	n/a

Burger King

Bacon Double Cheeseburger	507	30	53
Cheeseburger	318	15	42
Chicken BK Broiler Sandwich	267	8	27
Chunky Chicken Salad	142	4	25
Croissan'wich with Bacon	353	23	59
Croissan'wich with Ham	351	22	56
Croissan'wich with Sausage	534	40	67
French Fries, lightly salted, medium	372	20	48
French Toast Sticks, 1 order	538	32	54
Hamburger	272	11	36
Ocean Catch Fish Fillet	479	33	62
Onion Rings, 1 order	339	19	50
Pie, Apple	311	14	41
Salad, Chef	178	9	46
Whopper	614	36	53
Whopper with Cheese	706	44	56

Dairy Queen

Banana Split	510	11	19
Fish Fillet sandwich	370	16	39
Fish Fillet with Cheese sandwich	420	21	45
Grilled Chicken Fillet Sandwich	300	8	24
Hamburger, Single	310	13	38
Heath Blizzard, small	560	23	37
Malt, Regular Vanilla	610	14	21
Parfait, Peanut Butter	710	32	41
Shake, Regular, Chocolate	540	14	23
Sundae, Regular, Chocolate	300	7	21

Domino's

Pizza, Cheese, 2 slices	376	10	24
Pizza, Deluxe, 2 slices	498	20	36

Pizza, Double Cheese/Pepperoni, 2 slices	545	25	44
Pizza, Ham, 2 slices	417	11	24
Pizza, Pepperoni, 2 slices	460	18	35
Pizza, Sausage/Mushroom, 2 slices	430	16	33
Pizza, Veggie, 2 slices	498	19	34

Dunkin' Donuts

Apple Filled Cinnamon	190	9	43
Boston Kreme	240	11	41
Chocolate Frosted Yeast Ring	200	10	45
Glazed Yeast Ring	200	9	41
Honey Dipped Cruller	260	11	38
Jelly Filled	220	9	37
Plain Cake Ring	262	18	62
Powdered Cake Ring	270	16	53

Kentucky Fried Chicken

Buttermilk Biscuit, 2.3 oz	235	12	46
Coleslaw, 3.2 oz	114	6	47
Corn-on-the-Cob, 2.6 oz	90	2	20
Extra Tasty Crispy, center breast, 3.9 oz	344	21	55
Extra Tasty Crispy, drumstick, 2.4 oz	205	14	61
Extra Tasty Crispy, wing, 2 oz	231	17	66
French Fries, 2.7 oz	244	12	44
Hot & Spicy, center breast, 4.3 oz	382	25	59
Hot & Spicy, drumstick, 2.5 oz	207	14	61
Hot & Spicy, wing, 2.2 oz	244	18	66
Hot & Spicy, six wings, 4.8 oz	471	33	63
Kentucky Nuggets, six, 3.4 oz	284	18	57
Mashed Potatoes and Gravy, 3.5 oz	130	5	25
Sauce, Barbecue, 1 oz	5	1	26
Sauce, Sweet n' Sour, 1 oz	58	1	16
Skinfree Crispy, center breast, 4 oz	296	16	49
Skinfree Crispy, thigh, 3 oz	256	17	60

Long John Silver's

Baked Chicken, Light Herb	130	4	28
Baked Fish, Lemon Crumb, 3 pieces	150	1	6
Baked Fish, Lemon Crumb, 2 pieces, Rice, and Small Salad (w/o dressing)	320	4	11
Baked Shrimp, Scampi Sauce	120	5	38
Cole Slaw	140	6	39
Rice Pilaf	210	2	9

Salad, Small (w/o dressing)	8	0	0

McDonald's

Big Mac	500	26	47
Biscuit with Bacon, Egg, and Cheese	440	26	53
Biscuit with Sausage	420	28	60
Biscuit with Sausage and Egg	505	33	59
Cheeseburger	305	13	38
Chicken McNuggets (6 pieces)	270	15	50
Cone, Lowfat Frozen Yogurt, Vanilla	105	1	9
Cookies, Chocolaty Chip, 1 box	330	15	41
Cookies, McDonaldland, 1 box	290	9	28
Danish, Apple	390	17	39
Danish, Cinnamon Raisin	440	21	43
Danish, Iced Cheese	390	21	48
Danish, Raspberry	410	16	35
Dressing, Lite Vinaigrette, 1 oz	24	1	38
Dressing, Ranch, 1 oz	110	10	82
Egg McMuffin	280	11	35
Eggs, Scrambled, 2 eggs	140	10	64
Filet-O-Fish sandwich	370	18	44
French Fries, small	220	12	49
Hamburger	255	9	32
Hashbrowns	130	7	48
Hotcakes with 2 pats margarine and 1½ oz syrup	440	12	25
McLean Deluxe	320	19	28
Milk Shake, Chocolate Low-fat	320	<2	5
Milk Shake, Strawberry Low-fat	320	2	4
Milk Shake, Vanilla, Low-fat	290	<2	4
Pie, Apple	260	15	52
Quarter Pounder	410	20	44
Quarter Pounder with Cheese	510	28	49
Salad, Chef	170	9	48
Salad, Chicken, Chunky	150	4	24
Salad, Garden	50	2	36
Sauce, Barbecue, 1 serving	50	<1	9
Sauce, Hot Mustard, 1 serving	70	4	51
Sauce, Sweet-n-Sour, 1 serving	60	<1	3
Sausage	160	15	84
Sausage McMuffin	345	20	52
Sausage McMuffin with Egg	430	25	52
Sundae, Hot Caramel, Low-fat Frozen Yogurt	270	3	10
Sundae, Hot Fudge, Low-fat Frozen Yogurt	240	3	11

Sundae, Strawberry, Low-fat Frozen Yogurt	210	1	4

Pizza Hut

Hand-Tossed, Cheese, 2 slices, medium (15-inch), 7.9 oz	518	20	35
Hand-Tossed, Supreme, 2 slices, medium (15-inch), 8.5 oz	540	26	43
Pan, Super Supreme, 2 slices, medium (15-inch), 9.2 oz	563	26	42
Pan, with cheese, 2 slices medium (15-inch), 7.3 oz	492	18	33
Personal Pan, Pepperoni, whole (5-inch), 9.1 oz	675	29	39
Personal Pan, Supreme, whole (5-inch), 9.4 oz	647	28	39
Thin 'n Crispy, Pepperoni, 2 slices, medium (15-inch), 5.2 oz	413	20	44
Thin 'n Crispy, Supreme, 2 slices, medium (15-inch), 7.1 oz	459	22	43

Subway

BMT Salad, small	369	30	73
BMT Sub, Italian Roll, 6-inch	491	28	51
Club Salad, small	225	13	52
Club Sub, Italian Roll, 6-inch	346	11	29
Cold Cut Combo Salad, small	305	26	77
Cold Cut Combo Sub, Italian Roll, 6-inch	427	20	42
Ham & Cheese Salad, small	200	12	54
Ham & Cheese Sub, Italian Roll, 6 inch	322	9	25
Meatball Sub, Italian Roll, 6-inch	459	22	43
Roast Beef Salad, small	222	10	41
Roast Beef Sub, Italian Roll, 6-inch	345	12	31
Seafood & Crab Salad, small	371	30	73
Seafood & Crab Sub, Italian Roll, 6-inch	493	28	51
Steak & Cheese Sub, Italian Roll, 6-inch	383	16	38
Tuna Salad, small	430	38	80
Tuna Sub, Italian Roll, 6-inch	551	36	59
Turkey Breast Salad, small	201	11	49
Turkey Breast Sub, Italian Roll, 6-inch	322	10	28
Veggies & Cheese Sub, Italian Roll, 6-inch	268	9	30

Taco Bell (all portions consist of one serving)

Burrito, Bean	447	14	28
Burrito, Beef	493	21	28
Burrito, Chicken	334	12	32
Burrito, Combo	407	16	35
Burrito Supreme	503	22	39

Cinnamon Twists	171	8	42
Meximelt, Beef	266	15	51
Meximelt, Chicken	257	15	53
Nachos	346	18	47
Nachos Bellgrande	649	35	49
Pintos & Cheese	190	9	43
Pizza, Mexican	575	37	58
Salad, Taco	905	61	61
Salad, Taco, w/o shell	484	31	59
Salsa	18	0	0
Sauce, Hot Taco, 1 packet	3	0	0

Fats and Oils

Margarine, regular, soft, 1 tbsp	100	11	99
Margarine, Soft, Parkay, 1 tbsp	100	11	99
Margarine, Soft, Parkay, Corn Oil, 1 tbsp	100	11	99
Margarine, Soft Diet, Parkay Reduced Calorie, 1 tbsp	50	6	100
Margarine, spread, hard, 1 tbsp (1/8 stick)	75	9	100
Margarine, spread, hard, approx 1 tsp	25	3	100
Margarine, Squeezable, Shedd's Spread Country Crock, 1 tbsp	80	9	100
Margarine, Squeeze Parkay, 1 tbsp	90	10	100
Margarine, Stick, Corn Mazola, 1 tbsp	100	11	99
Margarine, Stick Corn Oil, Fleischmann's, 1 tbsp	100	11	99
Margarine, Stick, Corn Oil, Mazola, 1 tbsp	100	11	99
Margarine, Stick, Soy Oil, Chiffon, 1 tbsp	100	11	99
Margarine, Stick, Soy Oil, Weight Watchers Reduced-Calorie, 1 tbsp	60	7	100
Margarine, Stick, Sunflower Oil, Promise, 1 tbsp	90	10	100
Margarine, Tub, Soy Oil, Chiffon, 1 tbsp	90	10	100
Margarine, Tub, Soy Oil, Weight Watchers Reduced-Calorie Light Spread, 1 tbsp	50	6	100
Margarine, Tub, Sunflower Oil, Promise, 1 tbsp	90	10	100
Oil, Canola, Crisco, Puritan, 1 tbsp	120	13	98
Oil, Corn, Mazola, 1 tbsp	120	14	100
Oil, Olive, Bertolli, 1 tbsp	120	14	100
Oil, peanut, 1 tbsp	125	14	100
Oil, Safflower, Hollywood, 1 tbsp	120	14	100
Oil, Soybean, Crisco, 1 tbsp	120	13	98
Oil, soybean-cottonseed blend, hydrogenated, 1 tbsp	125	14	100
Oil, sunflower, 1 tbsp	125	14	100
Oil, Sunflower, Sunlite, 1 tbsp	120	14	100
Oil, Vegetable, Crisco, 1 tbsp	120	14	100

Shortening, Vegetable, Crisco, 1 tbsp	110	12	98
Shortening, Vegetable, Crisco Butter Flavor, 1 tbsp	110	12	98
Spray, Cooking (Vegetable Oil), Pam, 2½-second spray	14	2	100
Spray, No-Stick (Vegetable) Mazola, 2½-second spray	6	1	100
Spread, 50% Fat, Parkay, 1 tbsp	60	7	100
Spread, Parkay (50% vegetable oil), 1 tbsp	60	7	100
Spread, Stick, Touch of Butter, Kraft, 1 tbsp	90	10	90
Spread, Tub (Vegetable), Shedd's 1 tbsp	70	7	90

Gravies and Sauces
Gravies

Beef, canned, 1 cup	125	5	36
Beef, Franco-American, 2 oz	35	2	51
Brown, from dry mix, 1 cup	80	2	23
Brown, with onions, HomeStyle, Heinz, 2 oz	25	1	36
Chicken, canned, 1 cup	190	14	66
Chicken, Franco-American, 2 oz	45	4	80
Chicken, from dry mix, 1 cup	85	2	21
Turkey, canned, Heinz, Homestyle, 2 oz	25	1	36

Sauces

Cheese, from dry mix, prepared with milk, 1 cup	305	17	50
Hollandaise, prepared with water, 2 tbsp	30	3	90
Picante Sauce, Old El Paso, 2 tbsp	12	0	0
Picante Sauce, Pace, 2 tbsp	9	0	0
Soy Sauce, see Baking Products and Condiments			
Spaghetti, Chunky Garden Style, with Mushrooms and Green Peppers, Ragu, 4 oz	70	3	39
Spaghetti, Extra Chunky, Garden Tomato with Mushrooms, Prego, 4 oz	100	6	54
Spaghetti, Extra Chunky, Mushroom and Tomato, Prego, 4 oz	110	5	41
Spaghetti, Extra Chunky, Tomato and Onion, Prego, 4 oz	140	6	39
Spaghetti, Plain, Prego, 4 oz	140	5	32
Spaghetti, Ragu, 4 oz	80	3	34
Spaghetti, Thick & Hearty, Ragu, 4 oz	140	5	32
Spaghetti, with Meat, Homestyle, Ragu, 4 oz	70	2	26
Spaghetti, with Meat, Prego, 4 oz	150	6	36
Spaghetti, with Mushrooms, Prego, 4 oz	140	5	32
Spaghetti, with Mushrooms, Ragu, 4 oz	80	4	45
Spaghetti, with Mushrooms, Thick & Hearty, Ragu, 4 oz	140	5	32

White, prepared with milk, 1 cup	240	13	49

Packaged Entrees

Beef Noodle, Hamburger Helper, prepared with meat, 1 cup	320	15	42
Beef Stew, Dinty Moore, 10 oz	270	13	43
Cheeseburger Macaroni, Hamburger Helper, prepared with meat, 1 cup	370	19	46
Chicken, Sweet & Sour, La Choy, ¾ cup	230	2	8
Chili con carne w/ beans, canned, 1 cup	286	13	41
Chow Mein, Beef La Choy, ¾ cup	60	1	15
Chow Mein, Chicken, La Choy, ¾ cup	80	3	34
Egg Noodle and Cheese Dinner, Kraft, ¾ cup	340	17	45
Egg Noodle and Chicken Dinner, Kraft, ¾ cup	240	9	34
Lasagna, Hamburger Helper, prepared with meat, 1 cup	340	14	37
Macaroni and Cheese Deluxe Dinner, Kraft, ¾ cup	260	8	28
Macaroni and Cheese Dinner, Original, Kraft, ¾ cup prepared	290	13	40
Shells and Cheese Dinner, Velveeta, ½ cup	210	8	34
Spaghetti, Mild American Style Dinner, Kraft, 1 cup	300	7	21
Spaghetti Dinner, Tangy Italian Style, Kraft, 1 cup	310	48	23
Spaghetti in tomato sauce with cheese, canned, 1 cup	190	2	9
Spaghetti with Meat Sauce, Top Shelf 2 Minute Entrée, Hormel, 10 oz	260	6	21
Spaghetti with Meat Sauce Dinner, Kraft, 1 cup	360	14	35

Salad Dressings

Bacon, Creamy, Reduced Calorie, Kraft, 1 tbsp	30	2	60
Bacon & Tomato, Kraft, 1 tbsp	70	7	90
Blue Cheese, Chunky, Kraft, 1 tbsp	60	6	90
Blue Cheese, Chunky, Reduced Calorie, Kraft, 1 tbsp	30	2	60
Blue Cheese, Lite, Less Oil, Wish-Bone, 1 tbsp	40	4	90

CHAPTER TEN

Eating for Success

Counting Calories

E nergy in Foods

Counting calories sounds simple enough. The calories we get are found not only in the solid foods we eat, but also in the beverages we drink. Avoiding beverages with "bad fructose" will go a long way toward lowering your calorie intake from beverages. Early in my career, I had not learned about the problem the body has in recognizing "liquid calories" in soft drinks and fruit drinks—the calories provided by sugar or HFCS. I have since learned this important lesson. The "liquid calories" in soft drinks and fruit drinks do not lower the intake of solid foods enough to balance food intake over the day. In my early years, however, I needed to find out these things for myself.

I figured that counting calories presented the obvious solution for people who wanted to manage their weight. If I could just teach my patients to count their calories each day, I was sure they would have a firm grasp of their eating habits and be able to lose weight. So I tried it myself. I bought an accurate scale and an accurate measuring cup. First I estimated the portion size, and then I weighed the foods to see how accurately I had estimated them.

Much to my disappointment, my estimates were usually wrong one way or the other—either too high or too low. Round fruits and vegetables were a particular problem. I never realized when I took geometry in high school that the principles taught there would apply to nutrition. But here it was, staring me right in the face. A round fruit or vegetable, such as an apple, orange, or potato, changes in weight (and in calories) by a function of the

183

cube of the radius. For example, an orange that is only 10% larger across (in diameter) than another one has almost 33% more calories due to the increased weight and volume. It was apparent to me that calorie counting required a great deal of care and persistence.

Still, I figured that with the proper motivation, I could walk my patients through this approach. But one evening as I walked to one of my group meetings, I could see some of the participants in their cars hurriedly making entries in their calorie diaries.

For them, calorie counting was hopeless. But for some people, it was amazingly successful. Only you know whether you were born to be a calorie counter. If you think so, the next section may be all you need. Make no mistake about it: Calorie counting is a sure-fire method for managing your weight if it is approached with diligence and care. But if the thought of weighing and measuring foods turns your stomach, so to speak, then move on to the next section. This part of the chapter is not for you.

But first, let me share one piece of advice. No matter what approach you choose, skipping meals is not an effective or healthy way to avoid calories and manage your weight. Eat breakfast, lunch, and dinner, and possibly even a snack. Avoid the "bad fructose"-containing beverages and "bad fructose" in solid foods. Keep fat intake under control—remember, fat and fructose combined are a real problem (the "deadly duo"). In addition to improving your performance at work or in school, eating regularly goes a long way toward reducing hunger at night. Studies have shown that people who eat their food in several meals each day as opposed to eating one or two large meals are less likely to be overweight.[1] Based on my own work with this problem, I encourage all my patients to eat several meals a day. This may mean a change in your lifestyle. But so is losing weight. Change is essential, and changing the frequency with which you eat is one of those important changes on the road to success.

Before we go any further, let me put a bit more information on the road map of nutrition I gave you earlier. "Energy" is the ability to do work. The energy your body needs comes from the food you eat, as shown in the left-hand bar of Figure 1. Your body uses only what it needs to do its daily work (right-hand bar of Figure 1). This includes basal metabolism, which constitutes approximately two-thirds of your total energy needs, including energy to digest food, make and destroy cells, remove waste, breathe, circulate the blood, and maintain your body temperature. Any extra energy above what is needed is stored as fat. Those people walking around who do not have weight problems and who are not dieting are able to balance, over months and years, the calories in what they eat with the calories their bodies need. Avoiding the "bad fructose" (HFCS and sugar (sucrose))-containing beverages and foods, eating low-fat foods, and avoiding large portions will give your body a better chance to make the right adjustments over time.

When we eat, there is an increase in our metabolism. This is referred to as the "thermic effect of food" (shown as "TEF" on the right side of Figure 1). This effect is larger with protein and carbohydrate than with fat. TEF represents about 10% of our total daily energy production.

Activity, such as moving, talking, chewing, and running, is variable and uses approximately one-third of the total energy each day. This energy use is directly related to your body weight (if you weigh more, you use more calories for a particular activity) and increases with the amount of exercise or activity.

If you eat less food energy than you need, your body will call on the energy stored in your fat. This is the way you lose weight. This idea of a balance between what you eat and what you need, with your body fat serving as a buffer, is depicted below.

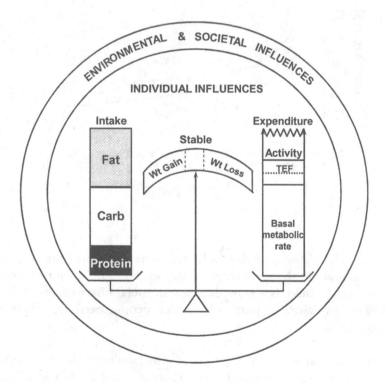

Figure 1. A diagram of energy balance and factors influencing it. In the center is a "balance," which will tip depending on the balance between the food intake in the left column and the energy expenditure in the right column. This balance is influenced by both individual factors and by a variety of environmental and social factors, represented by the circles that surround the energy-balance platform.

185

Basal metabolism, on the right side of the figure, is affected by various factors. It decreases as we get older (Figure 2). Males have a higher basal metabolism than do females. Hormones, such as thyroid hormones, can influence basal metabolism. A cold environment can increase it.

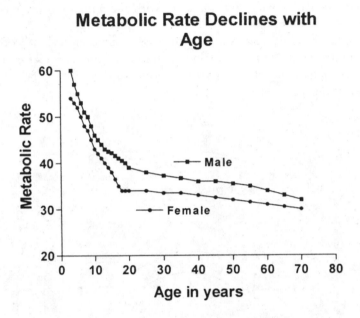

Metabolic Rate Declines with Age

Figure 2. The changes in metabolic rate with age. The highest rates of metabolism are in the early years of life, with a rapid drop to about age 20. Thereafter there is a slow decrease in metabolism of about 1% per year. This explains, in part, why older people need less food than younger ones.

Any food that is eaten and not used for metabolism or work is STORED as FAT. Normally, approximately 15–30% in men and 25–40% in women of body weight is fat. It serves as insulation, cushioning, and for emergency energy needs.

When you eat LESS food than your body needs, the deficit is made up from your internal or stored energy. During starvation, your stored fat is broken down and used for fuel.

Energy needs are continuous, but meals are intermittent. Thus there is a constant shift of energy into and out of fat cells and other storage sites in your body to fuel moving, digesting, making cells, destroying cells, removing wastes, breathing, and circulating the blood, among others.

Energy is measured as calories. But what is a calorie? It is the amount of heat required to raise 1 gram (about 5 grams in 1 teaspoon) of water 1 degree Centigrade (from 15 to 16 degrees). The caloric value of food tells you the amount of energy or heat your body will get when that food is used in your body.

To reiterate, daily calorie needs change:

- They decline with age.
- They increase with body size and weight.
- They are higher in men than women of the same age, height, and weight because men have more muscle mass.
- They are modified by glandular function.

Most adults require between 1,500 and 2,500 calories per day. The National Academy of Sciences[2] estimates that an average female, 5' 4" tall, age 19–22 years, weighing 120 lb (55 kg), needs 2,100 calories per day. The average male, 5' 10" tall, age 19–22 years, weighing 154 lb (70 kg), needs 2,900 calories per day.

As you know by now, one pound of body fat contains 3,500 calories. This means that to lose one pound of body fat, you must burn up 3,500 more calories than you eat. During one year, a woman consumes roughly 700,000 calories and a man consumes about 1 million calories. Failing to burn up only 1% of those calories can result in a weight gain of 2 to 3 pounds per year.

Worse yet, consider what will happen if we eat and store 100 calories more each day than we burn up. It's not that difficult. Look at the following list of foods that contain approximately 100 calories:

Table 1. Portions of Food with 100 Calories

Apple, 2¾" diameter	Good choice
Applesauce, 1 cup unsweetened	Good choice
Bacon, 2 slices, fried crisp	Poor choice
Butter, 1 Tablespoon	Poor choice
Hershey's milk chocolate bar, without nuts, 2/3 oz	Avoid
Pepsi Cola, 8 oz (almost unavailable in this size)	Avoid
Cookies: 2 chocolate chip	Avoid
6 ginger snaps	Avoid
6 vanilla wafers	Avoid
Green beans, fresh, 3 cups	Good Choice
Ham, fresh, lean, marbled, cooked, 1 oz	Fair Choice
Roast chicken: light meat, no skin, 2 oz	Good Choice

That extra 100 calories per day for thirty-five days will result in a weight gain of one pound. If this continues for a year, you will gain 10 pounds. In ten years, you will gain 100 pounds! The bottom line of weight loss is that you must either decrease the number of calories you are eating or increase the number you are burning up. Better yet, do both at the same time. Simply put, we must eat less *and* be more active. *Tip*: Do a bit of each.

Since any method of managing your weight must either decrease calorie intake, increase calorie output, or both, we could simply say eat less and exercise more. This is easier said than done, however. We know that wild animals seem to keep their body weight constant with a balanced storage of energy.[3] They eat only when fuel is needed (as signaled by hunger). Intuitively, they know that otherwise they might become less agile and end up as some other animal's dinner.

With "civilization," we have changed our ways of living. Humans eat for reasons other than the simple need for food. Thus to control calories, you must either directly focus on them, as I am doing with you in this chapter, or by indirectly focusing on where, when, and how you eat (see Chapter 8).

To lose weight permanently, you must permanently reduce the amount of stored energy. There are two factors on the diagram of energy balance that you can control: food intake and physical activity or movement.

Here's a more "positive" look at the function of calories and energy balance. If you require 1,800 calories per day for your normal bodily functions but eat only 1,300 calories per day, this equals a calorie "deficit" of 500 calories. That adds up to 3,500 calories in a week, or one pound of weight lost. One pound a week equals 52 pounds by this time next year.

Let's remember that water weight can confound some of these calculations. The weight of the water produced when you burn fat is more than the weight of the fat that is burned. Over short periods of time, it is possible to eat fewer calories than you need and still gain weight from the water produced by burning up this fat. A patient of mine illustrated this point most dramatically. She was staying in our metabolic unit while we studied her weight loss. She was an older woman and had few visitors. She was eating only 800 calories per day, and for nearly 30 days she didn't lose weight. We were measuring her metabolism and knew she was burning up over 1500 calories per day—so why no weight loss? Finally she began to get rid of the extra water and her weight declined to what we had anticipated it would be. But as the days went by before this happened, she got ever more discouraged.[4] Don't be discouraged or alarmed. This is only a short-term process. Your body will sooner or later shed this extra water, and your hard work will show up on the scale. We only hope it is sooner. *Tip*: Weigh yourself regularly at the same time of day and before eating.

If your caloric intake is 1000 calories/day less than you need for a week, you can expect to lose 2 pounds (7000 calories) of fat from your fat tissue that week.

To reiterate: To lose weight, you must decrease caloric INTAKE below expenditure or increase caloric OUTPUT above intake. If you need 1,800 calories each day and you take in 1,300 calories a day, there is a deficit of 500 calories per day. Over a 7-day period, this equals 3,500 calories or the equivalent of 1 pound per week of weight loss.

The Calories You Eat

To track the calories you eat, you will use a Bray Plan Monitor form like the one below. Each and every time you eat, including all meals and snacks, write down the food eaten. Also record, as accurately as possible, the amount that is eaten. Use whatever measurement is most familiar to you. Aim for the greatest possible accuracy. At least once a day, look up the number of calories that correspond to the amount of each food you ate.

Bray Plan Monitor **MONITOR FOR CALORIES**			
Day		Calories Consumed	
Food Eaten	Amount Eaten	Solid	Liquid

Figure 3. Bray Plan Calorie Monitor. This 3×5-inch form can be duplicated to allow you to record the foods you eat and their calorie content.

I have provided you with a list that has the calorie content of many commonly eaten foods on it (Appendix 1). Other lists and books are available at your bookstore or online. The data from the U.S. Department of Agriculture provides the basis for most books: 1) The U.S. Department of Agriculture Handbook No. 8, entitled *Composition of Foods: Raw, Processed, Prepared*, and its updates.[5] website: *http://www.nal.usda.gov/fnic/ food-comp/search/*.

The book *Bowes and Church's Food Values of Portions Commonly Used*, by Jean A.T. Pennington and Jean S. Douglass, 18th ed, published by Lippincott, Wilkins and Wilkins, 2004,[6] is also a useful source and for calories and carbohydrates, the book *Calories and Carbohydrates*, by B. Kraus and M. Reilly-Pardo,[7] is particularly useful because it contains information on many brand-name and packaged foods. If you can find one of these, there are many others to choose from.

Record the calories under liquid (if liquid food) or solid. When you have completed the calorie monitors for seven days, you will be ready to evaluate your calorie intake.

Analysis of Caloric Intake

Now that you have completed recording your calorie intake and the foods you have eaten for the past week, it is time to analyze the results. Place your seven daily Bray Plan Calorie Monitor cards in front of you.

Bray Plan Monitor ANALYSIS CALORIE INTAKE								
	Day							
	1	2	3	4	5	6	7	Grand Total
Solid								
Liquid								
Combined								

Figure 4. Bray Plan Analysis of Calorie Intake Form. This form will provide you the space to analyze your intake of calories from both liquid and solid sources.

Step 1.	Add up total caloric intake ingested as liquids for Day 1. Record that total in the column marked "Liquid" on the line for Day 1 using the form below or one of the 3×5 cards you bought.
Step 2.	Then add up total calorie intake for the solid food eaten on Day 1. Record this total under "Solids" on Day 1.
Step 3.	Repeat above steps for each of the seven days of your Bray Plan Monitor.
Step 4.	On the far-right lines, record the daily calorie intake by adding Liquids and Solids for each day.

You may want to do this by transferring your numbers to a spreadsheet. Here is an example from one of my patients.

Now let's take a look at what the numbers tell you. You may be surprised by the low-calorie totals. Many people don't seem to need much food because they are relatively inactive. They may also have not recorded all of the food they ate, however, we know that most people under-report by about 30%, and people with a weight problem may under-report even more.

Bray Plan Monitor **ANALYSIS CALORIE INTAKE**								
Day								
	1	2	3	4	5	6	7	Grand Total
Solid	1200	1000	1500	1450	1550	1000	1250	8950
Liquid	200	150	300	100	150	100	150	1150
Combined	1400	1150	1800	1550	1700	1100	1400	10,100

You may also be surprised at the low number of "liquid" calories in a society where soft drinks are so heavily advertised. One possibility is that this individual was drinking a lot of water. There may also be a wide variation from day to day.[8] This indicates a need for pre-planning your day's menu to help you better control your eating. It emphasizes the importance of recognizing how you might respond to certain events during the week.

If you are getting a large number of calories from beverages with "bad fructose," you may have identified the problem. Soft drinks and alcoholic beverages are the usual culprits. Here is where watching out for "bad fructose" comes in. Alcoholic beverages may also be a problem for some people.

If your daily totals are between 1,000 to 1,200 calories, you should be losing weight. If not, you may need a more careful way of measuring the amounts of food you eat or in recording every time you eat. As I've pointed out, calorie counting is hard to do. To succeed, I encourage you to purchase a small scale, which will weigh up to one pound. You can get one at most stationery and variety stores. With such a scale on your shelf, you can keep an accurate record of the calories contained in the foods you eat.

You have now learned what I have learned. Calorie counting is difficult, but it may be your cup of tea, so to speak. Here are some reasons it can be hard to do:

1. It is difficult to estimate portion sizes accurately.
2. Food combinations can be difficult to estimate unless there is a Nutrition Facts label with calories on it.
3. The caloric contents of food in restaurants and cafeterias can be difficult to obtain.

At this point, you may like counting calories. If so, keep it up. It can be a winner for you. If you don't like this method of counting calories, never fear. There are other ways you can get the information you need about your energy intake.

I have already described one way of monitoring your calorie intake. Now I would like to suggest other ways of making calorie counting simpler and more fun. Let's try the use of nutrition labels, the calorie glass, calorie scale, and food models.

Nutrition Labels and Calories

Nutrition labels with Nutrition Facts on canned and packaged foods are an important outgrowth of the efforts of nutritionists on behalf of the consumers around the country. All packaged food in your grocery store must have a nutrition label. A sample of the current format for nutrition labels is shown below. This one is from a cereal package.

The food label contains four important pieces of information for you: 1) It shows the serving size used in the package and the number of servings contained in that package; 2) it tells you the number of calories and amount of major macronutrients that are present in a serving; 3) it lists vitamins and minerals; and 4) it lists all of the ingredients in that food, starting with the one in highest quantity and then in decreasing order.

The calories are listed just after the serving size. This is followed by the number of calories from total fat. Then come saturated fat, *trans* fats, cholesterol, sodium, total carbohydrate, dietary fiber, sugars, and finally protein. From what you have learned about nutrition, you know that a gram of protein contains 4 calories, a gram of carbohydrate 4 calories, and a gram of fat 9 calories. It tells you this again on the label. With these figures, you can calculate approximately how many calories are in the serving, and you will find they are in agreement with what is printed on the nutrition label. In addition, the label contains information on the percentage of selected macronutrients that are present in the food based on the daily value for a 2000-calorie diet. Then come the ingredients in the food. I use this part of the label to identify foods that contain "bad fructose" (HFCS or sugar (sucrose)). If they do, I move on to the next food choice, if available.

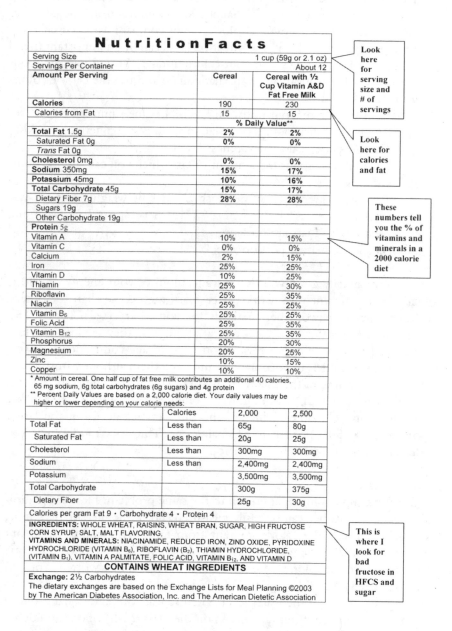

N u t r i t i o n F a c t s			Look here for serving size and # of servings
Serving Size		1 cup (59g or 2.1 oz)	
Servings Per Container		About 12	
Amount Per Serving	Cereal	Cereal with ½ Cup Vitamin A&D Fat Free Milk	
Calories	190	230	
Calories from Fat	15	15	
		% Daily Value**	
Total Fat 1.5g	2%	2%	Look here for calories and fat
Saturated Fat 0g	0%	0%	
Trans Fat 0g			
Cholesterol 0mg	0%	0%	
Sodium 350mg	15%	17%	
Potassium 45mg	10%	16%	
Total Carbohydrate 45g	15%	17%	
Dietary Fiber 7g	28%	28%	
Sugars 19g			
Other Carbohydrate 19g			
Protein 5g			These numbers tell you the % of vitamins and minerals in a 2000 calorie diet
Vitamin A	10%	15%	
Vitamin C	0%	0%	
Calcium	2%	15%	
Iron	25%	25%	
Vitamin D	10%	25%	
Thiamin	25%	30%	
Riboflavin	25%	35%	
Niacin	25%	25%	
Vitamin B$_6$	25%	25%	
Folic Acid	25%	35%	
Vitamin B$_{12}$	25%	35%	
Phosphorus	20%	30%	
Magnesium	20%	25%	
Zinc	10%	15%	
Copper	10%	10%	

* Amount in cereal. One half cup of fat free milk contributes an additional 40 calories, 65 mg sodium, 6g total carbohydrates (6g sugars) and 4g protein

** Percent Daily Values are based on a 2,000 calorie diet. Your daily values may be higher or lower depending on your calorie needs:

	Calories	2,000	2,500
Total Fat	Less than	65g	80g
Saturated Fat	Less than	20g	25g
Cholesterol	Less than	300mg	300mg
Sodium	Less than	2,400mg	2,400mg
Potassium		3,500mg	3,500mg
Total Carbohydrate		300g	375g
Dietary Fiber		25g	30g

Calories per gram Fat 9 · Carbohydrate 4 · Protein 4

INGREDIENTS: WHOLE WHEAT, RAISINS, WHEAT BRAN, SUGAR, HIGH FRUCTOSE CORN SYRUP, SALT, MALT FLAVORING,
VITAMINS AND MINERALS: NIACINAMIDE, REDUCED IRON, ZIND OXIDE, PYRIDOXINE HYDROCHLORIDE (VITAMIN B$_6$), RIBOFLAVIN (B$_2$), THIAMIN HYDROCHLORIDE, (VITAMIN B$_1$), VITAMIN A PALMITATE, FOLIC ACID, VITAMIN B$_{12}$, AND VITAMIN D
CONTAINS WHEAT INGREDIENTS

Exchange: 2½ Carbohydrates
The dietary exchanges are based on the Exchange Lists for Meal Planning ©2003 by The American Diabetes Association, Inc. and The American Dietetic Association

This is where I look for bad fructose in HFCS and sugar

Figure 5. Nutrition Facts Label. This is the nutrition label that is used on all packaged goods in your grocery store. Become familiar with it. It can help you keep track of your calories.

Now that you know what a nutrition label looks like, make use of it. I want you to start reading nutrition labels. Keep samples from the packages you bring home, and see how the calorie values compare with our charts.

Once you get in the habit, the nutrition label can be an important friend in helping you keep an "eye" on your calorie intake. Write down the foods you eat for which nutrition labels are inadequate and use the calorie counting form to help you.

What did you learn about nutrition labels? Let me summarize.

- Labels tell you about serving size in various containers.
- They increase "calorie awareness."
- They tell you about the amount of fat, which you can use in counting fat grams.
- They list ingredients (in decreasing order by weight) and tell you whether there is "bad fructose" (HFCS or sugar (sucrose)) and what kinds of fats are present.
- Aids in estimating portion size.

We have already given you two ways to monitor your energy or calorie intake. Since different ways work better for some people than for others, however, there are two other methods for you to try (see Chapter 15). Unless the food portions you eat are carefully chosen, they can lead you into a lot of calorie confusion. For this reason I encourage you to purchase of a few of the food models in portion sizes and keep them at home. In this way, you can get a feeling of the "size" of the food you are buying or preparing.

To illustrate this: If you bought two oranges, one of which is 2 inches in diameter and the other 3 inches, the number of calories in the larger orange is almost 50% more than the smaller one. Thus food models help you understand what is meant by a "portion."

Calorie Glass

A measuring cup is another approach to the same problem. Liquids are difficult to weigh, but they can be easily measured. From the measured volume, you can determine the calorie content from tables (Appendix 1). In our search for an alternative way to solve this problem, we developed a Calorie Glass, on which the calorie values of several liquids can be written. You can make one from an ordinary glass. Pour 2 ounces of water into the glass and place a piece of tape at the water level. Then repeat with additional 2-ounce portions until you have four tape marks on the glass. Many of our liquids are measured in ½ cup (4 oz) or 1 cup (8 oz). You can then easily get an idea of how much milk or soft drink you pour in the glass. This will make it easier to record your liquid calories. If you do this, I suggest you use a tall, thin glass rather than a short, squatty one. There is convincing evidence that when asked to pour the same amount into these glasses, people pour more into the short, squatty glass than into the tall, thin glass.[9] This gives you an idea about how to buy for your kitchen as well. As you need to replace your glassware, do so with taller, thinner ones and let the shorter, squattier ones go.

Each time you pour one of the liquids into the Calorie Glass, you will now have a readout of the amount you are about to ingest. With a glass for juices and a glass for other beverages such as milk, soft drinks, etc., you can get a pretty good idea of the calories you are drinking.

A third and final way to deal with calories is to purchase a small scale for weights up to one pound. With such a scale on your shelf, you can keep accurate records of the calories contained in the foods you eat. These scales are available in most health food stores and many stationery stores.

CHAPTER ELEVEN

Eating for Success

MyPyramid Food Guide and Energy Density

MyPyramid Food Guide

One simple way of evaluating food intake is to use the MyPyramid food guide and the **Nutrition Facts** label on most foods developed by the United States Department of Agriculture. MyPyramid uses a pyramid with vertical stripes up the side to represent the groups of foods (Chapter 4) and a staircase to the left to emphasize the importance of movement and physical activity. The food groups are identified at the base of the pyramid to provide a basic guide to good nutrition. The accompanying table lists these food groups along with serving sizes and the nutrients they contain.

Table 1. My Pyramid List of Food Groups

Grains	Vegetables	Fruits	Milk	Meat & Beans
Eat at least 3 ounces of whole-grain cereals, breads, crackers, rice or pasta every day. 1 oz is about 1 slice of bread, 1 cup of cereal, 1/2 cup of cooked rice, cereal, or pasta	Eat more dark-green veggies such as broccoli, spinach, and other dark leafy greens. Eat more orange veggies such as carrots and sweet potatoes. Eat more dry beans and peas such as pinto beans, kidney beans, and lentils.	Eat a variety of fruits. Choose fresh, frozen, canned (light syrup or water pack). Go easy on fruit juices.	Use low-fat or fat-free milk, yogurt, and other milk products. If you don't or can't consume milk, choose lactose-free products or other calcium sources, such as fortified foods and beverages.	Choose low-fat or lean meats and poultry. Bake it, broil it, grill it. Vary your protein routine - choose more fish, beans, peas, nuts, and seeds.
Eat a total of 6 oz every day.	Eat 2½ cups every day.	Eat 2 cups every day.	Eat 3 cups every day (for kids 2-8 years, it's 2 cups).	Eat 5½ oz every day.

Group 1: Grains: This group includes bread, cereal, rice, and pasta. MyPyramid recommends that whole-grain products make up at least half of the total eaten from this group. This group provides B vitamins and fiber for your diet. The range of calories in foods of this group is small: from 60 to 120 calories per serving. Since you have a weight problem, you may want to choose more servings per day rather than less. Most importantly, focus on whole-grain bread and those with fewer calories per serving. Whole-wheat bread is a good example since it is usually pre-sliced and thus portion-controlled (Chapter 14). Also available are whole-wheat "double fiber" breads, which may be even a better choice. Consider this: Large muffins available at the supermarket may have 200–250 calories per serving, but one muffin may actually contain 2–3 servings, for a total ranging from 400 to 750 calories! Muffins, rolls, and many other foods in this group can have a lot of "hidden fat."

Group 2: Vegetables: My motto is "vary your veggies." The colors of vegetables vary from dark green to orange. Eating such items as spinach, broccoli, carrots, and sweet potatoes will cover all your bases. You get not only important vitamins and fiber from veggies, you get those vital minerals. For adults, 2½ servings of vegetables daily are desirable. One serving of raw greens contains 20 or 30 calories, while a potato can be 80 calories (without butter or margarine). For people with a weight problem, emphasizing this group is particularly important because of the low calorie content of most vegetables. Potatoes may also not be your best choice because they have a high glycemic index.

Group 3: Fruits: Fruits, rather than fruit juices, are recommended for both meals and snacks. Two cups of whole or sliced fruits per day, which contain "good fructose," are recommended. Their main nutritional contribution is vitamins, minerals and, in some fruits, fiber. Note that there is considerable variation in the calorie or energy density (calories/g). It is better to eat either fresh or frozen fruits; with canned fruit, water-packed is preferable since syrup contains "bad fructose." Go easy on the fruit juice (4 oz or 120 ml), and avoid "fruit drinks," which are often not much more than "bad fructose" (sugar or HFCS) and water without much fruit or fiber. One serving of cantaloupe contains 20 to 30 calories, while an apple or banana can be 80 calories. For people with a weight problem, emphasizing this group is also important. In addition, fruits and vegetables can help lower blood pressure.[1,2]

Group 4: Milk: Milk, yogurt, and cheese make up this group. These products are good sources of calcium and vitamin D, which can help build and maintain strong bones. Two cups per day for adults and three cups per day for children, preferably fat-free or low-fat, are recommended. You have already seen the same nutritional value can be obtained from 8 ounces of skim milk as from two cups of ice cream, yet one cup of skim milk contains

90 calories and the corresponding caloric value for ice cream is 380 calories. As consumption of "bad fructose"-containing drinks (soft drinks, sport drinks, and fruits drinks) has increased, milk intake by children has decreased, to their potential detriment.[3] My *Low-Fructose Approach to Weight Control* could lead to an increase in milk consumption as a healthy alternative beverage.

Group 5: Meat and Beans: This group includes red meat, poultry, fish, dry beans, eggs, and nuts. Five and one-half ounces each day are recommended from this group. These protein-rich foods provide the amino acid building blocks your body needs to make its own protein. Meat is also a good source of vitamin B_{12}. Low-calorie items in this group have less than 50 calories per ounce. If nuts or peanut butter are being used to obtain the nutritional value from this group, calories can range as high as 400 to 500 calories per serving. Eat lean or low-fat meat, and eat more dry beans and peas.

Group 6: Oils, Sugar, and Alcohol: Here is where the *Low-Fructose Approach to Weight Loss* applies most, and here is where you need to read your food labels to see what kind of ingredients the food makers have used. If a food has "bad fructose" (HFCS) listed on the label, you know it is highly processed. There is no HFCS in nature—it is manmade. I try to avoid "bad fructose" (HFCS or sugar (sucrose)). Sugar- or HFCS-sweetened beverages and sugar-sweetened gelatins, candies, pastries, and cakes (fat and "bad fructose") provide more calories and little or no nutrition other than calories. Avoid the "bad fructose"!

We need oils, but you should get yours from fish, nuts, and liquid oils such as corn, soybean, canola, and olive oil, rather than from butter or margarine. *Trans*-fatty acids are the product of hydrogenation of liquid fats to make them solid. *Trans* fats are particularly risky with respect to heart disease and are currently being removed from the food supply. Read your food labels to avoid *trans* fats wherever possible. Cooking oil, mayonnaise, and snacks such as potato chips have fat but little or no other nutritional value. Wine, beer, and other alcoholic beverages are also part of this group. *Tip*: This is the group to avoid.

Bray Plan Monitor **MONITOR FOR FOOD GROUPS**						
Day						
Food Eaten	Veg	Fruit	Bread Grain	Milk Yogurt Cheese	Meat Fish Poultry Beans	Other

Self-Monitoring of Food Groups
Figure 1. Bray Plan Monitor for Food Groups. For the next week, record the foods that are eaten each day by the food group to which they belong. For prepared foods, you may need to list them in more than one group.

For the next week, identify the food groups to which the foods you eat belong, using the sample of the Bray Plan Pyramid Group Monitor shown here. On the left is a place for you to write down the foods you eat. On the right are six columns, one for each of the five food groups and one for the miscellaneous or "other" group. Every time you eat, take out the card and immediately write down the food groups that are on your plate. At the end of the week, we will examine your nutrition by food groups.

Now that we have completed a week of recording the MyPyramid foods you have eaten, let's analyze them. The procedure is similar to the one you have used before. The recording form is shown below. For each day, check off a box for each time you ate a serving of food from that food group. Record the miscellaneous or "other" group under the headings of fat, sugar, and alcohol by checking off the boxes.

With this information in front of you, you can tell which groups did best and which did worst. Equally important, you can get an idea of the number of times you ate something you recorded in the miscellaneous or "other" group. Now you are ready to begin to control the foods in the latter group.

Bray Plan Monitor **ANALYSIS OF FOOD GROUPS**																
Number of Times a Food Is Eaten																
	1	2	3	4	5	6	7	8	9	10	11	12	13	14	Add'l	Total
Bread and Grain																
Fruit and Vegetables																
Milk and Cheese																
Meat-Fish and Poultry																
Fat																
Sugar																
Alcohol																

Figure 2. Bray Plan Analysis of Food Groups Form. With this form, you can check off the number of times a given group of foods were eaten. An example from one of my patients is shown below.

Bray Plan Monitor **ANALYSIS OF FOOD GROUPS**																
Number of Times a Food Is Eaten																
	1	2	3	4	5	6	7	8	9	10	11	12	13	14	Add'l	Total
Bread and Grain	■	■	■	■	■	■	■									7
Fruit and Vegetables	■	■	■	■	■	■	■	■	■	■	■	■	■	■	+ 6	20
Milk and Cheese	■	■	■	■	■											5
Meat-Fish and Poultry	■	■	■	■	■	■	■	■	■	■	■	■	■	■	+ 3	17
Fat																
Sugar																
Alcohol																

Figure 3. This figure shows how one of my patients filled in this form.

Calories and Energy Density

Now let's examine the relationship between calories and the so-called "energy density" of foods. In the Nutrition Chapter (Chapter 4), I showed you that most of the energy we get comes from the fat, carbohydrate, and protein in your foods, and if you drink alcoholic beverages, some comes from the alcohol. In the adjacent Figure 4, I introduce the idea of energy density. Water on the left side has no energy, and fat, on the right side, is the most "energy-dense" food, having 9 calories per gram. All other foods fall in between. It is obvious the best way to lower the energy density of the foods you eat is to remove the fat or add water. These are the techniques food manufacturers use to lower energy density.

Energy Density

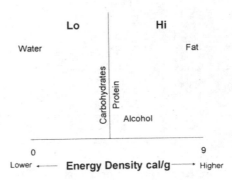

Figure 4. A diagram of energy density. Energy density expresses the number of calories a food has in relation to its weight (grams). Water has no calories and is at the left. Protein and carbohydrate are similar at 4 calories per gram and are near the middle. Alcohol has about 7 calories per gram. Anchoring the right side is fat, which is highest in energy density at 9 calories per gram.

When you count calories, you include calories from fat, carbohydrate, protein, and beverages. When you count fat grams, which are at the far right of this figure, you focus on just the fat.

For the rest of this chapter, we will focus on the use of a Hi-Lo Calorie Food Chart that will help you evaluate the relative amounts of calories or energy density. It can be used in shopping and to help control calories and select foods you choose to eat when you eat away from home. It is an easy way to help you select lower-calorie foods within each food group.

The idea is simple: Foods are divided into whether they are higher or lower in energy within each of the food groups in MyPyramid. If you select more of the low-energy foods from each group, you will get fewer calories, whether fat protein or carbohydrate calories. This chart divides foods into higher- and lower-calorie food categories according to MyPyramid Food Groups.

Food Group Servings	Relative Caloric Value				Calories used to split group
Vegetables	**Low**		**High**		50 kcal/100 g
	Asparagus	Greens	Lima beans	Potatoes	
	Beets	Lettuce	Peas	Sweet potatoes	
	Broccoli	Mushrooms			
	Cabbage	Pickles (Dill or Sour)			
	Celery	Summer squash			
	Chard/Spinach	Tomatoes			
	Cucumber	Turnips			
	Green beans	Winter squash			
Fruits	**Low**		**High**		50/kcal/100 g
	Apple	Gooseberries	Apple Juice	Mango	
	Apricots	Grapefruit	Bananas	Pears	
	Cantaloupe	Orange	Cherries	Pineapple	
	Berries	Papayas	Grape juice	Plums	
	Boysenberries	Peaches	Grapes	Prunes	
	Cranberries	Strawberries	Guava	Raspberries	
	Lemon	Watermelon			
Bread and Cereal	**Low**		**High**		75 kcal/100 g
	Bread (Choose whole grain)		Biscuits	Cookies	
	Melba toast		Muffins	Pie	
	Dry non-sugared cereals		Rolls	Pasta (macaroni)	
	Cooked plain cereal				
	Some saltine crackers		Corn	Tortillas	
			bread		
			Crackers	Doughnuts	
Milk	**Low**		**High**		60 kcal/100g
	Skim milk		Cottage Cheese		
	Low-fat milk		Whole milk		
	Buttermilk		Ice cream		
	Yogurt (skim milk no fruit)		Evaporated milk		
			Goat milk		
			Cheese		
Meat, Fish, Poultry & Beans	**Low**		**High**		150 kcal/100 g
	Liver	Abalone	Beef	Herring	
	Chicken	Bass	Ham	Sardines	
	Shell fish	Cod	Lamb	Trout	
	Shrimp	Flounder	Pork	Tuna (in oil)	
	Crab	Pike	Bologna	Salmon	
	Clams	Halibut	Hot dogs	Whitefish	
	Oyster	Swordfish	Turkey	Egg	
	Lobster	Tuna (in water)	Veal		
	Perch	Haddock			
	Trout				

This list is divided into the food groups we described earlier (far-left side). The foods in the list are split into those with high- and those with low-caloric values.

The left-hand side of the list contains the low-calorie foods, and the right-hand side of the list contains the high-calorie foods. I have made the exact divisions on a somewhat arbitrary basis, but they can be helpful in making shopping choices.

In the fruit group, the lower-calorie items are generally the berries and cantaloupe. In the vegetable group, it is tomatoes and the chewy or leafy vegetables such as celery, broccoli, or lettuce. The high-calorie fruits and vegetables tend to include those that are soft and easy to chew, such as bananas, cherries, dried fruits, watermelons, and sweet potatoes.

In the grain group, simple pieces of bread, toast, and saltine crackers are in the low-calorie group, while those made with higher fat content, such as pastries, pies, rolls, muffins, most crackers, and biscuits are included in the high-calorie group.

On the low-calorie side in the milk group are the foods from which the butterfat has been removed, such as skim milk or low-fat yogurt.

In the meat group, the foods on the low-calorie side are poultry, liver, veal, and most fish, all of which have less fat. High-calorie meats include most of the red meats, frankfurters, processed meats, and the redder fishes.

The miscellaneous group contains fats, sugars, and alcohol. There are no low-calorie items in this group, and they often contain "bad fructose." For those wishing a more detailed explanation, the separation was done in this way:

Group 1.	Grains and cereals: The lower-calorie designation has 75 calories or less per serving. The higher-calorie serving has more than 75 calories.
Group 2.	Vegetables are divided up using a half-cup measure. The lower-calorie foods are those with less than 50 calories per half-cup, and higher-calorie ones have values above 50 calories per half-cup.
Group 3.	Fruits, like vegetables, are divided using the half-cup measure. The lower-calorie foods are those with less than 50 calories per half-cup, and higher-calorie ones have values above 50 calories per half-cup.
Group 4.	Milk group: Lower-calorie items are those with less than 100 calories per serving (skim milk). The higher-calorie foods have more than 100 calories per serving (8 oz).
Group 5.	Meat, fish, poultry, and bean group: The lower-calorie items have less than 50 calories per ounce,

and some (the shellfish) have 50 calories in 2 ounces. The higher-calorie items contain 75 calories per ounce, except for luncheon meats, duck, goose, and sweetbreads.

Group 6.   Oil, sugar, and alcohol: The oil-containing foods include butter, margarine, cooking oil, mayonnaise, and potato chips. All these have little nutritional value other than calories. This group also contains foods that contain predominantly "bad fructose" (HFCS or sugar (sucrose)), i.e., sugar-sweetened beverages, candies, pastries, cakes, etc. Finally, all alcoholic beverages are in this group. There is no high-low separation here.

Monitoring for Energy Density: The Hi-Lo Approach

Now let's see if this idea can help you with your weight. In the space below is a Bray Plan Monitor, which you can use for recording food groups and the high-low calorie nutrients you eat for the next week.

Bray Plan Monitor MONITOR FOR HI-LO FOOD GROUPS			
Day			
Food Eaten	Food Group	High	Low

Figure 3. Bray Plan Monitor for High-Calorie/Low-Calorie Food Groups, which is similar to the ones you have used before.

Keep a list of the foods you eat on the Bray Plan High-Low Monitor like the one shown here. Divide them up by food groups as outlined above, and whether they are from the high or low part of the chart. Analyze the seven days of records on the form below, which gives you a way of recording number of foods that are high or low in calories from each group you ate on each day. A sample is shown below. After seeing the breakdown, you can decide how you can change the foods you eat in order to increase the number of lower-calorie foods.

Bray Plan Monitor **ANALYSIS OF HI-LO FOOD GROUPS**																
Number of Times a Food Is Eaten																
		1	2	3	4	5	6	7	8	9	10	11	12	13	Add'l	Total
Bread and Grain	Hi																
	Lo																
Fruit and Vegetables	Hi																
	Lo																
Milk and Cheese	Hi																
	Lo																
Meat-Fish and Poultry	Hi																
	Lo																
Fat																	
Sugar																	
Alcohol																	

Figure 4. Bray Plan Analysis Form for High-Calorie and Low-Calorie Food Groups. This is the form you will use to fill in the relative calorie value of the foods you have eaten using the high and low divisions described here. Below is an example from one of my patients.

Bray Plan Monitor **ANALYSIS OF HI-LO FOOD GROUPS**																
Number of Times a Food Is Eaten																
		1	2	3	4	5	6	7	8	9	10	11	12	13	Add'l	Total
Bread and Grain	Hi																6
	Lo																12
Fruit and Vegetables	Hi																9
	Lo															+4	17
Milk and Cheese	Hi																1
	Lo																8
Meat-Fish and Poultry	Hi																11
	Lo																6
Fat																	
Sugar																	
Alcohol																	

Figure 5. This is an example of a form filled in by one of my patients.

Now you are ready to apply the ideas of energy density in the Hi-Lo Food Group system to your own shopping and eating.

CHAPTER TWELVE

Eating for Successs

The Menumax® Nutrient Density Diet

Alphabet Soup

"Bad fructose" found in table sugar (sucrose) and HFCS can be sneaky. Like fats, it can get into your body without you even noticing. In the U.S., our consumption of fat and sugar has gone up sharply and has been doing so for years. Look at Table 1, which shows the increase in sugar (sucrose) and "bad fructose." For more than two hundred years, there has been a steady increase in both. The increase has been more than five hundred-fold in these two hundred years. In the last thirty years, as the number of overweight people has increased so rapidly, the world sugar (sucrose) production has risen nearly two fold.

Table 1. Sugar (sucrose) production in millions of tons per year for each of the years listed. The "bad fructose" represents the half of the sugar (sucrose) molecule that is fructose.

Year	Sugar (sucrose Production)	"Bad Fructose"
1800	0.25	0.125
1850	1.5	0.75
1880	3.8	1.9
1890	5.2	2.6
1900	11.0	5.5
1950	35.0	17.5
1970	70.0	35.0
1990	110.0	55.0
2000	128.0	64.0

Source: Yudkin 1986[1]; www. illovosugar.com/sordofsugar[2]

As sugar production increases, so does our weight. These two trends may well be related. Desserts, fried foods, cheeseburgers, and many other dishes we have learned to love are high in fat and "bad fructose" from either sugar (sucrose) or HFCS. But the fats and "bad fructose" we eat often have no other nutrients with them. They are nutrient-poor. This contrasts with fruits, which have "good fructose" but also contain vitamins and minerals and are naturally nutrient-rich. The same goes for fish, vegetables, and lean meats. In general, when there is less fat and less "bad fructose" (sugar (sucrose) or HFCS) in a food, then there will be greater amounts of other nutrients we need for good health. The idea of comparing nutrient content to fat and sugar content or to the total amount of energy is known as "nutrient density." I will use this idea in this chapter to give you my way of planning nutritious and nutrient-dense, or naturally nutrient-rich, meals.

As we have already discussed, to manage your weight, you need to eat less energy in the form of fat, protein, and carbohydrate than you burn up. But there is an important difference in the amount of energy contained in an equal amount of fat versus protein or carbohydrate. Fat has more than twice as much energy (9 calories per gram) as protein or carbohydrate (4 calories per gram), and it is often associated with less overall nutrition. When you are gaining weight, fat provides nearly three times as much energy. This means that eating fat is the quickest and most efficient way to gain weight.

The typical American receives 34–37% of his or her daily calories from fat. Women participating in a study in which they ate diets containing an average of only 21% fat lost nearly seven pounds without even trying.[3] You can, too. The less fat you eat, the more you lose. At the same time, you will increase the nutrient density of your diet and give your body more of the vitamins and minerals it needs.

The first step is to learn what kinds of foods have fat. We did this earlier by counting fat grams (Chapter 9). Fruits and vegetables, as a rule, have little or no fat. That is one reason why you don't see many obese vegetarians. A diet high in fresh fruits and vegetables is also believed to reduce the risk of heart disease,[4] to lower blood pressure,[5] and to prevent cancer.[6] It seems your mother was right after all: Eat your fruits and vegetables.

Menumax Nutrient and Energy Density Plan

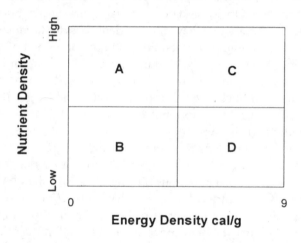

Figure 1. Diagram showing energy density and nutrient density. The letters A, B, C, and D refer to the relative nutrient and energy density values used for scoring foods in the MENU MAX nutrient density diet.

The idea of nutrient density or how many of the good vitamins and minerals are in food provides and its relation to energy density (Chapter 11) is presented graphically here. Energy density, which ranges from 0 (water) to 9 cal/gram for fat, is shown across the bottom. On the side is "nutrient" density ranging from none in the case of water (water is a nutrient but should have nothing else in it) to the fruits, vegetables, milk, and meat/poultry/eggs that occur naturally and provide nutrient rich sources of foods.

To compare the nutritional values of various foods more clearly, I have ranked items within each food group by their nutrient density. To do this, I picked the familiar A, B, C, and D grading system we use in schools. Foods with less energy density and more nutrient density earn an obvious "A." Foods with lots of energy, but very few if any nutrients, are again an obvious "D." Good examples of this are the soft drinks and most fruit drinks, which have "bad fructose" (HFCS or sugar (sucrose)), and high-fat foods. When you weigh food, as we did in the calorie-counting section, the number of calories relates to the energy content of the food. Foods with more fat or "bad fructose" (HFCS or sugar (sucrose)) per unit of weight have more energy (calories) and often less nutrition. Carbohydrate and protein also contribute to the amount of energy per unit weight of food.

In addition to the fat, carbohydrate, and protein in foods, there are other important components to consider, such as vitamins and minerals. The more vitamins and minerals per unit of the food, the better its overall nutrient density. These vitamins and minerals are often present in high-protein, high-fiber foods and in fresh fruits and vegetables. There you have the concept of nutrient density. Obviously, such high-fat items as lard, butter, vegetable shortening, and margarine have few nutrients besides fat unless added in processing, such as vitamin D or vitamin E. On the other end of the spectrum, fresh fruits, vegetables, whole grains, skim milk, fish, and skinless chicken have a very high nutrient density. In other words, there's a lot of bang for your nutrition buck in each of these foods. The longer the bar in figures in the appendix are, the more nutritious the food. You get more for your nutritional dollar from these foods.

To identify the nutrient density of foods quickly, we rated foods with the highest nutrient density as "A" and those with the lowest nutrient density as "D." "B"-rated foods are also nutritious but slightly less so than "A"s. "C"-rated foods are not so nutritious but better than "D"s. On top of an A-D rating system, we also provide insight into the fat content by using a color scale. An "A"-rated food is the big winner in our system. On the other hand, a "D"-rated food flunks our test. Table 2 is a short list of the nutrient density of foods using the A, B, C, and D system.

The Menumax® Meal Planner uses this system to help you develop your own menus, control your calories, reduce fat, and obtain good nutrition, all at the same time.

You already know the amount of nutrition in a food and its caloric value are not necessarily related. We used this concept earlier in developing the High-Low Food Guide for shopping and choosing foods.

You are also familiar with the idea of calories in foods and the use MyPyramid as a way of dividing foods into groups to improve selecting a variety of foods. The Menumax® Meal Planning System uses the same ideas but in a different way.

Menumax Food Planner
Table 2. The short version of the Menumax® Food Guide with Foods Rated A through D

BREADS AND CEREALS

A	B	C	D
Bran Flakes	Brown Bread,	Biscuits	Bread, French
Bread,	Boston,	Bread, Raisin	Toast
Cracked Wheat, Rye	Bread, French,	Crackers, soda	Cakes, all types
and Whole Wheat	Vienna, and White	Rice, White	Cookies, all types
Cornflakes	Cornbread	Crackers, Whole	
Noodles	Crackers, Saltines	Wheat	
Oatmeal	Farina, Enriched	Pretzels	
Rolls, Whole	Macaroni	Rice, Instant	
Spaghetti	Muffins,	Rolls, Danish,	
		Enriched Flour or	
		Rolled Oats	
		Pancakes	
		Pizza with cheese	
		Rice, Brown	
		Rolls, Hard Roll	

FRUITS

A	B	C	D
Boysenberries	Apricots, Raw	Bananas, Raw	Apple, Fresh
Gooseberries	Cherries, Sour	Blackberries	Apple Juice
Rhubarb	Grapefruit	Blueberries	Applesauce
Tomato Juice	Melon,	Cherries, Sweet	Coconut
Cantaloupe	Cranberries	Figs, Raw	Grape Juice
Oranges, Raw	Currants, Black	Grapes	Drink
Orange Juice,	Grapefruit	Grape Juice (100%)	("bad" Fructose)
Fresh or Frozen	Juice (100%)	Peaches, packed	
Papayas	Lemons	in syrup	
Peaches,	Loganberries		
Peaches, Canned	Melon, Muskmelon		
in water	and Honeydew		
Persimmons	Plums, raw		
Pineapple, Fresh	black		
Canned in water			
Strawberry			

Tangerines
Watermelon

VEGETABLES

A	B	C	D
Asparagus	Beans, yellow	Beans, Lima	Bean, white
Broccoli	Brussels sprouts	Beets, Red,	Corn, on or
Chard, Swiss	Cauliflower	Cooked	off the cob
Beans, green	Celery	Cabbage	Lentils
Kale	Cucumbers	Carrots	Pickles, sweet
Lettuce,	Peppers, green	Coleslaw	Potatoes, French
Mustard greens	or chili	Kohlrabi	fried
Okra, Pickles, dill	Onions		scalloped
Parsley, Pumpkin, raw	Peas, green		with cheese
Spinach	Pickles, sour		Mashed from
	Potatoes, raw		flakes
	baked, or boiled		
	Pumpkin, canned		
	Rutabagas		
	Squash, winter		
	acorn		
	butternut		
	Sweet potatoes		
	Turnips		

MEAT, FISH, POULTRY AND BEANS

A	B	C	D
Meat			
Beef, arm	Beef, round	Bacon, Canadian	Bacon, cured
Flank steak	dried & cooked	Beef, rib	Beef,
Hamburger,	Lamb, leg	Pork	Chuck ribs
Lean liver, calf	Fresh Picnic	Porterhouse	T-Bone steak
Pork,	Pork,	Spareribs	steak
Fresh Ham	Fresh loin	Lunch meat	Club steak
Lean only	Rib (lean)	Meat loaf	Rib eye
Sausage		Sausage	Corned beef hash
Liverwurst		Polish style	Lamb, loin rib
Veal, Chuck		Salami	Sausage, blood
			Bologna
			Frankfurters, pork

A	B	C	D

Fish

A	B	C	D
Abalone	Pompano	Lobster newburg	Tuna in oil
Clams, raw meat	Salmon, fresh	Oysters	
Crab, steamed	Shad	(high sodium)	
Halibut	Haddock, fried		
Mussels, meat	Mackerel		
Whitefish only	Smelt		
Lobster	Ocean perch		
Pollack	Bluefish		
Rockfish	Tuna in water		
Snail			
Sturgeon			
Sword fish			
Cod, (raw, fresh)			
Flounder			
Scallops			

Poultry

A	B	C	D
Chicken,	Chicken,	Chicken a la King	
Light meat	Dark meat		
Breast	Drumstick		
Liver			
Eggs, any style			
Turkey, roasted			
light or dark meat			

MILK AND CHEESE

A	B	C	D
Skim milk	Milk ½%,	Milk, whole	Butter Milk
	1%, or 2%	Margarine	Cheese, blue or
	Cheese, cottage	Cheese,	roquefort,
	low fat milk	Cottage,	camembert, cream
	Yogurt,	creamed,	Cream, whipping
	low fat milk	Cheddar,	Cream, Half & half
		American	Ice cream,
		Processed,	regular or rich
		American	
		Yogurt,	
		whole milk	
		Ice milk	

1. Food Groups

All foods in the Menumax® system have been divided up into five food groups and the miscellaneous group. The calorie values for each of the groups that were used to divide them into higher-calorie or lower-calorie groups are listed in Table 2.

Table 3. Calorie values for each of the food groups used in the Menumax® system.

Food Group	Calories per Serving
Bread and Cereal	75
Fruits	50
Vegetables	50
Meat/Fish and Poultry	75
Milk and Cheese	100
Miscellaneous (Other)	50

2. Rating Foods

In addition to the calorie values listed in Table 2, the food items in the Menumax® system have been rated by a computer program to give me an indication of their nutritional value. I chose a familiar grading system like that used in schools: A for best choice, B for good choice, C for fair choice, and D for poor choice. A list of the grades for some of the common foods is shown in Table 2. This table is a shortened list of all of the foods in the figures above. It can be used for shopping and eating out.

3. Free Foods

In addition to these lists of foods, there are several foods you can eat in essentially unlimited amounts, as well as seasonings that can make foods taste better. These are the "free foods" shown in Table 12-2.

Table 3. Free Foods You May Add to Your Diet As Desired

Coffee, without sugar, cream, or milk
Tea, without sugar, cream, or milk
Clear broth
Bouillon (has high salt content)
Consommé
Lemon
Gelatin (unsweetened)
Pepper
Spices and seasonings
Vinegar

Vegetables (when eaten raw):
Asparagus
Broccoli
Cabbage
Cauliflower
Celery
Cucumber
Greens (beet, chard, dandelion, kale)
Lettuce
Mushrooms
Peppers
Radishes
Sauerkraut
Spinach
Watercress

The following general guidelines will also help you shop and prepare foods from which you can get the most nutrition with the least calories.

4. **Tips for Food Preparation**
   * Shop from a prepared list.
   * Shop after you have eaten.
   * Buy only the foods you list.
   * Buy lean cuts of meat. When layers of fat are visible, remove them before cooking.
   * Boil, broil, or bake foods (do not fry or sauté).
   * Substitute fresh fruits and fruits canned in water for fruits packed in sugar or syrup—a source of "bad fructose."
   * Use imitation or low-fat mayonnaise rather than real mayonnaise.
   * When cooking oil is needed, use canola (or similar) oil rather than other shortenings, butter, or lard.
   * When selecting cheese, choose from those made with partially skimmed milk. These include Jarlsberg, Esrom, Tilsit, Samsoe, Danbo, Loraine Cheddar, and Valembert, as well as 2% milk versions of cheddar, jack, and Swiss.
   * In cooking, make use of stock prepared from meat or chicken.
   * Substitute tangy spices, bay leaf, caraway seed, chives, and cloves for salt in cooking.
   * As a before-dinner beverage, try lemon juice or lime juice with a twist of lemon on ice with soda water or a dash of white wine rather than beverages with "bad fructose."

5. Tips for Shopping

- Buy 100% fruit juices preferably NOT made from concentrate. Avoid fruit drinks, which are a source of "bad fructose" (HFCS is a dead giveaway—if present, I walk away) water, and flavorings with vitamins added.
- Steam or cook vegetables only until they are crisp and tender to save vitamins and minerals. Undercook rather than overcook.
- Buy skim milk rather than whole milk. Use evaporated skim milk instead of cream.
- Add your own fresh fruit to low-fat yogurt to give a variety of flavors.
- Use margarine instead of butter. Choose a high-quality margarine, which may have less trans-fatty acids. Even such giants as McDonald's and KFC are eliminating trans-fats from the foods they fry.
- Choose ice milk, which is lower in calories than ice cream.
- Use the Nutrition Facts labels of foods to get the most nutrition from your foods.
- Check newspaper ads for foods on sale.

Now that you have some idea of how to shop for foods using the food lists and nutritional ratings, you can begin planning individual meals that will maximize the nutrition in your menu while pleasing your tastebuds. This is the idea behind the Menumax® system.

Each day there are a minimum number of servings from each food group to give you all the nutrition you need, except calories. When your total calorie intake is below 1,200 calories per day, it is difficult, if not impossible, to get all the vitamins and minerals you need from the food alone. For this reason, I recommend taking supplemental vitamins and minerals. Any vitamin with 100% of the Recommended Daily Intake (RDI)[7] for vitamins and minerals will do.

Table 4 below contains the number of servings from each food group that are needed to provide the number of calories listed on the left.

Table 4. Servings needed from each food group to get the calorie level listed

Calorie Level	Bread/ Cereal	Fruits	Vegetables	Meat/ Fish/Poultry	Milk/ Cheese
Number of Servings at each calorie level					
800	2	2	2	5	1
1,000	2½	3	3	5	1½
1,200	3	4	3	6	2
1,500	4	4	4	7	3
1,800	5	5	5	8	3½

A serving of the bread group = 75 cal; a serving of fruit, 50 cal; a serving of vegetables, 50 cal; a serving of meat/fish or poultry, 75 cal; and a serving of milk, 100 cal.

Now let me show you how to plan your own menus. First, select the desired number of calories you want to eat. In general, a 1,200-calorie diet for women and a 1,500-calorie diet for men are good choices. For Table 5, I have selected a 1,200-calorie diet. You may wish to start at a higher or lower level. Remember that to lose 1 pound per week, you should select a calorie level that is 500 calories per day below your estimated energy need. The total number of servings is 3 for bread/cereal, 4 of fruits, 3 of vegetables, 6 of meat/fish/poultry, and 2 from the milk/cheese group.

Table 5. Sample 1200-Calorie Menumax® Food Servings

Servings Per Day	Bread/ Cereal	Fruits	Vegetables	Meat/ Fish/Poultry	Milk/ Cheese
	3	4	3	6	2
Distribution of the servings by meal					
Breakfast	1	1			1
Snack		½			
Lunch	1		1	1	
Snack		½			
Dinner	1	1	2	4	1
Snack		1			

Next, under the food groups, list the number of servings shown in Table 4 needed to get this number of calories. Finally, select foods you like from the lists. You are better off choosing more foods with the "A" and "B" ratings than foods with "C" and "D" ratings.

Substitutions can be made between the various groups, particularly when the total number of calories is above 1,200 per day. You may wish to rearrange the times at which you eat the various servings from a particular food group. This is perfectly all right.

With this guide in front of you, you are ready to use the Menumax® Meal Planner to plan other menus and select the appropriate portion sizes.

On the next page is space for you to plan the first week's menu from the Menumax® Meal Planner guide. When the entire week is ready, you will have learned about the ways in which substitutions can be made and how to select more foods with high nutritional value. From the preceding lists, you can see how easy it is to plan other meals.

George A. Bray, MD

MENUMAX® MEAL PLANNER
1200-CALORIE DIET

	Bread/ Cereal	Fruits	Vegetables	Meat/Fish Poultry	Milk/ Cheese
Breakfast No. of servings	1	1			1
Foods Selected	1 oz. dry cereal	Strawberries (1 cup)			½ cup skim milk
Snack No. of servings					
Foods Selected					
Lunch No. of servings	2	1	1	2	
Foods Selected	2 slices Whole Wheat Bread	Apple	2 Carrots	Tuna (water packed)	
Snack No. of servings					
Food Selected					
Dinner No. of servings		1	2	4	
Foods Selected		Plum	Broccoli (1 cup)	Lean hamburger (1 patty 4" diameter)	milk in coffee
Snack No. of servings		1			1
Food Selected		Banana			½ cup skim milk

You are now ready to monitor your nutritional choices. For the next week, keep track of what you actually eat, the quantity of food you eat, and whether it is an "A," "B," "C," "D," or "M" (miscellaneous) food. The form we want you to use is shown below.

MENUMAX® MEAL PLANNER

Calorie Level

	Bread/ Cereal	Fruits	Vegetables	Meat/Fish Poultry	Milk/ Cheese
Breakfast No. of servings					
Foods Selected					
Snack No. of servings					
Foods Selected					
Lunch No. of servings					
Foods Selected					
Snack No. of servings					
Food Selected					
Dinner No. of servings					
Foods Selected					
Snack No. of servings					

Now that you have completed the exercise, here is the summary table for several calorie levels.

Table 6. Serving sizes from various food groups for different calorie levels

Food Group	Calorie Level							
	1000		1,200		1,500		1,800	
	# Serv	Cal	# Serv	Cal	# Serv	Cal	# Serv	Cal
Bread	2½	170	3	210	4	280	5	350
Fruits	3	150	4	200	4	200	5	250
Vegetables	3	150	3	150	4	200	5	250
Meat/Fish/Poultry	5	450	6	450	7	525	8	600
Milk/Cheese	1½	200	2	200	3	300	3½	350

Now let's see how well it works for you. The next form is to prepare your own Menumax® diet to carry with you. It is a 3×5-inch card with the good groups and the meals on it. List the number of servings in the appropriate box for the day meal and food group. On the next form, monitor what you ate from that menu plan according to whether it was in the A, B, C, or D group of foods.

Bray Plan Monitor **PLANNER FOR MENUMAX DIET**						
Day	Number of Servings Consumed					
Meal	Vegetables	Fruits	Bread/ Grain	Milk/ Yogurt/ Cheese	Meat/ Fish/Beans Poultry	Other
Breakfast						
Snack						
Lunch						
Snack						
Dinner						
Snack						

This form is to record the types of foods you ate in each serving size. Following a week of recording your intake of A, B, C, and D foods, we will mark up an analysis form to see how you have done.

Bray Plan Monitor
MONITOR FOR RATING FOODS USING THE A, B, C, D SYSTEM

Day

Food Eaten	Veg	Fruit	Bread Grain	Milk Yogurt Cheese	Meat Fish Poultry Beans	Other

Bray Plan Monitor
ANALYSIS FOR RATING FOODS USING THE A, B, C, D SYSTEM

Day								Number of Servings							
Food Group	Rating	1	2	3	4	5	6	7	8	9	10	11	12	Add'l	Total
Vegetables	A & B														
	C & D														
Fruits	A & B														
	C & D														
Bread/Grain	A & B														
	C & D														
Milk/Yogurt/ Cheese	A & B														
	C & D														
Meat/Fish	A & B														
	C & D														
Other																

With this food monitor, you will be making the same sort of recordings you used with several other parts of this book. Remember to write down everything you eat on your Bray Plan Monitor as soon after you have eaten it as possible. Don't fill in the monitor from memory; do it on the spot. Be honest with yourself because you have only yourself to help, and the fat is yours to lose or keep. You can add the A, B, C, or D values if you have correctly listed the foods.

Now that you have recorded your food choices and their nutritional values for a week, you are ready to see for yourself how much you have learned about nutrition. Lay the monitors for the past week out on the table in front of you. For each day, record from left to right, under each of the food groupings, the number of servings that were "A" or "B" on the top half and the ones that were "C" and "D" on the lower half. When you have recorded all of the food items eaten, you can immediately see whether you were maximizing your menu choices. Since peoples' food choices will vary from time to time, there are no forbidden foods; however, your nutrition will be improved if more of the choices you make are from the "A" and "B" lists than from the "C" and "D" lists.

At the end of this chapter are the major food groups divided using the energy density (calories per gram and nutrient density (A, B, C, D) system) I have developed in this chapter. The longer the bar, the larger the amount you need to eat to get the calories listed at the bottom. The evaluation I have assigned to the food is listed on the left as A, B, C, and D.

The Menumax® Meal Planning System
Food Groups

Group Number	Food Items	Calories per Serving
1	Bread and Cereals	75
2	Fruits	50
3	Vegetables	50
4	Meat, Fish, Poultry	75
5	Milk and Cheese	100
6	Miscellaneous (fat sugar, and alcohol)	50

All foods in the Menumax® system have been divided up into six food groups as used in MyPyramid. These six food groups are:

Menumax® 1000-Calorie Diet

(Numbers in parentheses identify a recipe listed after the weekly menus.)

Menumax® Meals for Week 1

Monday

Breakfast
1 poached egg
1 slice cracked wheat toast
½ of a 4" grapefruit
4 oz skim milk
Coffee or tea with artificial sweetener

Lunch
Vegetable soup (Campbell's), 7 oz
½ Tuna Salad Sandwich on cracked wheat bread with lettuce (26)
2 plums (2" diameter)
4 oz skim milk
No-calorie beverage or iced tea

Dinner
Roast beef (very lean), 3 oz
Parslied boiled potato, 1 medium
Asparagus a la Lemon (1) ½ cup
4 oz skim milk
Strawberry Fruited Jell-O Mold (23)
No-calorie beverage or iced tea

Calories: 990
Protein: 55 grams

Tuesday

Breakfast
4 oz fresh orange juice
¾ cup corn flakes with ½ cup strawberries
4 oz skim milk
Coffee or tea with artificial sweetener

Lunch
Gumbo Creole Soup (Heinz) 7 oz

Chef Salad (5) with 2 tbsp Creamy Lo-Cal Dressing (7)
Saltines; 2
Peach, fresh, 2½" diameter
4 oz skim milk
No-calorie beverage or iced tea

Dinner
Roast chicken (white meat, no skin) 2½ oz
Fluffy brown rice, ½ cup
Seasoned broccoli with mushrooms
4 oz skim milk
Raspberries, fresh, ½ cup
Coffee or tea with artificial sweetener

Calories: 990
Protein: 55 grams

Wednesday

Breakfast
Cantaloupe, ¼ of 5" diameter
Oatmeal, ½ cup
4 oz skim milk
Coffee or tea with artificial sweetener

Lunch
Old Fashioned Hamburger Patty (16)
Zucchini, steamed, ½ cup
Carrots, steamed, ½ cup
4 oz skim milk
Pear, ¾ of a large fruit
No-calorie beverage or iced tea

Dinner
Baked fresh ham, 1 slice, 4¼" × 4" × 1/8"
Black-eyed peas, ¼ cup
Collard greens, ½ cup
Cornbread, 2" square
Tapioca pudding, ½ cup
No-calorie beverage or iced tea

Calories: 990
Protein: 59 grams

Thursday

Breakfast
Tomato-Mushroom (25) or Onion-Mushroom Omelette (17) made with 1 egg
Whole wheat toast, 1 slice
4 oz grapefruit juice
Coffee or tea with artificial sweetener

Lunch
Tomato soup (made with water), 7 oz
Grilled cheese sandwich: 1 slice whole wheat bread and ½ slice cheese
Honeydew melon, 2" wedge
4 oz skim milk
No-calorie beverage or iced tea

Dinner
Veal Parmesan, 2½ oz (27)
Parslied noodles
Spinach Salad (22) with 2 tbsp Dilly Dressing (9)
Apricots, 3 medium
4 oz skim milk
Coffee or tea with artificial sweetener

Calories: 1005
Protein: 42 grams

Friday

Breakfast
Orange juice, fresh, 4 oz
Bran flakes, ¾ cup with banana, ½ medium, sliced
4 oz skim milk
Coffee or tea with artificial sweetener

Lunch
Cottage cheese (low fat), 6 level tbsp
Strawberries, fresh, ½ cup
Pear halves, water-packed, 2
Tangerine, 2½" diameter, diced
Bed of lettuce
Whole wheat roll, 1
Margarine, 1 tsp

Vanilla wafers, 3
Iced tea or no-calorie beverage

Dinner
Broiled halibut, 3 oz
Parslied brown rice, ½ cup
Seasoned green beans, ½ cup
Sherbet, ½ cup
4 oz skim milk

Calories: 1000
Protein: 50 grams

Saturday

Breakfast
Grapefruit, ½ of 4" diameter
Farina, ½ cup
4 oz skim milk
Coffee or tea with artificial sweetener

Lunch
Chicken-Rice Soup (Heinz), 7 oz
Liverwurst sandwich: 1 slice rye bread; 1 slice (1 oz) liverwurst; mustard
Watermelon, ½ slice, ¾" thick
4 oz skim milk
Iced tea
Dinner
Fiesta Taco (11)
Triple Bean Salad (25)
Tangerine, 2½" diameter
4 oz skim milk

Calories: 980
Protein: 48 grams

Sunday

Breakfast
Tomato juice, 8 oz
Scrambled egg, 1
Whole wheat toast, 1 slice
4 oz skim milk

Lunch
Swiss cheese sandwich: 1 slice rye bread; ½ oz Swiss cheese; mustard; lettuce
Cabbage salad with boiled dressing
Plum, 1, 2" diameter
4 oz skim milk

Dinner
Roast turkey, 3 oz
Seasoned boiled potato, 1 medium
Winter squash, mashed, ½ cup
Tossed green salad, ½ cup with 2 tbsp Dilly Dressing (9)
Pound cake, 1 slice, 2¾" × 3" × 5/8"
4 oz skim milk
Coffee or tea with artificial sweetener

Calories: 1000
Protein: 54 grams

Menumax® Meals for Week 2

Monday

Breakfast
Fresh orange juice, 4 oz
Buckwheat pancake, ¼" diameter
Maple syrup, 2 tbsp
4 oz skim milk
Coffee or tea with artificial sweetener

Lunch
Cottage cheese, low fat, ½ cup
Tuna Salad (26), ½ cup on lettuce bed
Carrot sticks, 2
Grapes, ½ cup
Iced tea or no-calorie beverage

Dinner
Oriental Chicken and Broccoli (18)
Fluffy brown rice, ½ cup
Pineapple slices, water packed, 2
4 oz skim milk
Coffee or tea with artificial sweetener
Calories: 1000
Protein: 47 grams

Tuesday

Breakfast
Grapefruit, ½ of a 4" diameter
Corn flakes, ¾ cup
Peach, fresh, sliced (3-3/8" diameter)
4 oz skim milk
Coffee or tea with artificial sweetener

Lunch
Consommé, 7 oz
Ham sandwich: 1 slice rye bread; 1 oz boiled ham; mustard; lettuce
Chilled asparagus spears, ½ cup, with 2 tbsp Dilly Dressing (9)
Cantaloupe, ¼ of 5" diameter
4 oz skim milk
Dinner

Meatloaf (14), 2 oz, with 1 tbsp catsup
Baked potato (small) with chives and 1 tbsp sour cream
Seasoned beets, ½ cup
Spinach Salad (22), ½ cup, with 2 tbsp creamy lo-cal dressing
Apricots, ½ cup, fresh or water packed
4 oz skim milk
Coffee or tea with artificial sweetener

Calories: 995
Protein: 43 grams

Wednesday

Breakfast
Tomato juice, 8 oz
Oatmeal, ½ cup
4 oz skim milk
Coffee or tea with artificial sweetener

Lunch
Chicken Noodle Soup (Campbell's), 7 oz
Peanut butter and jelly sandwich: 1 slice whole wheat bread; 1 tbsp peanut butter; 1 tsp jelly
Celery and carrot sticks, 2 each
Orange, fresh, 1, 3–3/8" diameter
4 oz skim milk

Dinner
Mediterranean Pork Chop (15), 1
Mashed potato (with milk, margarine), ½ cup
Strawberries, fresh, 1 cup
4 oz skim milk
Coffee or tea with artificial sweetener

Calorie: 995
Protein: 48 grams

Thursday

Breakfast
Tomato-Mushroom (25) or Onion-Mushroom Omelette (17) made with 1 egg
Whole wheat toast, 1 slice

4 oz grapefruit juice
Coffee or tea with artificial sweetener

Lunch
Tomato soup (made with water), 7 oz
Grilled cheese sandwich: 1 slice whole wheat bread and ½ slice cheese
Honeydew melon, 2" wedge
4 oz skim milk
No-calorie beverage or iced tea

Dinner
Veal Parmesan, 2½ oz (27)
Parslied noodles
Spinach Salad (22) with 2 tbsp Dilly Dressing (9)
Apricots, 3 medium
4 oz skim milk
Coffee or tea with artificial sweetener

Calories: 1005
Protein: 42 grams

Friday

Breakfast
Pineapple juice, 4 oz
Farina, ½ cup
4 oz skim milk
Coffee or tea with artificial sweetener

Lunch
Consommé, 7 oz
Chef salad (5) with 2 tbsp Creamy Lo-Cal Dressing (7)
Bran muffin, 1 average
Peach, fresh, 2½" diameter
4 oz skim milk
No-calorie beverage or iced tea

Dinner
Baked Orange Halibut (2), 3 oz
Parslied brown rice, ½ cup
Brussels sprouts, ½ cup
4 oz skim milk
Vanilla wafers, 3

Coffee or tea with artificial sweetener

Calories: 1000
Protein: 55 grams

Saturday

Breakfast
Tomato juice, 8 oz
Corn flakes, ¾ cup with ½ cup blueberries
4 oz skim milk
Coffee or tea with artificial sweetener

Lunch
Vegetable Soup (Campbell's), 7 oz
Tuna Salad Sandwich (26), ½, on whole wheat bread
Apple, 2½" diameter
4 oz skim milk

Dinner
Baked calf liver and onions, 3 oz
Parslied noodles, ½ cup
Seasoned carrots, ½ cup
Tossed salad, ½ cup, with 2 tbsp Creamy Lo-Cal Dressing (7)
Watermelon, ½ slice, ¾" thick
4 oz skim milk
Coffee or tea with artificial sweetener

Calories: 960
Protein: 48 grams

Sunday

Breakfast
Grapefruit, ½ of 4" diameter
Soft cooked egg on whole wheat toast
4 oz skim milk
Coffee or tea with artificial sweetener

Lunch
Cottage cheese, low fat, 6 tbsp
Cantaloupe, ¼ of 5" diameter, sliced
Plum, 1 sliced

Angel food cake, 1/10 of cake
Iced tea or no-calorie beverage

Dinner
Spaghetti with Meat Sauce (21)
Green beans, ½ cup
Lettuce salad, ½ cup, with Dilly Dressing (9)
French bread, 1 slice
Margarine, ½ tsp
Tangerine, 2½"
4 oz skim milk
Coffee or tea with artificial sweetener

Calories: 990
Protein: 46 grams

Menumax® Meals for Week 3

Monday

Breakfast
Pineapple, sliced, 2 large (fresh or water packed)
Oatmeal, ½ cup
4 oz skim milk
Coffee or tea with artificial sweetener

Lunch
Tomato soup, 7 oz
Liverwurst sandwich: 1 slice rye bread; 1 slice (1 oz) liverwurst; mustard; lettuce
Lime fruit dessert
4 oz skim milk

Dinner
Bueno Tostada (4)
Honeydew melon, 2" slice
8 oz skim milk
Coffee or tea with artificial sweetener

Calories: 1000
Protein: 45 grams

Tuesday

Breakfast
Orange juice, fresh, 4 oz
Tomato-Mushroom (24) or Onion-Mushroom Omelette (17), 1 egg
Whole wheat English muffin, ½
4 oz skim milk
Coffee or tea with artificial sweetener

Lunch
Beef noodle soup, 7 oz
Swiss cheese sandwich: 1 slice rye bread; ½ oz Swiss cheese; mustard; lettuce
Apple, 2½" diameter
4 oz skim milk

Dinner
Southern Stewed Chicken (20), 3 oz vegetables
Fluffy brown rice
Pear, 1 large
4 oz skim milk
Coffee or tea with artificial sweetener

Calories: 970
Protein: 52 grams

Wednesday

Breakfast
Tomato juice, 8 oz
Puffed rice, 1 cup with ½ cup banana slices
4 oz skim milk
Coffee or tea with artificial sweetener

Lunch
Old Fashioned Hamburger Patty (16)
Asparagus, ½ cup
Seasoned carrots, ½ cup
Cinnamon applesauce (unsweetened), ½ cup
4 oz skim milk

Dinner
Baked beef tongue with mustard
Green peas with mushrooms, ½ cup
Stewed tomatoes, ½ cup
Lettuce salad, ½ cup with 1 tbsp Creamy Lo-Cal Dressing
Peach shortcake: 2 peach halves (water packed); biscuit, ½ medium;
Cool Whip, 1 tbsp
4 oz skim milk
Coffee or tea with artificial sweetener

Calories: 1000
Protein: 59 grams

Thursday

Breakfast
Grapefruit-orange juice, unsweetened, 4 oz
Farina, ½ cup

4 oz skim milk
Coffee or tea with artificial sweetener

Lunch
Salad plate: Tuna Salad (26), ¼ cup; cottage cheese, low fat, ¼ cup; fruit salad, ½ cup strawberries and ¼ cup diced pear; on a lettuce bed
Vanilla wafers, 3
4 oz skim milk

Dinner
Veal Parmesan (27), 2½ oz
Parslied noodles, ½ cup
Spinach salad, ½ cup with 1 tbsp Creamy Lo-Cal Dressing (7)
Apricots, ½ cup fresh or water packed
4 oz skim milk
Coffee or tea with artificial sweetener

Calories: 1000
Protein: 48 grams

Friday

Breakfast
Grapefruit, ½ of 4" diameter
Scrambled egg, 1
Bran muffin, 1 medium
4 oz skim milk
Coffee or tea with artificial sweetener

Lunch
Vegetable Soup, Campbell's, 7 oz
Chicken Salad Sandwich (6): 1 slice whole wheat bread; chicken salad, 2 oz; lettuce
Grapes, ½ cup
4 oz skim milk

Dinner
Herbed Fish Bake (12) Halibut, 3 oz
Brown rice pilaf (with parsley and mushrooms)
Steamed broccoli, ½ cup
Pineapple slice, 1 large
4 oz skim milk
Coffee or tea with artificial sweetener

Calories: 990
Protein: 60 grams

Saturday

Breakfast
Orange juice, fresh, 4 oz
Bran flakes, ¾ cup with ½ cup boysenberries
4 oz skim milk
Coffee or tea with artificial sweetener

Lunch
Gumbo Creole Soup (Heinz), 7 oz
Egg Salad (10) Sandwich: 1 slice whole wheat bread; egg salad; lettuce
Carrot and celery sticks, 2 each
Plum, 1
4 oz skim milk

Dinner
New England Boiled Dinner: Ham, fresh, baked, 3 oz; seasoned cab-
bage, ½ cup; parslied carrots, ½ cup; boiled potato, 1 medium
Sherbet, ½ cup
4 oz skim milk
Coffee or tea with artificial sweetener

Calories: 985
Protein: 44 grams

Sunday

Breakfast
Tomato juice, 8 oz
Honeydew melon, 2" slice
Oatmeal, ½ cup
4 oz skim milk
Coffee or tea with artificial sweetener

Lunch
Salad: 1½ cup mixed greens; ¼ cup flaked tuna; 2 tbsp Creamy Lo-Cal
Dressing
Saltines, 4
Strawberries, ½ cup
4 oz skim milk

Dinner
Roast beef, very lean, 3 oz
Seasoned green peas, ½ cup
Sliced tomato salad, 1 medium
Whole wheat roll, 1
Margarine, 1 tsp
Peaches, 2 halves, water packed
4 oz skim milk
Coffee or tea with artificial sweetener

Calories: 985
Protein: 49 grams

Menumax® Meals for Week 4

Monday

Breakfast
Grapefruit juice, 4 oz
Wheaties, 1 cup with ½ cup red raspberries
4 oz skim milk
Coffee or tea with artificial sweetener

Lunch
Chicken Noodle Soup (Campbell's), 7 oz
Cottage Cheese Fruit Plate: cottage cheese, low fat, 6 tbsp; apricots, sliced, fresh or water packed, ½ cup; grapes, ½ cup
Saltines, 4
Pound cake, 1 slice, 2¾" × 3" × 5/8"
4 oz skim milk

Dinner
Broiled veal cutlet, not breaded, very lean, 1 slice, 3" × 4" × ¼" with lemon and capers
Baked potato with chives, 1 small
Seasoned beets, ½ cup
4 oz skim milk
Coffee or tea with artificial sweetener

Calories: 1005
Protein: 45 grams

Tuesday

Breakfast
Orange juice, fresh, 4 oz
Poached egg, 1 on 1 slice whole wheat toast
4 oz skim milk
Coffee or tea with artificial sweetener

Lunch
Consommé, 7 oz
Chef Salad (5) with 2 tbsp Dilly Dressing (9)
Cantaloupe, ½ of 5" diameter
4 oz skim milk

Dinner
Oriental Chicken and Broccoli (18)
Fluffy brown rice, ½ cup
Pineapple, 1 large slice, fresh or water packed
4 oz skim milk
Coffer or tea with artificial sweetener

Calories: 1010
Protein: 58 grams

Wednesday

Breakfast
Grapefruit, ½ of 4" diameter
Cream of Wheat, ½ cup
4 oz skim milk
Coffee or tea with artificial sweetener

Lunch
Chicken Gumbo Soup (Campbell's), 7 oz
Grilled cheese sandwich: 1 slice whole wheat bread; ½ slice American cheese
Sliced tomato, 1 medium
Vanilla ice cream, 3 oz
4 oz skim milk

Dinner
Spaghetti with Meat Sauce (21)
Seasoned spinach, ½ cup
French bread, 1 slice
Margarine, 1 tsp
Plum, 1
4 oz skim milk
Coffee or tea with artificial sweetener

Calories: 1000
Protein: 45 grams

Thursday

Breakfast
Tomato-Mushroom (25) or Onion-Mushroom Omelette (17) made with 1 egg

Whole wheat toast, 1 slice
4 oz grapefruit juice
Coffee or tea with artificial sweetener

Lunch
Tomato soup (made with water), 7 oz
Grilled cheese sandwich: 1 slice whole wheat bread and ½ slice cheese
Honeydew melon, 2" wedge
4 oz skim milk
No-calorie beverage or iced tea

Dinner
Veal Parmesan, 2½ oz (27)
Parslied noodles
Spinach Salad (22) with 2 tbsp Dilly Dressing (9)
Apricots, 3 medium
4 oz skim milk
Coffee or tea with artificial sweetener

Calories: 1005
Protein: 42 grams

Friday

Breakfast
Orange juice, fresh, 4 oz
Buckwheat pancake, 1
Maple syrup, 2 tbsp
Soft-cooked egg
Coffee or tea with artificial sweetener

Lunch
Liverwurst sandwich: 1 slice rye bread; 1 slice (1 oz) liverwurst; mustard; lettuce
Carrot and celery sticks, 2 each
Pear, ½ large
4 oz skim milk

Dinner
Baked Orange halibut (2)
Green peas with mushrooms, ½ cup
Cabbage-carrot slaw with boiled dressing
Watermelon, ½ slice, ¾" thick

4 oz skim milk
Coffee or tea with artificial sweetener

Calories: 985
Protein: 45 grams

Saturday

Breakfast
Cantaloupe, ½ of 5" diameter
Bran flakes, ¾ cup
4 oz skim milk
Coffee or tea with artificial sweetener

Lunch
Tomato soup, 7 oz
Chicken Salad (6) on lettuce bed
Whole wheat bread, 1 slice
Margarine, ½ tsp
Boysenberries, ½ cup
4 oz skim milk

Dinner
Southern Oven-Fried Chicken (19), 3 oz
Black-eyed peas, ¼ cup
Mustard greens, ½ cup
Sherbet, ¼ cup
4 oz skim milk
Coffee or tea with artificial sweetener

Calories: 1005
Protein: 55 grams

Sunday

Breakfast
Tomato juice, 8 oz
Oatmeal, ½ cup
Nectarine, 1 large
4 oz skim milk
Coffee or tea with artificial sweetener

Lunch
Beef Patty Creole (3)
Spinach salad, ½ cup, with 1 tbsp Creamy Lo-Cal Dressing
Seasoned Carrots
Honeydew melon, 2" wedge
4 oz skim milk

Dinner

Mediterranean Pork Chop (15), 1
Boiled parslied potato, 1 medium
Broccoli with mushrooms, ½ cup
Apple, 2½" diameter
4 oz skim milk
Coffee or tea with artificial sweetener

Calories: 980
Protein: 60 grams

Recipes for Menumax® 1000

1. Asparagus a la Lemon
2. Baked Orange Halibut
3. Beef Patty Creole
4. Buena Tostada
5. Chef Salad
6. Chicken Salad
7. Creamy Low-Calorie Dressing
8. Creole Sauce
9. Dilly Dressing
10. Egg Salad
11. Fiesta Taco
12. Herbed Fish Bake
13. Lime Fruit Dessert
14. Meat Loaf
15. Mediterranean Pork Chop
16. Old-Fashioned Hamburger Patty
17. Onion-Mushroom Omelette
18. Oriental Chicken and Broccoli
19. Southern Oven-Fried Chicken
20. Southern Stewed Chicken
21. Spaghetti with Meat Sauce
22. Spinach Salad
23. Strawberry Fruited Jell-O
24. Tomato-Mushroom Omelette
25. Triple Bean Salad
26. Tuna Salad
27. Veal Parmesan

Number 1. Asparagus a la Lemon

½ cup asparagus
1 small clove garlic, minced
2 slices onion
1 chicken bouillon cube
Grated peel and juice of ½ lemon

Place asparagus, onion, garlic, and bouillon cube into a Teflon-coated pan. Stir fry until asparagus is crisp-tender, about 5 minutes. Stir in lemon peel and juice and heat through.

25 calories

Number 2. Baked Orange Halibut

4 oz halibut
½ tbsp orange juice concentrate, thawed
¼ tbsp chopped parsley
¼ tbsp lemon juice
1/8 tsp dill weed
½ cup water

Preheat broiler. Place fish in shallow pan. Combine orange juice concentrate, parsley, lemon juice, dill weed, and water and mix well. Pour over fish. Marinate 30 minutes, turning once. Remove fish and place on broiler pan coated with vegetable spray. Broil for 6 minutes, 3" from heat. Turn and broil until fish flakes easily, about 5–6 minutes. Baste with reserved marinade; brush with more marinade on top just before serving.

150 calories per serving

Number 3. Beef Patty Creole

3 oz very lean ground beef
Place beef patty on foil in oven and bake at 350°. When almost cooked, top with Creole sauce and heat through.

Number 4. Bueno Tostada

Lightly toast one corn tortilla until crisp. Top with one cup of chopped lettuce. Sprinkle 3 oz lean, cooked, drained ground beef over the lettuce. Top with ½ cup canned tomatoes spiced with a small amount of chili powder.

270 calories

Number 5. Chef Salad

½ of a 4" head of lettuce
½ raw cucumber, sliced
½ raw green pepper, diced

½ cup grated carrot
1 slice boiled ham, sliced
1 oz Swiss cheese, diced

Mix all ingredients together. Serve with dressing indicated.

290 calories

Number 6. Chicken Salad

2 oz lean chicken, no skin, diced
½ cup diced celery
2 tsp mayonnaise substitute

Mix and serve chilled on lettuce bed or in a sandwich.

180 calories per serving

Number 7. Creamy Low-Calorie Dressing

½ cup buttermilk
2 tbsp prepared mustard
1 tbsp vinegar
1 tbsp vegetable oil

Mix all ingredients and serve.

16 calories per tablespoon

Number 8. Creole Sauce

½ cup canned or fresh tomatoes, chopped
2 tbsp chopped onion
2 tbsp celery
2 tbsp chopped green pepper
¼ tsp oregano
Dash of black pepper

190 calories per serving

Number 9. Dilly Dressing

1 cup tomato juice
1 tsp grated lemon peel
2 tbsp lemon juice
½ tsp salt (optional)
½ tsp dill weed
½ tsp dry mustard
¼ tsp sugar substitute

Mix all ingredients together and shake well.

5 calories per tablespoon

Number 10. Egg Salad

1 egg, cooked hard
1 tsp mayonnaise
2 tbsp chopped celery
2 tsp pickle relish

Mix all ingredients and chill.

110 calories per recipe

Number 11. Fiesta Taco

1 corn tortilla, toasted and folded in half
3 oz very lean ground beef
2 tbsp chopped onion
2 tbsp chopped green pepper
Pinch of garlic powder
½ tsp chili powder
½ cup shredded lettuce
¼ cup chopped tomatoes
½ oz grated cheddar cheese

Cook ground beef in Teflon-coated pan until browned, chopping through meat to prevent clumping. Add onion and green pepper until tender. Drain excess fat very well. Add garlic powder and stir. Fill taco shell and top with lettuce, tomatoes, and grated cheese.

300 calories per taco

Number 12. Herbed Fish Bake

3 oz lean fish
1 tbsp parsley
1 tsp tarragon

Sprinkle herbs over fish and bake at 375° until flaky.

150 calories per 3 oz

Number 13. Lime Fruit Dessert

Prepare Lime Jell-O according to package directions. When tightly set, add 1 cup of fresh diced fruit. Place in refrigerator until set.

90 calories per ½ cup

Number 14. Meat Loaf (8 2-oz servings)

½ cup skim milk
2 tbsp catsup
1 slice bread, broken into pieces
1 lb very lean ground beef
2 egg whites, slightly beaten
⅛ tsp dry mustard powder
½ cup chopped onion
⅛ tsp sage
2 tsp chopped celery
⅛ tsp garlic powder
1 medium tomato peeled and chopped
1 tbsp lemon juice
⅛ tsp pepper

Pour milk over bread and allow to stand 5 minutes. Mix in remaining ingredients. Form into a loaf and place on a rack in a shallow roasting pan. Bake at 375° for 1–½ hours.

135 calories per 2-oz serving

Number 15. Mediterranean Pork Chop

1 loin pork chop, very lean, ½" thick, well trimmed
¼ tsp oil
½ tsp marjoram
⅛ tsp garlic powder
⅛ tsp pepper
½ cup water

Brown chop in oil in skillet. Pour off fat. Mix seasonings together and sprinkle over chops. Add water and cover tightly. Reduce heat and simmer over low heat until tender, about 45 minutes.

125 calories per serving

Number 16. Old-Fashioned Hamburger Patty

3½ oz lean ground beef patty (before cooking)
½ medium onion
½ cup sliced mushrooms

Quickly brown mushrooms and onion in a Teflon-coated pan. Remove. Place hamburger into oven preheated to 375° until cooked. Top with mushrooms and onion and heat through.

180 calories per 3-oz patty

Number 17. Onion-Mushroom Omelette

1 egg, beaten
¼ cup chopped onions
½ cup sliced mushrooms

Quickly brown onion and mushrooms in a Teflon-coated pan without oil, butter, or margarine. Remove from pan and mix with the egg. Place mixture into Teflon-coated pan and cook until done. Fold and serve.

115 calories per omelette

Number 18. Oriental Chicken and Broccoli

3 oz white meat of chicken, diced, no skin
1½ cups broccoli, cut into bite-sized pieces
½ cup sliced mushrooms
½ tsp ginger
½ tsp garlic

Sauce Mixture
1 tbsp soy sauce
1 tbsp water
½ tsp cornstarch

Heat Teflon-coated pan. Add diced chicken and toss until lightly browned, about 5–7 minutes. Add broccoli, mushrooms, ginger, and garlic, and stir until crisp-tender. Add sauce mixture and heat through.

250 calories per recipe

Number 19. Southern Oven-Fried Chicken

3 oz chicken, white meat
2 tbsp Shake 'n Bake for Chicken

Coat chicken with Shake 'n Bake and bake at 375° for about 30 minutes.

185 calories per 3-oz serving

Number 20. Southern Stewed Chicken

1 chicken breast
1 cup canned tomatoes
1 cup chicken bouillon
1 small onion chopped
½ green pepper, chopped
2 carrots, chopped
1 small stalk celery, chopped
1 clove garlic, split
1 small bay leaf
2 tsp chili powder

Cover chicken with tomatoes and chicken bouillon. Bring to a boil and boil for about 15 minutes. Add the remaining ingredients. Cover and simmer until tender.

Serving size: 3 oz white chicken meat, without skin, plus vegetables.

210 calories per recipe

Number 21. Spaghetti with Meat Sauce

½ cup spaghetti, cooked tender
3 oz very lean ground beef, cooked and crumbled, with excess fat drained off
¼ cup Low-Calorie Tomato Sauce

Low-Calorie Tomato Sauce

2 cans (6 oz each) tomato paste
3 cups water
¼ cup finely chopped onion
1 garlic clove, minced
2 tbsp lemon juice
Dash of Tabasco sauce
¼ tsp basil
⅛ tsp pepper

Combine all ingredients and mix well. Simmer over low heat for 30 minutes, stirring constantly.

275 calories (½ cup spaghetti, 3 oz meat, 1¼ cup sauce)

Number 22. Spinach Salad

½ cup fresh spinach
4 small radishes, sliced
1 oz bean sprouts
¼ cup fresh sliced mushrooms

45 calories per ½-cup serving

Number 23. Strawberry Fruited Jell-O

Prepare Strawberry Jell-O according to package directions. When slightly set, add a cup of fresh diced fruit. Place into refrigerator until set.

90 calories per ½ cup

Number 24. Tomato-Mushroom Omelette

1 egg, beaten
½ cup mushrooms
¾ of a medium tomato, diced

Stir mushrooms and tomato lightly in Teflon-coated pan without any oil, butter, or margarine. Remove. Add the beaten egg and cook over low heat until done. Top one half of the omelette with the mushroom and tomato mixture and fold omelette over. Heat through for about 3–5 minutes over a very low flame.

115 calories per omelette

Number 25. Triple Bean Salad

2 tbsp kidney beans, cooked
¼ cup cooked green beans
¼ cup cooked yellow wax beans
2 tbsp vinegar
1 tsp corn oil
1 clove garlic
1 slice of onion
Pepper

Toss and serve on a bed of lettuce.

110 calories per ½-cup serving

Number 26. Tuna Salad

½ cup water-packed tuna
2 tbsp diced celery

1 tbsp sweet pickle relish
1 tbsp mayonnaise

Mix well and chill. Use only one half of the mixture when preparing a half sandwich or salad plate.

240 calories per ½-cup serving; 120 calories per ¼-cup serving

Number 27. Veal Parmesan

1 veal cutlet, breaded (4"×2¼"×½" or 2½ oz)
½ cup Tomato Sauce
½ oz grated Parmesan cheese

Place breaded veal cutlet into oven heated to 375°. Bake 20–30 minutes. Top with Tomato Sauce and grated cheese and heat until warmed through.

315 calories per serving

Bread, Cereal, Rice and Pasta

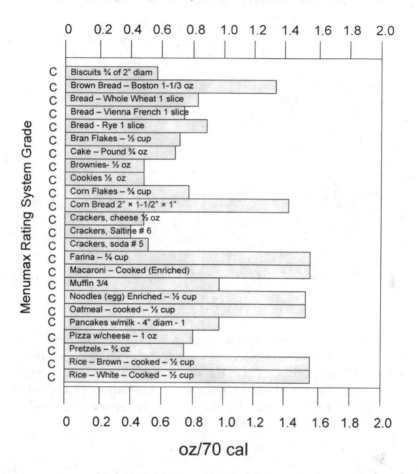

Figure 1. Rating of foods within food groups using nutrient density. The relative values of various foods have been rated and assigned "A" for best, "B" for next best, "C" for somewhat less good, and "D" for lower choice. The length of each bar is an indication of the nutrient density. The longer the bar, the better the nutrition per food unit. Select more foods with longer bars.

Bread, Cereal, Rice and Pasta - II

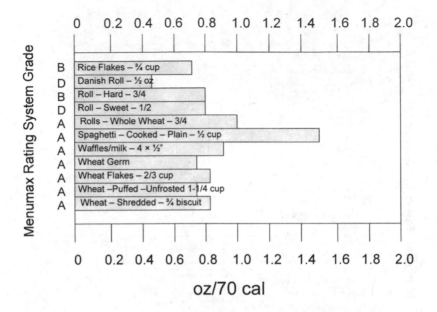

Figure 2. Rating of foods within food groups using nutrient density. The relative values of various foods have been rated and assigned "A" for best, "B" for next best, "C" for somewhat less good, and "D" for lower choice. The length of each bar is an indication of the nutrient density. The longer the bar, the better the nutrition per food unit. Select more foods with longer bars.

Fruits

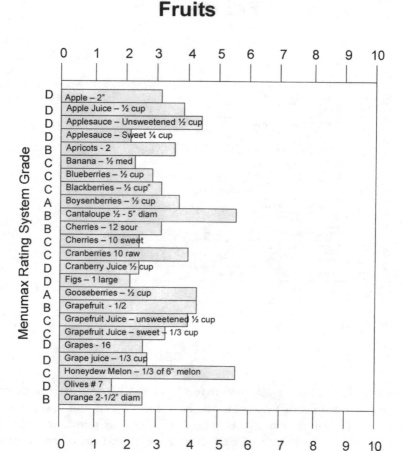

Figure 3. Rating of foods within food groups using nutrient density. The relative values of various foods have been rated and assigned "A" for best, "B" for next best, "C" for somewhat less good, and "D" for lower choice. The length of each bar is an indication of the nutrient density. The longer the bar, the better the nutrition per food unit. Select more foods with longer bars.

Fruits - II

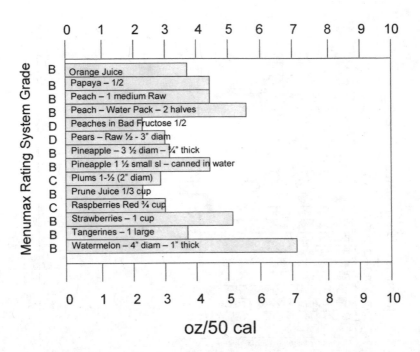

Figure 4. Rating of foods within food groups using nutrient density. The relative values of various foods have been rated and assigned "A" for best, "B" for next best, "C" for somewhat less good, and "D" for lower choice. The length of each bar is an indication of the nutrient density. The longer the bar, the better the nutrition per food unit. Select more foods with longer bars.

Vegetables

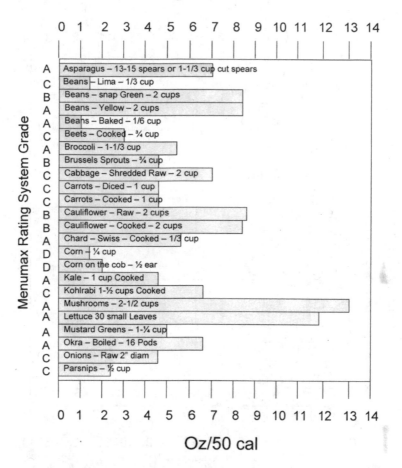

Figure 5. Rating of foods within food groups using nutrient density. The relative values of various foods have been rated and assigned "A" for best, "B" for next best, "C" for somewhat less good, and "D" for lower choice. The length of each bar is an indication of the nutrient density. The longer the bar, the better the nutrition per food unit. Select more foods with longer bars.

Vegetables - II

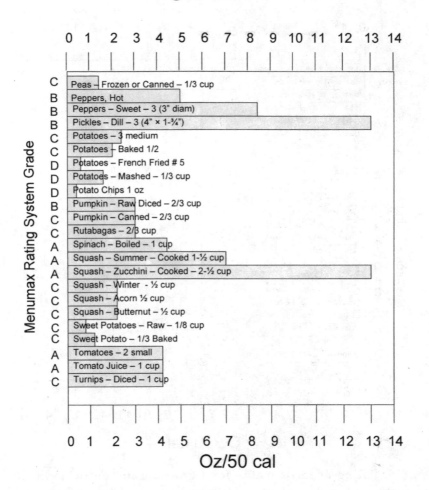

Milk, Yogurt, Cheese and Eggs

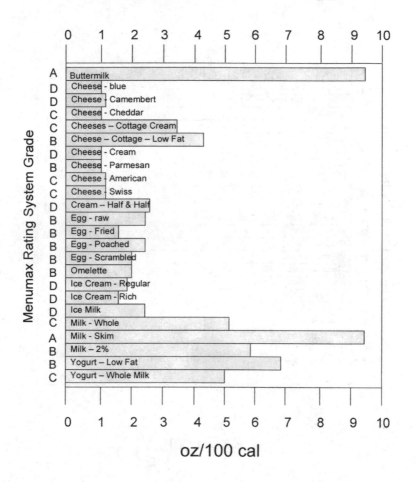

oz/100 cal

Fish, Poultry & Meat

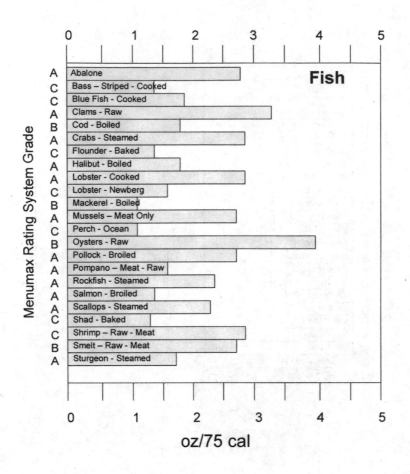

Fish, Poultry & Meat - II

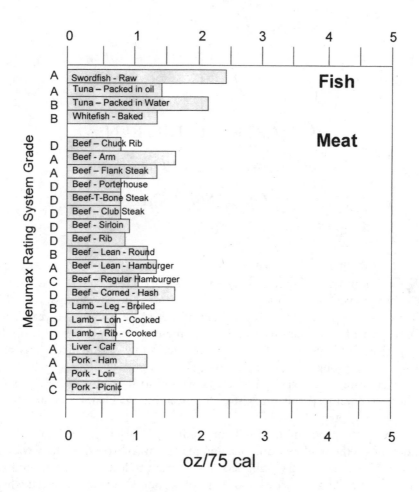

CHAPTER THIRTEEN

The Menumax® 800 Diet Plan

A Quick-Start Diet

Y ou now know there are many ways to succeed at weight loss. If you want a very low-calorie diet for rapid, short-term weight loss, then this chapter is for you. I first used this kind of diet some twenty-five years ago. It was part of a program to evaluate treatments for weight loss. I thought my patients would not be able to stick to such a low-calorie diet. I was surprised—and wrong. As they came in for their regular weighing each week, they were often overjoyed at the rate of weight loss. From these early experiences, I developed this diet using the Menumax® planning system presented in Chapter 12.

This is the program for you if you want *rapid weight loss*. It is an *optional* detour on the roadmap, and one you may want to bypass. We have found, however, that many overweight people who want to lose weight want to lose it now. The feeling of success and sense of accomplishment generated when weight is lost rapidly and steadily can help you deal better with later portions of the program, which are designed to re-educate and reshape you and your eating patterns. If this doesn't appeal to you, you may choose the 1200-calorie Menumax® diet you just planned.

To beat an old horse, so to speak, let me just reiterate that more rapid weight loss means you must eat fewer calories each day. When you eat less than 1,200 calories of food energy per day, however, you may not be getting all of the nutrients your body needs. Because of this, any diet with less than 1,200 calories of energy per day should, in my view, be supplemented with vitamins and minerals to provide the additional nutrients your body needs. We will examine those extra nutrients after describing the diet.

THE Menumax®-800 DIET

The diet I have formulated for rapid weight loss is recommended for the first four weeks only.

Table 1. Composition of Menumax®-800 Diet

Component	Amount per Day	Calories per Day
Protein	75 g/d (grams per day)	300 kcal
Carbohydrates	75 g/d (grams per day)	300 kcal
Fat	22 g/d (grams per day)	180 kcal

This diet is designed to provide the major nutrients each day. It is very low in calories. This is the reason you lose weight more rapidly. You are eating less energy than your body is using, and the extra energy is being drawn from the energy warehouses in your fat cells.

My first consideration in designing this diet was to select a *low calorie level*. Obviously, the lowest level is fasting. The experience I have had with total fasting indicates it is not a sensible way to lose weight, except in a hospital.[1] From my experience, I have found this Menumax®-800 diet can be followed safely for four weeks or more of rapid weight loss.

My second consideration in designing this diet was to provide a more than adequate intake of protein. Protein is important to your nutrition, particularly for the young and for the elderly. Protein is essential for the amino acids needed to rebuild body proteins and for all of the functions of our daily metabolism. The Food and Nutrition Board of the National Academy of Science[2] has recommended an intake of 44 to 50 grams per day of protein for women and an intake of 59 to 63 grams for men. To be well on the safe side during a time when the total caloric intake is restricted, I chose 75 grams per day.

Protein intake constitutes 40% of the total calories each day you remain on the diet. In addition to providing the building blocks for the body tissues, protein helps satisfy the body after a meal. This "satiety" value of proteins can be important in helping you control your hunger.

Although I provided more protein than you need, the Menumax®-800 diet obviously does not provide all of the carbohydrate and fat that are needed to maintain your weight. That is why you lose weight. We had to make a choice between carbohydrates and fat. Glucose from carbohydrate can stimulate the sympathetic nervous system and increase triiodothyronine or prevent its fall.[3] We selected a diet with 75 grams of carbohydrate. This will yield 300 calories when metabolized in your body.

Certain fats are also essential for proper function of the body.[4] They are involved in keeping the skin and red blood corpuscles in good condition, as well as the proper working of the nervous system, and other nervous tissues. The body cannot make these essential fatty acids, which we have to obtain from the diet. Such fats as corn oil provide an adequate amount of most of these fatty acids, and we have included 22 grams per day of fat in the diet in order to meet this need.

Any diet should also provide all of the vitamins and minerals our bodies need.[2] A diet of food providing 800 calories will not give you all of the nutrients you need. For that reason, I recommend that you take a multi-vitamin tablet with minerals while you are on this diet.

In planning the menus for the first phase of the Menumax®-800 Diet, I have used the techniques for calorie exchange described earlier. With this material as your guide, you can plan your own alternatives to the ones I have included; however, I have provided four weeks of menus for you if you wish to use them.

Using the food groups I described earlier, I laid out the meal plan as shown in this and the next table.

Table 2. Construction of the Menumax®-800 Diet

Food Group	Calories/Unit	Total No. of Units Each Day	Calories/Day
Meat/Fish/Poultry	75	4	300
Vegetables	75	2	150
Fruit	50	2	100
Bread/Cereals	75	1	75
Milk	100	2	200

Table 3. Division of the Food Groups between Three Meals Each Day

Group	Meal Breakfast	Lunch	Dinner
Meat/Fish/Poultry		1	3
Vegetables		1 (when no fruit)	1
Fruit	1	1 (sometimes)	1
Bread/Cereal	1		
Milk (skim)	½		

In addition to the amount of skim or ½% or 1% milk listed above, water, sparkling water with ice and lemon, or non-caloric beverages such as coffee or tea can be consumed as desired. At least 6–8 glasses of water or calorie-free beverages should be consumed each day. Because the meals provide so few calories, I also took into account the need some dieters have for between-meal snacks. Foods and beverages from the accompanying table may be used as desired.

Table of Food You May Add to Your Diet As Desired
Coffee, without sugar, cream or milk
Tea, without sugar, cream or milk
Clear broth
Bouillon
Consommé
Lemon
Gelatin (unsweetened)
Pepper
Spices and seasonings
Vinegar
Vegetables:
    Asparagus
    Broccoli
    Cabbage
    Cauliflower
    Celery
    Cucumber
    Greens (beet, chard, dandelion, kale)
    Lettuce
    Mushrooms
    Peppers
    Radishes
    Sauerkraut
    Spinach
    Watercress

Menumax®-800 MEAL PLAN FOR WEEK 1

(Recipes identified by number are in Chapter 12)

MONDAY
Breakfast

Toast 1 slice
Grapefruit ½ of a 4" fruit
Coffee or tea with artificial sweetener

Lunch

Tuna (water packed) 2 oz with diced pickles and celery on lettuce leaves
Sliced tomatoes ½ cup
Coffee, tea, or other calorie-free beverage

Dinner

Chicken (white meat), 4 oz
Broccoli ½ cups with lemon juice
Apple 2" in diameter
No-calorie beverage, iced tea, coffee

TUESDAY
Breakfast

Cereal (corn flakes or equivalent) ¾ cup
Tomato juice 8 oz
Skim milk 2 oz

Lunch

Omelette (made with 1 egg)
Green peas ½ cup
No-calorie beverage

Dinner

Veal (1 slice 3×4 inches and ½ inch thick) broiled or baked
Green beans ½ cup
Sparkling water with ice and lemon or no-calorie beverage

WEDNESDAY
Breakfast

Toast 1 slice
Orange juice 4 oz
Coffee or tea with artificial sweetener

Lunch

Tuna 2 oz with pickles and celery on lettuce
Mushrooms 2 cups
No-calorie beverage

Dinner

Fish (except salmon) 2–3 oz baked or broiled with lemon
Potato ½ of a medium with chives
Sparkling water with ice and lemon juice, or no-calorie beverage
Cantaloupe ½ of a 5" fruit

THURSDAY
Breakfast

Cereal (bran flakes) ⅞ cup
Milk (skim) 2 oz
Tomato juice 8 oz

Lunch

Chicken salad ½ oz on lettuce with celery
Carrots 2
No-calorie beverage

Dinner

Lean ground beef patty 3 oz broiled
Green peas ½ cup
Sparkling water with lemon and ice or no-calorie beverage
Pear ½ of a large

FRIDAY
Breakfast

Toast 1 slice
Grapefruit ½ of a 4"
Coffee, tea with artificial sweetener

Lunch

Omelette 1 egg
Beets ⅔ of a cup
Apple 2-inch diameter
No-calorie beverage or black coffee or iced tea

Dinner

Chicken 4 oz
Tomatoes 1 cup canned
Cantaloupe ½ of a 5"
No-calorie beverage or black coffee or tea

SATURDAY
Breakfast

Cereal (⅔ cup cooked)
Milk ¼ cup (2 oz)
Cantaloupe ½ of a 5"
Coffee, tea with artificial sweetener

Lunch

Tuna (water packed) 2 oz on lettuce
Carrots 2 to 3
No-calorie beverage

Dinner

Fish 3 oz baked or broiled
Green beans ½ cup
Berries 2 cup (except strawberries, 1 cup)
Sparkling water with lemon and ice, coffee or tea with artificial sweetener

SUNDAY

Breakfast

Toast 1 slice
Tomato juice 8 oz
Coffee, tea, etc. with artificial sweetener

Lunch

Chicken salad ½ oz with pickles and celery on lettuce
Mushrooms 2 cups
No-calorie beverage or coffee or tea

Dinner

Ground beef 3 oz broiled or baked
Green peas ½ cup
Pear ½ large

MENUS FOR WEEK 2

MONDAY
Breakfast

Dry, unsweetened cereal, ¾ cup
4 oz skim milk
4 oz orange juice
Coffee or tea with artificial sweetener

Lunch

3 oz cottage cheese (Low fat) on lettuce bed
1 cup sliced strawberries
½ of a 3-inch orange
No-calorie beverage or iced tea or coffee

Dinner

Broiled Veal (1 slice 3x4 inches and ½ inch thick)
Herbed tomato halves or ½ cups Broccoli
Honeydew melon 2" wedge
Sparkling water with ice and lemon juice or no-calorie beverage

TUESDAY
Breakfast

Toast 1 slice
4 oz skim milk
4 oz grapefruit juice
No-calorie beverage, iced tea or coffee

Lunch

Shrimp, 2 oz boiled, with pickles and celery on lettuce bed
2 cups mushrooms
No-calorie beverage, iced tea, or coffee with artificial sweetener

Dinner

Bueno Tostada (4)
Cantaloupe ½ of 5" diameter

Sparkling water with ice and lemon juice or no-calorie beverage

WEDNESDAY
Breakfast

Cooked cereal, ½ cup
4 oz skim milk
4 oz orange juice
Coffee or tea with artificial sweetener

Lunch

Omelette (made with 1 egg)
Asparagus a la Lemon (1), 1½ cups
Apple 2" diameter
No-calorie beverage or iced tea

Dinner

Broiled fish with lemon wedge (3 oz fish)
Green peas with mushrooms, ½ cup
Pear, ½ large

THURSDAY
Breakfast

Dry, unsweetened cereal, ¾ cup
4 oz skim milk
½ of 4" grapefruit
Coffee or tea with artificial sweetener

Lunch
Flaked Tuna (2 oz water-pack) on tossed salad greens (1 cup) with lemon juice
½ cup raspberries
No-calorie beverage or iced tea

Dinner

Lean ground beef patty (3 oz), baked with mushrooms
Beets, ⅔ cup
Blueberries, 2 cup

FRIDAY
Breakfast

Toast, 1 slice
4 oz milk, skim
8 oz tomato juice
Coffee or tea with artificial sweetener

Lunch

Tomato-Mushroom Omelette (made with 1 egg)(24)
OR
Onion-Mushroom Omelette (17)
Green beans, ½ cup
Tangerine, 1½ " diameter
No-calorie beverage or iced tea or coffee

Dinner

Oriental Chicken and Broccoli (18) (use exact quantities in recipe)
Strawberries, ½ cup sliced
Sparkling water with ice and lemon juice or no-calorie beverage

SATURDAY
Breakfast

Cooked cereal, ½ cup
4 oz skim milk
4 oz orange juice
Coffee or tea with artificial sweetener

Lunch

3 oz cottage cheese (low-fat) on lettuce bed
½ of a 2" apple, diced
½ of a large pear, diced
No-calorie beverage or iced tea

Dinner

Broiled Veal (1 slice, 3"×4"×½") with lemon and capers
½ cup asparagus

Honeydew Melon, 2" wedge
Coffee or tea

SUNDAY
Breakfast

Toast, 1 slice
4 oz skim milk
Cantaloupe, ½ of 5" diameter
Coffee or tea with artificial sweetener

Lunch

Flaked Tuna, 2 oz on 1 cup tossed salad greens with lemon juice
Orange, ½ of 3" diameter
No-calorie beverage or iced tea

Dinner

Herb Fish Bake (12) 3 oz
Potato, ½ of a medium with chives
Strawberries, 1 cup
Sparkling water with ice and lemon or iced tea

MENUS FOR WEEK 3

MONDAY
Breakfast

Dry, unsweetened cereal, ¾ cup
4 oz skim milk
4 oz grapefruit juice
Coffee or tea with artificial sweetener

Lunch

Chicken salad, 1½ oz on lettuce with celery
Sliced tomatoes (1 large) with Dilly Dressing (6)(2 T)
No-calorie beverage or iced tea

Dinner

Lean ground beef patty (3 oz)
Caraway Cabbage (5) (2 cups)
Apple, 2" diameter
Sparkling water with ice and lemon or no-calorie beverage

TUESDAY
Breakfast

Toast, 1 slice
4 oz skim milk
4 oz orange juice
Coffee or tea with artificial sweetener

Lunch

Shrimp, 2 oz boiled, with pickles and celery on lettuce bed
Mushrooms, 2 cups
No-calorie beverage or iced tea

Dinner

Baked Veal (1 slice, 3"×4"×½")
Green Peas, ½ cup
Orange, ½ of 3" diameter

Sparkling water with ice and lemon juice or iced tea or coffee

WEDNESDAY
Breakfast

Cooked cereal, ½ cup
Honeydew melon, 2" wedge
Coffee or tea with artificial sweetener

Lunch

Poached egg (1) on Toast, 1 slice
Raspberries, ½ cup
No-calorie beverage or iced tea

Dinner

Southern Stewed Chicken (20) (3 oz.)
Pear, ½ of a large
Sparkling water with ice and lemon juice or iced tea or coffee

THURSDAY
Breakfast

Dry, unsweetened cereal, ¾ cup
Strawberries, ½ cup
4 oz skim milk
Coffee or tea with artificial sweetener

Lunch

3 oz cottage cheese (low-fat) on lettuce bed
1½" Tangerine
Pear, ½ of a large
No-calorie beverage or iced tea

Dinner

Fish, 3 oz Baked or broiled
Potato, ½ of a medium with parsley
Blueberries, ½ cup
No-calorie beverage

FRIDAY
Breakfast

Toast, 1 slice
4 oz skim milk
8 oz tomato juice
Coffee or tea with artificial sweetener

Lunch

Flaked Tuna (2 oz water-pack) on lettuce
Cold asparagus spears with Dilly Dressing (6)(1½ cups with 2 Tbsp Dressing)
No-calorie beverage or iced tea

Dinner

Stove Top Chiles Rellenos (made with 1 egg) (14)
Green Beans, 1½ cups
Apple, 2" diameter
Sparkling water with ice and lemon juice or no-calorie beverage

SATURDAY
Breakfast

Cooked cereal, ½ cup
4 oz skim milk
Cantaloupe, ½ of a 5" diameter
Coffee or tea with artificial sweetener

Lunch

Diced Chicken, 1½ oz on 1 cup lettuce with lemon and tarragon
Tangerine, 1½" diameter
No-calorie beverage or iced tea

Dinner

Baked Meatballs, 2 (each 1½ oz)
Beets, ⅔ cup
Pear, ½ of a large
Sparkling water with lemon juice or iced tea or coffee

SUNDAY
Breakfast

Dry, unsweetened cereal, ¾ cup
4 oz skim milk
Grapefruit, ½ of a 4" diameter
Coffee or tea with artificial sweetener

Lunch

3 oz cottage cheese (low-fat) on lettuce bed
Raspberries, ½ cup
Apple, ½ of a 2" diameter
No-calorie beverage or iced tea

Dinner

Herb Chicken (light meat, no skin, 3 oz) (8)
Broccoli, 1½ cups
Honeydew Melon, 2" wedge
Sparkling water with ice and lemon juice or iced tea

MENUS FOR WEEK 4

MONDAY
Breakfast

Toast, 1 slice
4 oz skim milk
4 oz grapefruit juice
Coffee or tea with artificial sweetener

Lunch

Tomato-Mushroom Omelette (made with 1 egg)(24)
OR
Onion Mushroom Omelette (17)
Green peas, ½ cup
Tossed salad (1 cup) with Dilly Dressing, 2 Tbsp dressing (9)
No-calorie beverage or iced tea

Dinner

Broiled fish with lemon wedge (3 oz)
Carrots, steamed, 2–3
Blackberries, ½ cup
Sparkling water with ice and lemon juice or iced tea

TUESDAY
Breakfast

Cooked cereal, ½ cup
4 oz skim milk
4 oz orange juice
Coffee or tea with artificial sweetener

Lunch

Shrimp, 3 oz boiled with pickles and celery on lettuce bed
2 cups mushrooms
No-calorie beverage or iced tea

Dinner

Broiled Veal (3"×4"×2", 1 slice) with lemon and capers
Potato, ½ of a medium with chives
Strawberries, ½ cup
Sparkling water with ice and lemon juice or iced tea or coffee

WEDNESDAY
Breakfast

Dry, unsweetened cereal, ¾ cup
4 oz skim milk
Grapefruit, ½ of a 4" diameter
Coffee or tea with artificial sweetener

Lunch

3 oz cottage cheese (low fat) on lettuce bed
Cantaloupe, ½ of a 5" diameter
Apple, 2" diameter
No-calorie beverage or iced tea

Dinner

Beef Patty Creole, 3 oz (Lean) (3)
OR
Old Fashioned Hamburger Patty (16)
Asparagus, 1½ cups
Orange, ½ of a 3" diameter
Sparkling water with ice or lemon juice or iced tea

THURSDAY
Breakfast

Toast, 1 slice
4 oz skim milk
8 oz tomato juice
Coffee or tea with artificial sweetener

Lunch

Flaked tuna, 2 oz on mixed salad greens with lemon juice
Pear, 2 of a large
No-calorie beverage or iced tea

Dinner

Bueno Tostada (4)
Honeydew Melon, 2" wedge
Sparkling water with ice and lemon juice or iced tea or coffee

FRIDAY
Breakfast

Cooked cereal, ½ cup
4 oz skim milk
4 oz grapefruit juice
Coffee or tea with artificial sweetener

Lunch

Omelette, plain (made with 1 egg)
Herbed Broiled Tomato Halves
Blueberries, ½ cup

Dinner

Oriental Chicken and Broccoli (18) (use exact quantities in recipe)
Apple, 2" diameter

SATURDAY
Breakfast
Dry cereal, unsweetened, 3/4 cup
4 oz skim milk
Strawberries, ½ cup
Coffee or tea with artificial sweetener

Lunch

Chicken Salad, 1½ oz on lettuce with celery
Carrots, 2–3
No-calorie beverage or iced tea

Dinner

Veal with Tomatoes Baked (1 slice 3"x4"x½")
OR
Broiled Veal plus Tossed salad with Lemon Juice

Potato, ½ of a medium with chives
Tangerine, 1½"
Sparkling water with ice and lemon juice or iced tea

SUNDAY

Breakfast

Toast, 1 slice
4 oz skim milk
Grapefruit juice, 4 oz
Coffee or tea with artificial sweetener

Lunch

3 oz cottage cheese (low-fat) on lettuce bed
Pear, ½ of a large
Cantaloupe, ½ of a 5" diameter
No-calorie beverage or iced tea

Dinner

Herbed Fish Bake, 3 oz
Beets, 2/3 cup
Honeydew Melon, 2" wedge
Sparkling water with ice and lemon juice or iced tea or coffee

CHAPTER FOURTEEN

Eating for Success

The Portion-Control Strategy:

An Alternative to the Menumax® 800 Diet Plan

Diet Shakes
Portion control means controlling the portion sizes of the foods you eat. The use of portion control got off to a rocky start. More recently, however, there have been important advances you may want to incorporate into your own nutrition plan.

Portion control and calorie control go hand-in-hand. Almost everyone who has dieted has tried to lose weight with some kind of diet plan. When I started to practice, I was given a package of "tear-off" diet sheets by one of the pharmaceutical companies to give to my patients. Many doctors continue to do this—it is simple (for the physician). One problem with diet sheets is that patients have to buy and prepare foods in just the right amount. If you carefully follow any diet, however, you will lose weight. Here I want to talk about portion control as a way to make your nutritional choices easier.

The simplest form of portion control is a glass of milk. An 8-oz glass of skim milk has 90 calories. It has protein and calcium and added vitamin D. Many "formula diets" are similar to milk but add other ingredients, and they are often called "shakes." The first product in this category I remember was called Metrecal. I used it when I brought my patients into the hospital for fasting or for low-calorie dieting. Metrecal was a liquid formula diet in a can. It contained all of the nutrients that were known to be needed and had only 225 calories in each can. Metrecal means "metered calories." It was developed by a research hospital in New York and then sold to the public in the 1960s. Metrecal succeeded spectacularly, and other formula diets in a can followed rapidly. The result was a wave of weight loss and weight regain—our friend weight cycling. Weight control is a chronic problem, and when people finished the Metrecal diet, they returned to eating the way they had eaten before, with the inevitable result: weight regain. Following the initial hype over Metrecal and related products, portion-controlled diets largely disappeared.

The rebirth of portion control occurred in the early 1970s with very low-calorie formula diets. These too were developed in research hospitals. But they were popularized by the daily newspapers. The newspaper and glamour magazine stories helped boost sales spectacularly. Then came "The Last Chance Diet," which popularized a formula diet with a large amount of collagen as the protein component.[1] To the regret of many, this formula proved very popular but hazardous to their health. Following numerous reports of problems and a number of deaths,[2] the U.S. Food and Drug Administration withdrew this dietary formulation.

It was some years before another formula diet appeared. This time it was the Cambridge Diet. The Cambridge Diet swept the United States and made its developers very rich. This formula diet was based on the work of Dr. Alan Howard.[3] It was a 320-calorie/day formula bought by millions of people. Although marketed through a "counselor" system, these counselors did not have sufficient training to provide the kind of service group leaders provide in most behavioral weight-control programs. After a spectacular burst of sales, the original Cambridge Diet Company in the United States went bankrupt.[4]

It is hard to keep a good idea down, and portion control was reborn again in two different forms. The very low-calorie diet formulations became part of medically managed weight-loss programs.[5] Optifast and Medifast were among the leaders. Use of the Optifast program by national celebrities helped catapult it into the public arena. Once again, weight cycling and the concern about "fairness in advertising" led to Congressional hearings and a decline in the sales of Optifast and other similar formula diets.[6]

Diet and Your Metabolism
Does a 320-calorie diet or a 400-calorie-per-day diet produce quicker weight loss than an 800-calorie-per-day formula diet? You would think so, based on our discussion of energy balance. If you eat fewer calories, you should lose weight faster, all other things being equal. Not so! "Things" turn out not to be equal. Surprising as it may seem, the rate of weight loss with the 800-calorie-per-day diet was just as rapid as with the other two lower-calorie diets.[7]

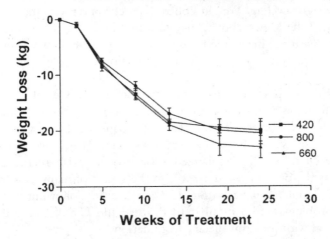

Comparison of 420kcal, 660 kcal and 800 kcal Formulas

Figure 1. Weight losses of subjects in the three dietary conditions during treatment. Subjects consumed either a 420-kcal/d, 660-kcal/d, or 800-kcal/d diet during weeks 2–13, a re-feeding diet during weeks 14–19, and a 1200- to 1500-kcal/d diet for the remainder of treatment.[7]

How can this be? If you eat fewer calories you should lose faster, right? Not always. It depends on how your body responds to the low-calorie diets.

It has been known for years that low-calorie diets lower energy needs. This was one of my first research findings.[8] I took several of my patients onto our hospital ward. During the first few days, they ate the food they claimed they had been eating at home. Surprisingly, they each lost weight. To stop the weight loss, we increased their food so weight loss stopped. After a few days with a stable weight, I reduced their food intake to 450 calories per day. Each day, I measured the amount of energy they were burning using a metabolism machine. Each one of my patients showed a decrease in the amount of energy s/he needed. They reduced their metabolism by about 15%. They had become metabolically "more efficient."

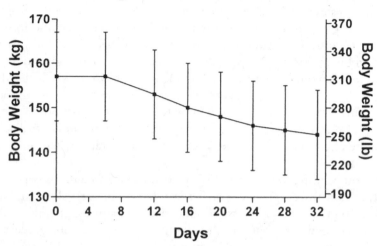

Figure 2. Effect of caloric intake on body weight and energy expenditure of six obese patients.[8]

This means that if you eat a very low-calorie diet, you may lose less weight than you expected.[9] This can be frustrating. One reason that weight loss during the 320-calorie diet was no faster than during the 800-calorie diet may be this increased metabolic "efficiency." The body simply adjusts by lowering its metabolism.

Do all diets lower metabolism? No. Only the diets with less than 800 calories appear to do this. Your metabolism will drop more if the very low-calorie diet is also low in carbohydrate. The fact is that carbohydrate will keep you from becoming more efficient when following a very low-calorie diet,[10] and this is why we used sufficient carbohydrate in planning the Menumax® diets. Diets that are too low in carbohydrate lower the active form of your thyroid hormone, which is essential for keeping up your metabolic rate. Low-carbohydrate diets can lower the activity of your sympathetic nervous system and lead to the loss of sodium from your body. Leptin also decreases with reduced-calorie diets.[11] When you lose sodium, you lose water. You do not want to lose water unless you are already overloaded with water. You want to lose fat. Losing water is a quick way of losing weight. It is the basis for most "quick weight-loss diets" and is the reason why quick weight gain usually follows such diets.

Frozen Meals

Back to portion control. The use of formula diets or nutrition bars for one or two meals each day makes sense to me, and I use this approach from time to time. It can provide an easy way to regulate the number of calories you get. I find yogurt a particularly tasty way to do this. If the formula tastes good and is easy to make up, it can be used at breakfast and, if desired, at lunch, too. In contrast with a total diet made up of formulas, which I do not favor, I think that for some people replacing one or two meals with a portion-controlled meal may be a good way to control the portions they eat. In a long-term four-year study, this strategy of using portion-controlled diets was quite effective.[12] I favor a replacement at lunch rather than breakfast or later in the day.

If you want to control the portions you eat at some meals with a shake or other non-frozen product, what should you choose? There are several products on the shelf, and some commercial programs use them, too. Most, if not all of them, are found in the pharmacy section of your grocery store or in the drug store. Ultra Slim-Fast occupied most of the shelf space when I visited my pharmacy. Ultra Slim-Fast comes in many flavors. There were a number of different flavors in a powdered form to make your own shake. Or there are ready-to-drink formulas in cans. In addition to the shakes, there were five different kinds of chocolate refreshment bars.

Glucerna, Optifast, and Slim-Fast were the three canned formulas we used at the Pennington Biomedical Research Center in one of our large NIH-funded clinical studies.[13] After enrolling in the study, people were offered a choice among these three dietary formulations. People liked them all, but the favorites were Glucerna and Optifast. We have also found Glucerna to be useful in treating some of our diabetic patients who tend to gain weight.[14] There are a number of solid portion-controlled Glucerna foods, including puddings and soups. Nestlé produces several kinds of powdered shake mixes under the name "Sweet Success." Ultra Diet Quick was similar to the Ultra Slim-Fast but only comes in a powdered form. Dynatrim, California Slim, Palm Springs Elite Total Diet Plan, and Cybergenics Quick Trim were also available. Herbalife provides similar products through their distributor system.

Frozen foods make portion control easy at the evening meal. The freezers of most supermarkets have several different brands of "portion-controlled" meals. Weight Watchers frozen foods grew out of the Weight Watchers weight-control program. There are more than thirty entrees available under the Weight Watchers label. "Healthy Choice" is manufactured by ConAgra, one of the world's largest food manufacturers. There are more than forty entrees to choose from under the Healthy Choice label. "Lean Cuisine" is the label used by Nestlé/Stouffer foods for their frozen portion-controlled meals. There are more than twenty entrees available in this line as well. Another smaller line of portion-controlled foods has the label "Budget Gourmet Light and Healthy" and is produced by the All-American Gourmet Company. Again, there are more than twenty entrees in this line. Both the Banquet label and the Tyson label have nutritional foods but not necessarily calorie- or portion-controlled foods. Their brands are Healthy Balance for the Banquet line and Healthy Portion for the Tyson line.

A generous variety of meals is available. If you use portion control, you need to pick those meals from those brands you like best. The nice thing about them is they are easy to prepare and have the calories printed on the package. They also help with controlling fat intake, since they are usually lower in fat. The drawback is the higher salt content and sometimes the presence of "bad fructose" as HFCS or sucrose.

A plan for using a portion-controlled diet incorporates the shake concept for breakfast and a frozen dinner. In addition, it adds two servings of fruit, one slice of bread or toast, and an 8-oz glass of skim milk to complement the other items. A frozen breakfast or lunch could also be used, and meal-replacement bars or soups could also be substituted. The choice is yours. Since you are seeking the healthiest choices, read the label to see whether "bad fructose" (HFCS or sucrose) is added. If so, try to find something where it is not. Plan to eat 1200 to 1500 calories each day.

A large variety of foods can pose a problem, and I have a suggestion for you: Try to limit your choices. Most of us like a variety of foods and tend to eat them with a frequency that is related to our likes and dislikes. Let's say you gave me a list of the foods you like. I then prepared samples of a half-dozen of these and let you taste a bite of each and give me a rating of how much you liked each one. Your ratings would all be high, since I picked foods you like. Next I let you eat an entire lunch of one of those foods and then come back and have you taste and rate all your favorite foods again. The food you ate for lunch would not be rated as highly as the other foods on your list. This is called "sensory-specific satiety." It explains why even if we are full, we still have room for dessert. We can put this principle to work for us in portion control.

Using the space below, list your ten favorites from the list of portion-controlled foods in Table 1:

1. _____

2. _____

3. _____

4. _____

5. _____

6. _____

7. _____

8. _____

9. _____

10. _____

Make sure your list is in the order of your preference, with the one you like most at the top of the list, your second preference is number 2, and so on. Now let's focus on the top five items. Buy three weeks' worth of dinner meals from these top five. To do this, purchase five of your #1 choice and four each from your choices # 2, 3, 4, and 5, for a total of twenty-one meals. Now for the next three weeks, eat whichever of the entrees you like each night. With a five-day choice, you will find they begin to become monotonous. My wife taught me this by giving me peppermint-stick ice cream with chocolate sauce every night for so long that I don't care if I ever see either peppermint-stick ice cream or chocolate sauce again. This also happened to the children when they got bologna sandwiches every day for weeks in a row. They never care to see a bologna sandwich again.

There is a good reason for limiting our food choices. When we give animals that are susceptible to becoming overweight a variety of foods, they will overeat. When they have the same diet every day, this doesn't happen. It is this principle I am having you use in keeping your choice of portion-controlled entrees to a limited number.

Breakfast
One Shake or Breakfast Bar
+
One Slice of Toast
+
Coffee, tea

One 8-oz liquid diet drink, made with skim milk. One slice of toast with jelly.

Lunch
One Entrée or Breakfast Bar
Or
One Diet Shake
+
Diet soda, coffee, or tea

One Frozen Meal of about 300 calories
Or
One 8-oz liquid diet drink, made with skim milk.

Dinner
One Entrée
+
Two Vegetables
+
Two Fruits
+
Diet soda

One Frozen Meal with of about 300 calories
And
½ cup of 2 cooked vegetables. Fruits, choose two: apple, orange, banana, or ¾ cup of fruit juice or ½ cup of sliced fruit.

Bray Portion-Control Plan
Phase I. Intervention Diet (approximately 1250 calories)
A scheme for using portion-control meals, formula diets, and selected food from the Menumax® meal-planning system.

Table 1. Portion-Controlled Meals

		per serving		
Liquid Diet Drinks	Calories	Fat, g	Chol, mg	Sodium, mg
Nestlé Sweet Success:				
Chocolate Raspberry Truffle	200	3	-	210
Creamy Milk Chocolate	200	3	-	230
Dark Chocolate Fudge	200	3	-	210
Rich Chocolate Almond	200	3	-	230
Ultra Slim Fast:				
Chocolate Royale	220	3	5	220
Coffee	200	3	5	300
French Vanilla	210	3	5	220
Powder Diet Drinks				
California Slim:				
Chocolate	220	3	-	190
Vanilla	220	3	-	190
Mix with Juice	220	<1	-	40
Nestlé Sweet Success:				
Creamy Milk Chocolate	180	2	-	280
Dark Chocolate Fudge	180	2	-	280
Twinfast:				
Vanilla	80	<1	-	180
Slim-Fast:				
Chocolate Malt	190	1	-	230
Ultra Slim-Fast:				
Mix with Juice	200	<1	-	80
Ultra Slim-Fast Plus:				
Café Mocha	180	<1	-	260
Chocolate Fantasy	250	2	-	330
Dutch Chocolate (99% lactose free)	190	2	-	200
Mix with juice	250	1	-	80
Strawberry	190	1	-	250
Vanilla	190	1	-	250

Commercial Portion-Controlled Entrees

Healthy Choice Dinners:	Serving (oz)	Calories	Fat (g)	Sat Fat (g)	Chol (mg)	Sodium (mg)
Beef Enchilada	13.4	370	5	2	30	450
Beef Pepper Steak	11	290	6	3	65	530
Beef Sirloin Tips	11.75	280	8	3	65	370
Breast of Turkey	10.5	290	5	2	45	420
Chicken and Pasta Divan	11.5	310	4	2	60	510
Chicken Dijon	11	260	3	1	45	420
Chicken Enchilada	13.4	340	5	2	30	470
Chicken Oriental	11.25	230	1	<1	45	460
Chicken Parmigiana	11.5	270	3	2	50	240
Herb Roasted Chicken	12.3	290	4	2	50	430
Lemon Pepper Fish	10.7	300	5	1	40	370
Mesquite Chicken	10.5	340	1	<1	45	290
Pasta Primavera	11	280	3	2	15	360
Salisbury Steak	11.5	300	7	3	50	480
Salsa Chicken	11.25	240	2	1	50	450
Shrimp Creole	11.25	230	2	<1	60	430
Shrimp Marinara	10.5	260	1	<1	60	320
Sirloin Beef w/ BBQ sauce	11	300	6	3	50	320
Sole au Gratin	11	270	5	3	55	470
Sweet and Sour Chicken	11.5	280	2	<1	50	260
Turkey Tetrazzini	12.6	340	6	3	40	490
Yankee Pot Roast	11	260	4	2	55	310
Healthy Choice Entrees						
Baked Cheese Ravioli	9	250	2	1	20	420
Baked Potato w/ Broccoli and Cheese Sauce	10	240	5	2	15	510
Beef Fajitas	7	210	4	2	35	250
Beef Pepper Steak	9.5	250	4	2	40	340
Cheese Manicotti	9.25	220	3	2	30	310
Chicken a l'Orange	9	240	2	<1	45	220
Chicken and Vegetables	11.5	210	1	<1	35	490
Chicken Chow Mein	8.5	220	3	1	45	440
Chicken Enchiladas	9.5	280	6	2	30	510
Chicken Fajitas	7	200	3	1	35	310
Chicken Fettuccini	8.5	240	4	2	45	370
Fettuccini Alfredo	8	240	7	2	45	370
Glazed Chicken	8.5	220	3	1	45	390
Lasagna with Meat Sauce	10	260	5	2	20	420

Linguini w/ Shrimp	9.5	230	2	1	60	420
Macaroni and Cheese	9	280	6	3	20	520
Macaroni and Cheese (17 oz)	8.5	260	5	2	15	490
Mandarin Chicken	11	260	2	<1	50	400
Rigatoni in Meat Sauce	9.5	260	6	2	30	540
Roasted Turkey and Mushroom in Gravy	8.5	200	3	1	40	380
Seafood Newburg	8	200	3	1	55	440
Sole w/ Lemon Butter Sauce	8.25	230	4	2	45	430
Spaghetti w/ Meat Sauce	10	280	6	2	20	480
Zucchini Lasagna	11.5	250	3	2	15	400

Weight Watchers Entrees	Serving, oz	Calorie	Fat, g	Sat fat, g	Chol, mg	Sodium, mg
Barbecue Glazed Chicken	7	200	6	3	30	450
Beef Sirloin Tips	7.5	210	6	3	30	560
Beef Stroganoff	8.5	280	9	1	30	590
Chicken a la King	9	230	4	1	30	460
Chicken a l'Orange	8	200	1	0	15	320
Chicken Chow Mein	9	200	1	0	20	480
Chicken Cordon Bleu	7.7	170	5	1	50	560
Chicken Francais	8.5	150	1	0	10	390
Chicken Kiev	7	190	5	2	15	470
Chicken Marsala	8	110	1	0	10	340
Chicken Mirabella	9.2	160	1	0	10	480
Chicken Nuggets	5.9	220	7	2	40	500
Fiesta Chicken	8	200	1	0.5	15	460
Grilled Chicken Suiza	8.5	240	6	2	35	590
Grilled Glazed Chicken	8	130	1	0	10	460
Homestyle Chicken/Noodles	9	240	7	2	30	450
Honey Mustard Chicken	7.5	140	1	0.5	15	340
Imperial Chicken	8.5	210	4	1	25	420
Lemon Herb Chicken Piccata	7.5	170	1	0	15	520
Tex-Mex Chicken	8.3	260	4	1.5	35	430
Grilled Salisbury Steak	8.5	250	9	3	30	590
London Broil	7.5	110	3	1	25	320
Fried Fillet of Fish	7.7	230	8	2.5	25	450
Oven Baked Fish	7	150	4	1	10	260
Southern Baked Chicken	6.3	170	7	2	45	520
Nacho Cheese Enchiladas	8.9	250	6	2.5	25	520
Nacho Grande Chicken Enchiladas	9	290	8	2.5	20	560
Shrimp Marinara	8	150	1	-	25	400

Roast Turkey Medallions	8.5	190	1	0	15	490
Stuffed Turkey Breast	8.5	270	8	3	60	520
Veal Patty Parmigiana	8.2	150	4	1	50	550

Weight Watchers Baked Potatoes:

Broccoli and Ham	11.5	240	5	3	15	520
Broccoli and Cheese	10.5	270	6	6	5	570
Chicken Divan	11.25	280	7	2	30	480
Homestyle Turkey	11.75	250	7	2	60	510
Vegetable Primavera	10	220	7	3	5	460

Weight Watchers Mexican

Beef Enchiladas Ranchero	9.12	190	5	2	20	500
Cheese Enchiladas Ranchero	8.87	260	10	2	25	550
Chicken Enchiladas Suiza	9	230	7	2	40	530
Chicken Fajitas	6.75	210	5	2	25	490

Weight Watchers Pasta

Angel Hair Pasta	10	200	4	1	10	330
Baked Cheese Ravioli	9	240	6	2	30	370
Cheese Manicotti	9.25	260	8	3	25	510
Cheese Tortellini	9	310	6	1	15	570
Chicken Fettuccini	8.25	280	9	3	40	590
Fettuccini Alfredo	8	230	7	2	25	550
Garden Lasagna	11	260	7	2	15	430
Italian Cheese Lasagna	11	290	7	2	20	510
Lasagna	10.25	270	6	2	5	510
Lasagna Florentine	10	190	1	0.5	10	420
Macaroni and Beef	9.5	230	5	1.5	15	540
Macaroni and Cheese	9	260	6	2	20	550
Pasta Portofino	9.5	150	1	0	0	270
Ravioli Florentine	8.5	170	1	0	10	530
Romanoff Supreme	9.5	240	8	3	25	570
Spaghetti with Meat Sauce	10	240	7	1	5	490
Swedish Meatballs	9	280	8	3	30	510
Three Cheese Rotini	9.5	270	9	3	10	460
Tuna Noodle Casserole	9.5	240	7	2.5	15	580

Weight Watchers Pizza

Cheese Pizza	6.03	300	7	2	10	310

Deluxe Combination Pizza	7.32	320	9	2	10	370
Deluxe French Bread Pizza	5.94	260	7	1	10	480
Pepperoni Pizza	6.08	320	8	2	15	550
Pizza Bianca	5.8	330	9	5	20	490
Sausage Pizza	6.43	340	10	2	10	380
Three Cheese Pizza	6.07	320	6	3	20	350

Weight Watchers Sandwiches

Chicken and Broccoli Pita	5.4	190	5	1	5	420
Grilled Chicken Sandwich	4	210	6	2	20	420
Handy Pocket-Cheese						
Sauce and Ham	4	200	6	2	5	490

Ultra Slim-Fast Entrees

Beef Pepper Oriental	12	320	3	2	35	840
Cheese Ravioli	12	330	3	2	40	770
Chicken Chow Mein	12	320	6	2	60	580
Chicken Fettuccini	12	390	11	4	65	960
Chicken and Vegetables	12	290	3	0	30	850
Country Style Vegetables						
and Beef Tips	12	210	5	2	50	930
Lasagna w/ Meat Sauce	12	330	9	3	55	980
Mesquite Chicken	12	440	1	0	45	370
Mushroom Gravy over						
Salisbury Steak	10.5	290	5	3	35	830
Roasted Chicken						
w/Rice Medley	12	270	3	1	50	740
Shrimp Creole	12	240	4	1	80	730
Shrimp Marinara	12	290	3	1	70	880
Spaghetti w/Beef and						
Mushroom Sauce	12	330	9	3	40	810
Sweet and Sour Chicken	12	320	1	0	40	470
Tomato Sauce over Meatloaf	10.5	340	9	3	35	780
Turkey Medallions						
in Herb Sauce	12	330	5	2	55	720
Turkey w/Glaze Sauce						
and Dressing	10.5	340	5	2	50	570
Vegetable Lasagna	12	240	4	2	15	730

Lean Cuisine Entrees:

Chicken Chow Mein	9	230	5	1	40	500
Chicken Italiano	9	270	6	1	40	590

Cheese Canoli	9.125	270	8	4	25	590
Fettuccini Alfredo	9	280	7	3	15	570
Fettuccini Primavera	10	260	7	2	20	580
Fiesta Chicken	8.5	240	5	2	40	560
Glazed Chicken and Rice	8.5	250	7	2	50	590
Homestyle Turkey	9.38	230	6	1.5	50	590
Honey Mustard Chicken	7.5	230	4	1	40	540
Broccoli/Cheese Potato	10.25	270	9	3	25	510
Chicken Fettuccini in Alfredo Sauce	10.25	240	6	2	35	540
Lasagna	10.25	280	6	3	25	560
Macaroni/Cheese/Broccoli	9.75	240	7	3	25	560
Mexican Rice w/Chicken	9.13	270	5	1	20	580
Mandarin Chicken	9	270	5	1	35	570
Pasta and Chicken Marinara	9.5	270	6	2	35	460
Teriyaki Stir-Fry	9	260	5	1	30	510
Macaroni and Cheese	9	240	7	3	25	560
Macaroni and Beef	10	250	6	1	25	540
Swedish Meatballs	9.125	290	8	3	55	550
Cheddar Bake w/ Pasta and Vegetables	9	230	7	2	15	540
Chicken Pie	9.5	310	10	2	40	590
Chicken Fettuccini w/ Broccoli	9	250	6	2.5	35	540
Chicken Enchilada Suiza	9	290	5	2	25	490
Marinara Twist	10	280	5	2	10	550
Spaghetti w/Meatballs	9.5	290	7	2	30	550
Oriental Beef	9	250	8	3	30	480

Budget Gourmet Entrees	Serving, oz	Calories	Fat, g	Sat Fat, g	Chol, mg	Sodium, mg
Chicken Breast Primavera	11					
Herb Chicken Breast and Fettuccini	11	280	8	3	55	620
Beef Sirloin Salisbury Steak	11	230	8	3	25	720
Sirloin Beef	10.1					
Beef Sirloin in Wine Sauce	11	280	8	2	25	560
Stir Fry Turkey Breast	11.1					
Teriyaki Chicken Breast	11	290	6	1	30	670
Beef Stroganoff	8.7					
Chicken Au Gratin	10					
French Chicken	10	200	8	3	30	950
Glazed Turkey	9	260	5	2	30	710

Ham/Asparagus	9				
Italian Vegetables and Chicken	10.25	310	8	2	30	690
Mandarin Chicken	10	250	5	1	40	550
Oriental Beef	10	290	8	3	30	670
Pasta/Chicken/Italian	10				
Salisbury Steak	9				
Beef Sirloin		1400	47	16	<300	<2400
Chicken Parmigiana	11	270	9	3	50	530
Stuffed Turkey Breast		240	6	1	30	610
Beef Stroganoff		230	7	3	30	520
Chicken Au Gratin		220	8	4	30	790
Spaghetti w/Chunky Tomato and Meat Sauce	10	300	8	2	35	470

Banquet-Healthy Balance:

Chicken Mesquite		260	6	2	45	600
Salisbury Steak		270	8	4	35	800
Turkey and Gravy w/Dressing		270	5	2	40	750

Le Menu:

Beef Sirloin Tips and Pasta		290	11	-	-	1030

Tyson:

Chicken Marsala	9	180	3	-	47	600
Grilled Chicken	7.75	220	3	-	55	520
Honey Roasted Chicken	9	220	4	-	48	500
Chicken Francais	9	270	11	-	-	790
Chicken Piccata	9	200	4	-	60	550
Chicken Mesquite	9	320	8	-	55	660
Grilled Italian Style Chicken	9	200	3	0	40	440
Chicken Supreme	9	230	6	-	51	480
Glazed Chicken w/Sauce	9.25	240	4	-	44	930

CHAPTER FIFTEEN

Group Support
Getting the Social and Family Support You Need

We all need support from our family and friends. This is particularly true when we are trying to do something difficult—like managing your weight and keeping it off. Over the past ten years at the Pennington Biomedical Research Center, I have been leading our efforts in three nationally funded research programs, where we are using weight loss to reduce health risks. The first study is the Diabetes Prevention Program. To join this program, you had to be at "high" risk for diabetes. We recruited nearly four thousand people nationwide over three years who met this criterion. In this study, participants met one-on-one with a counselor who helped them change their eating behaviors with a focus on losing weight.[1,2] These subjects lost an average of 7% of their body weight. This is about 15% of their excess weight. Many people have kept the weight off for over five years. This study also showed that weight loss could reduce a person's risk of developing diabetes over the first three years by nearly 60%—a great success.

In the second study, we enrolled over five thousand people who already had diabetes to find out whether a changing lifestyle in a weight-loss program could lower their risk of developing serious complications from diabetes.[3,4] In this study, we conducted the behavioral program in groups, rather than one-on-one, and used a portion-controlled diet like the ones described in Chapter 14. The participants lost 8.6% of their body weight in one year on average—nearly 25% of excess weight, which was slightly more weight after one year in this study[4] than in the study described earlier[1]—and many have kept the weight off for up to four years. Whether it was the group treatment or the addition of a portion-controlled diet, we don't know, but it is clear that the combination of strategies is better than either one alone—a point that has been shown time and again.[5,6] The important point is that *groups* appear to be as good as or better than individual support for individuals who are losing weight but that both can be successful. **Tip:** Use whatever support you have available.

Groups

Have you been to Weight Watchers? To Overeaters Anonymous? To a TOPS (Take Off Pounds Sensibly) Club meeting? Each of these programs is organized differently. One is commercial, the other two are non-commercial self-help clubs but with very different approaches.

The fact that each of these programs is doing well tells me there are "different strokes for different folks." You may be someone who benefits from a group setting when you are managing your weight. If so, this chapter is for you. On the other hand, you may be a do-it-yourself-er—someone who prefers to deal with your weight problem within the family or with a few friends. If so, you may want to skip this chapter.

I began to help patients manage their weight problems more than thirty years ago. Initially, I used the medical model. That is, I met with my patients individually, one-on-one. As I learned more about the problems of being overweight, I learned that some people did well this way but others did not. For the latter individuals, I tried a number of different things. This was at the time that behavior modification was first making its big splash, back in the 1970s.[7,8,9] I had an opportunity to test groups *versus* individual treatment when we were evaluating a new drug for weight loss. For some of the people, we organized groups, and for others, we used individual treatment. The behavioral program provided in groups was clearly helpful for people managing their weight.

Group support can also be found on the Internet. And the Internet can be used to deliver weight-loss programs.[10,11] The advantage of the Internet is that people don't have to get into their cars to drive to a meeting place. The downside of the Internet is that personal interaction is reduced or absent. As we have already learned, those people who actively participate in an Internet support program can do as well and sometimes better than those who do not.

We learned two important lessons here. First, we found that groups kept people coming for a longer period of time than did individual attention. Groups did not necessarily help them lose more weight, but they did keep them coming. And if people are not coming back for help, we cannot provide them with what they need. Adding individualized feedback to an Internet program and providing a chat room are helpful additions. Groups can be helpful in keeping people interested. This is, in part, because people develop sharing relationships, which helps with hard times and bumps in the road of weight management. Not everybody will have a good week or a bad week at the same time. Ups and downs are a part of life and a part of managing your weight. The support provided by the people who were "up" one week was important to the people who were "down" that week. In another week, the participants might reverse these roles. In addition to this support, groups provided opportunities for role-playing for those difficult situations that people managing their weight confront regularly.

We learned something else from these groups. Not all groups are the same. Both the leaders and members are important. Our initial group leaders were two physicians, a nurse, a dietitian, and a recent college graduate. We thought physicians might do better as group leaders because of the aura of authority they are supposed to have. No such luck. In fact, the groups led by the physicians were no better or worse than the other groups.

Group Leaders

Group leaders are important, however. There was a big difference among the three non-medical group leaders. One leader had fewer subjects at the end than the other two. The people in this group also lost less weight. Some people are just better at leading groups and providing the enthusiasm that gets people to return than are other leaders. Professional experience is not a necessary requirement. Our physicians weren't better than the non-physicians, and one dietitian was much better than the nurse and the college graduate. Then what is important, you might ask? I think it is empathy. Leaders who can empathize with you are much better. When I search for group leaders, I look for someone who has lost weight and has been successful in keeping the weight off. They know what they are talking about. They have "been there and done that" and can reach out from experience. As a result, they are better able to help you get there, too.

Each group has its own structure. Overeaters Anonymous was patterned after Alcoholics Anonymous. If you are the type of person who is excited by a "revival" type of commitment when you are managing your weight, then Overeaters Anonymous may be your cup of tea, so to speak. There are chapters of Overeaters Anonymous all over the United States. The headquarters is in Torrance, California.

Take Off Pounds Sensibly (TOPS) was organized in Milwaukee, Wisconsin, and that is where its headquarters are located. TOPS is a not-for-profit group that organizes "social" clubs and has weigh-ins. The support this approach provides may be for you. They do not subscribe to a specific program, and they do not have the "revival" atmosphere that goes with Overeaters Anonymous.

Weight Watchers is a commercial company formerly owned by Heinz Foods. The story of Weight Watchers has been chronicled many times. It began with an enthusiastic group formed in New York.[14] Their diet was based on the Prudent Diet developed by Dr. Norman Jolliffe.[15] I thoroughly recommend the dietary principles of Dr. Jolliffe, who was head of the New York Department of Health. Jean Nidetch, the founder of Weight Watchers, was using the Prudent Diet. She and a group of friends developed an effective support system for weight loss. Gradually they developed franchises in the United States and then around the world. Weight Watchers became both a national and then an international success. You can find groups in many cities. The Weight Watchers group leaders meet the criteria I described above. They have been overweight. They have lost weight. They have kept the weight off and have the empathy to develop groups.

The Weight Watchers program has changed over time. They have developed a line of foods, which are available in frozen food sections of supermarkets. This was the reason that Heinz Foods bought them. In addition to changing the diet with the times, Weight Watchers has added a behavior-modification program originally designed by one of the founders of behavior modification.[16] This, too, has evolved. The opinion of most experts is that Weight Watchers provides a valuable service to many people. There are also clinical trials showing the efficacy of the Weight Watchers program.[17,18]

Several other commercial programs are available, including Jenny Craig, Nutri-System, Herbalife, and LA Weight Loss, but clinical trials establishing the effectiveness of these programs have not been published.

There are many other groups for behavioral support during weight loss that I have not described because many of them are local. Your hospital or medical clinic may well have one. Others are run by psychologists, and still others are found in university clinics. The YMCA and the YWCA often have groups helping people manage their weight. With the facilities they have for exercise, this is often a good place to start looking. If you are a person who likes groups and can find one in your community, great.

A final option is to develop a group of your own based on the principles I present here. If you and a few friends read this book, you have the basis for developing your own support group. There are a number of options available.

CHAPTER SIXTEEN

Diets, Fads, and Residential Programs

Rating Diets

New Diets—New Diets. How can you tell which is for you? The list below will give you some guidelines. These guidelines were adapted from a book by Theodore Berland called *Consumer Guide: Rating the Diets* (Consumer Guide, 1975).[1] I think they provide a good basis for evaluating any weight-loss program, including the present one.

1. Has the author(s) of the diet tried it on hundreds, even thousands, of overweight people, objectively compared the results against a number of similar people on regular or other weight-reducing diets, and published the findings in a recognized and reputable medical journal?

2. Is the diet based on sound nutritional principles?
   √   The dietary plans described in this book are based on the advice of the National Research Council's Food and Nutrition Board.[2]

3. Is the diet based on some "secret" no one discovered before? If the answer is yes, move on. These secrets do not exist. Remember, though, you can lose weight, temporarily, on any diet. Just paying attention to what you eat will do it, at least for a while.
   √   But there are many useful eating habits that you can adopt, which I have outlined for you in this book.

4. Is the diet well balanced nutritionally? If the answer is no, be careful. Only well-balanced diets are safe.
   √   A well-balanced diet includes food from all of the MyPyramid basic food groups: grains, fruits, vegetables, meat/protein, and dairy. We focus here, however, on reducing fructose and fat (the "deadly duo"). Diets that are deficient in the amounts of food provided in

301

any of these groups are not balanced. Diets with fewer than about 800 calories a day should be medically supervised. Sound nutrition is the basis of our Menumax nutrient-density diets.

5. Is the person promoting the diet known, well respected, and knowledgeable in nutrition? If the answer is no, he or she may be a fast-buck artist who has no regard for your health and safety.

 √ While many physicians have published books on diets, simply being a physician does not qualify one in nutrition. My entire career of more than forty years has been spent working with overweight people and their problems, most recently as Executive Director of the Pennington Biomedical Research Center in Baton Rouge, Louisiana, where the study of obesity is one of the major areas of research. I have already published more than one thousand and six hundred papers, reviews, and abstracts, mostly on obesity.

6. How long has the diet been around? If less than five years, view it with suspicion. Anyone can invent a new diet, but only a few diets survive. At the same time, many bad old diets that have been resuscitated should have been left to their eternal rest. Examples are the high-fat and low-carbohydrate diets. Beware that longevity alone is not a guarantee.

 √ The basis for the Bray Plan Low-Fructose Approach diet was developed in the 1970s. It was selected for a training film by the American Medical Association in 1980 and has been used in a number of hospitals in Los Angeles and on the east coast for more than twenty-five years.

7. Is the proponent of the new diet challenging the recommendations of the best authorities? It's okay to challenge, but a valid challenge has to be backed up with new findings that should be available for scrutiny. Beware the diet huckster who challenges everything in sight but has no substantial scientific data.

8. Does the diet allow for individual preference, practice, and taste? The meal plan should be flexible and allow you to eat the foods you like and eat meals according to the rhythm of your life activities. Rigid diets that tell you what and when to eat and give you no nutritional information are doomed to fail in the longrun.

 √ In Chapter 7, I helped you identify your individual needs and then outlined a number of dietary plans, allowing you to choose what works best for you.

9. Could you live on this diet for the rest of your life? Weight management is a full-time, lifelong project. One-week or fourteen-day diets offer temporary weight loss, at best. Then what? You need to take weight off and keep it off. That means a full-time, full-life plan.

 √ The Menumax® meal planning system and Bray Plan Monitors for your activities are designed to do just these things for you.

10. Is the claim made that the diet is based on principles of another expert or a health association? If so, what do THEY think of this diet? More than one popular, best-selling diet book has been written by one person and based on another's research. In just about every case, the original proponent of the principle was not consulted and, in fact, would not have approved of the other's work, which often perverted sound principles.

√   The principles I have used in this book are solid and tested by my own experience over the past forty years.

These guidelines can help you evaluate any program, not just the Low-Fructose Approach outlined here. You can lose weight with any diet if you follow it faithfully. Eating fewer calories than you need will do it every time.[3] The question you should ask is whether the program can help you maintain the weight loss, if that is your goal. Here is where few programs meet their test.

The popular diets today focus on such plans as high-protein, low-fat, balanced reduction in energy, reduced glycemic index diet, or special diet fads, such as "eat all of the grapes you want." Is one combination of nutrients better than another? An analysis of popular diets[4] suggests they all end up producing about the same level of calorie intake, so one might guess they would produce similar weight losses. Two studies have compared four popular diets in a head-to-head trial. The first study was done in Boston.[5] The Atkins Diet,[6] the Ornish Diet,[7] the Protein Power Diet,[8] and the Weight Watchers diet[9] were used. About one hundred sixty men and women were included. On *average*, there was a modest weight loss with each diet. It was about five pounds after six months and was similar for all diets. What was remarkable was the wide variation in success with each diet. For each diet, there were some people who did very well indeed, while others did not. Those who did well were able to stick to that particular diet. Like any other "treatment," if you don't follow the diet precisely, it doesn't work as well. This study supports one of the pivotal points of this book—there are different strokes for different folks. I always enlist my patients' advice on what dietary plan they might want to try. If the things we develop together work, then I encourage them to stay with it. If they don't work, we always have something else to try.

The second head-to-head comparison was done at Stanford University in California.[10] Only premenopausal women were included. In this trial the Atkins low-carbohydrate diet,[6] the Ornish low-fat diet,[7] and the Protein Power[8] (high-protein) diet were compared to a LEARN Manual[11] for behavior weight loss. After six months, the women eating the Atkins diet were slightly but significantly lighter than the other three groups.

To decide for ourselves, a colleague at Harvard and I designed an even larger study that included eight hundred men and women.[12] The trial was done in Boston and Baton Rouge. There were four diets: high protein (25%)-high fat (40%), high protein (25%)-low fat (20%), low protein (15%)-high fat (40%), and low protein (15%)-low fat (20%). This combination of protein and fat produced four levels of carbohydrate intake: 35%, 45%, 55%, and 65%, providing a good range of values. The trial lasted for two years, twice as long as the other trials. In addition, all participants had the same behavioral and lifestyle group support as well as access to a computer tracking system from which they could get feedback on how well they were following their specific diet. After six months there was no difference in weight loss, and at two years with nearly 80% of the people reporting, weight losses were similar and not affected by the composition of the diet. From this study, I would conclude as I have that the type of macronutrients in the diet is not a deciding factor in whether you lose weight and how much.[13]

Fads: Hope Springs Eternal

It is the hope that the next diet will "cure my weight problem" that provides the market for the new crop of diet books that appear every year. By this time, you should realize there are no magic dietary combinations, but there are valuable things you can do to manage your weight.

The fact that hope springs eternal also provides a market for some of the most "imaginative" ideas around. For example, one advertisement I particularly like says "This is it! EternaSlim. The Complete One Night Weight Loss Program." The ad holds out the hope that you can lose weight at night by taking a special pill. We all lose weight during the night, however, since we are calling on our energy stores to provide the energy we need to fuel our body. This product promotes an amino acid that is alleged to release growth hormone, one of our natural hormones, and this will increase weight loss at night. We are already losing weight at night, however, and there is no evidence that this product adds to that weight loss. It is a clever but deceptive gimmick.

On the metabolic ward in the hospital where I trained, we had a bed that was mounted on a scale that was so sensitive it could weigh a nickel (5 grams). We had our overweight and normal-weight patients sleep in this bed. Every night, every patient lost weight! The reason is simple: Following the evening meal, they had to use the food they ate plus the food stored in fat from previous meals for their bodily needs. Everyone loses weight when asleep. Any treatment I give you will cause you to lose weight overnight. The question is whether the treatment caused you to lose more weight than if you had not used the treatment. This advertisement for EternaSlim does not tell us, but I doubt it.

Among the items that have been touted as aids to help you lose weight are "Cholecystokinin," Konjac Glucomannan, phenylalanine, arginine, and others. These are dealt with in Chapter 21.

Residential Programs

No two people are identical. What works for you may not work for another. What works for you now may not work for you at another time. The material I have presented in previous chapters gives you several options and ways of maintaining the success you achieve and new options to use when needed.

One of my first patients was a very heavy man.[14] He sold commercial real estate. He weighed over 400 pounds. Every other year he would make a trip to Dr. Kempner's Rice Diet program at Duke University. He would lose a large amount of weight and then return to his business. Over the next twelve to twenty-four months, he would regain all of the weight he had lost, to surpass his previous peak weight. He would then return for another period at the residential weight program. And so it went.

How good are residential weight-control programs? While you are there, they will help you lose weight. If the program is a good one, it will also help you with a number of aspects of your lifestyle that can help you remain thinner. This could include instruction in a lower-fat diet, learning how to become more active and how to optimize various areas of personal hygiene. You may also participate in groups for behavioral and lifestyle change. The rub comes when you leave. If the small amount of weight you lose is what you want, you may be fulfilled. If you are like my former patient, this may not be enough.

Select carefully. If you can afford a residential weight-control program, there are many to select from, but do it carefully. I prefer ones that are run by health professionals or that have a significant involvement of health professionals with an interest in weight loss. The materials the residential program sends should also tell you about the diet they use and other items in the program. Shop carefully.

CHAPTER SEVENTEEN

Cellulite and Spot Reducing

Spot Reducing

Do you have bumpy thighs? Most overweight women and many not-so-overweight ones do, particularly as they get older. Let me share with you a poem written at Christmas as a new cream designed to smooth your thighs was being released.

> *T'is the week before Christmas, I've tears in my eyes.*
> *Because you been so remiss with my thighs.*
> *My stockings are stuffed with pockets of fat*
> *But you still don't give a darn about that!!!*
> *But all the while I have this dream*
> *That under the tree will be a thigh cream*
> *That simply applied will melt away inches*
> *Making me gorgeous, encouraging clinches*
> *So be a friend, be a gent.*
> *This little gift won't cost you a cent.*
> *Get on the phone and scout up a jar*
> *Otherwise...I will blow up your car!*

A colleague of mine received this poem from a well-known actress and promptly called my office, where I was able to keep him from having his car blown up.

The idea of spot-reducing is as old as the cosmetic industry. Many things have been tried. You can get massages. You can use saunas. Herbs have been used. So have "slim jeans," tight jeans to compress the fat. In spite of all of the efforts, there was no real progress until we began to understand how fat cells work. When I first reviewed the treatments for spot-reducing about, there was nothing that was effective.

A lot has changed since then. First, we have learned a lot about how fat gets into and out of fat cells. We have also learned how fat cells are put together to make fat lobules—what you may call cellulite. Your individual fat cells (and you have more than forty to sixty billion of them, which is nearly ten times the world's population) are grouped together in golf ball-sized collections. Surrounding each of these collections is a connective tissue package, which holds them in place and anchors them to the skin. The dimpling you see on the skin of your thighs and buttocks results from the enlargement of individual fat cells, which stretches the connective tissue tight. When a number of golf ball-sized collections stretch their connections to the skin, the skin between these collections of fat is pulled in, producing the dimpling or "cellulite" appearance.

Once upon a time, I didn't believe in cellulite. Cellulite was a "different" kind of fat.[1] But we scientists believed that all fat cells are the same. I gave up that view in 1978, when the work on a treatment for cellulite began. I became a believer as I learned more about how fat cells work and the differences in their function in different locations on the body.

Thigh Cream for Cellulite

If you already know about fat cells, you don't need to read the next paragraph. Fat cells are the major storehouse for our body fat. They have many functions, but chief among them is storing fat. Fat storage is like a bank account. When you deposit money, your account balance increases. When you deposit fat, the fat account increases and the fat cell enlarges. When you withdraw money from your bank account, the balance declines. So, too, with fat cells. When the body is using fat for energy, it "withdraws" fat from your fat cells. Deposits and withdrawals of fat are occurring all the time.

The storage of fat in a fat cell is regulated by a delicate chemical balance. The principal actor is a factor that helps the fat cell take fat from the blood and deposit it in the fat cell. The hormone, insulin, which comes from your pancreas, plays an important role in this process. You know insulin through its relation to diabetes. When insulin is absent or relatively ineffective, people become diabetic.

The removal of fat from a fat cell is also a delicate balance. On the one hand are the various factors that stimulate or activate fat cells to release their fat stores. On the other side are factors that can slow down the release of fat. I had been working on the chemical messengers for the breakdown of fat for many years. In 1978 I took a leave of absence from my university to learn more about the process. By this time, it was clear that fat cells on the thigh and buttocks were different from those on the stomach area. Both were different from the fat cells that line the interior of the body. The differences lay in the way that fat breakdown was controlled. When you want to slow your car down, you can take your foot off the accelerator, you can use the brake pedal, you can shift to a lower gear, or you can use the hand-brake. Likewise, there are a number of different controls determining how fat is broken down, just like the many ways to stop your car.

Cells on the thighs and buttocks break down fat more slowly than those on the abdomen. This occurs because of a difference in the chemical balance of hormones that affect fat cells. I knew the kinds of chemical signals that could mobilize or break down fat, as well as the signals that stopped this process. I decided to try to reduce the "cellulite" deposits by directly applying the chemicals to the thigh in a formulation that could be absorbed by the cells just below the skin. As with many of my studies on patients, this work was conducted with my longtime friend and associate, Dr. Frank Greenway.

We decided to do our first study by giving the chemical by injection.[2] Women who were concerned about the dimpling of their cellulite were asked if they wanted to evaluate a new treatment that had been reviewed by the Food and Drug Administration and approved for an Investigational New Drug License. The volunteer women were treated with a number of small injections to each thigh. One thigh got the active chemical, and the other thigh an inactive one. As our earlier work in the test tube had predicted, the treated thigh became thinner, near the site of the injection.[2]

This was the beginning. Our predictions had worked. But certainly not many women were going to be interested in receiving a course of injections for their "cellulite." Could we deliver the chemicals to the skin with a cream? After some thinking, we decided we would broaden the search for treatments and use available agents that activated fat breakdown. We also planned tests for agents that would release the "brakes" on fat breakdown. Under the same Investigational New Drug License from the Food and Drug Administration, we developed three separate creams.[3] Patients who were concerned about their thigh dimpling again volunteered. Women's thighs are particularly good for these studies because each woman has two of them. One can serve as the "treated" side and the other as the "non-treated" side. A cream with active ingredients was applied to one thigh. The other thigh received the cream without active ingredients. We measured the size of each thigh before and during treatment. As predicted, each of the treatments reduced the size of the treated thigh.

So much for the early science of our discoveries. At this point, we published our results in a scientific journal and looked for someone to develop the idea. To our surprise, several major drug companies and cosmetic companies were not interested. We continued to conduct research on our idea. Finally in 1993, a fourth study was presented at a scientific meeting and received wide publicity.[4,5] From that point on, many different groups were interested.

The cosmetic element used in the cream has been available for many, many years. It is chemically similar to the caffeine in coffee or the theophylline in tea. Both of these chemicals have been in the food supply for a long time. The safety thus seemed to us to have been clearly established. The chemical we used is available as an over-the-counter agent for treatment of asthma. Why can't I take it by mouth, you ask? Simple. When you do that, it gets to all of the fat cells, and the net effect is zero. Only when it reaches the edges of those taut, golf ball-like lobules of fat can you reduce the tension of the part next to the skin and smooth the dimpling.

Removal of fat from the dimpled thighs will take a few weeks. Once removed, it will gradually reaccumulate if the treatment is stopped. Thus the treatment will need to be repeated at intervals.

CHAPTER EIGHTEEN

Success at Behavioral Control of Eating

Your Eating Behavior

- Eating is a habit; that is, we do it repeatedly, and often without giving much thought to it.
- Weight gain, for many people, results from overeating, and overeating is often due to poor eating habits that have developed over long periods of time.
- Weight may be controlled by identifying these "problem" habits and then changing them into new, more positive eating habits. We have already talked about thinking positively in Chapter 3. The changes can be permanent—a feature missing when you simply eliminate specific foods rather than changing your eating behavior.
- To make the changes, you must first systematically observe and become aware of the habits that control your eating patterns. Then you can identify and assume control over the problem areas. You may think you are aware of everything you eat now, but until you do it using the system I describe here, you will not have a realistic picture of your eating behavior.

What is the rationale for this behavioral approach to eating?

Behavior is produced by various cues or signals. There are many cues that may lead to eating, some of which are appropriate and some of which are not. For example, boredom, anxiety, depression, and the smell of food may be inappropriate cues for eating. Likewise, hunger, mealtimes, and certain social occasions are more appropriate cues. You must learn to identify the appropriate cues for eating and learn to substitute non-eating activities for those times when you respond to inappropriate cues.

You will discover the details of your own eating patterns in terms of what, why, when, where, and how you eat. We will examine each of these factors so you can become more fully aware of them.

Analyzing Your Eating

- Remember, eating is a behavior that is initiated by cues or triggers (stimuli) that lead to a response. This diagram in Figure 1 shows these relationships.
- An association between each of these cues and the response of eating develops because at some time the cue was rewarded by eating. Although the initial rewards may no longer exist, the response of eating continues because of the earlier associations.

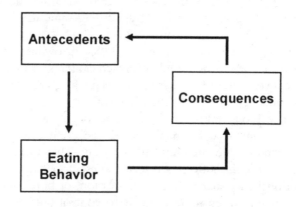

Chain of Behaviors

Component	Elements
Antecedents	The events that are associated with and that can serve as triggers for eating events.
Behaviors of eating	The time and place of eating. The rate of eating. The amount eaten.
Consequences of eating	Using rewards for modifying antecedents and eating behaviors, such as point systems.

311

Figure 1. The relation of antecedents of eating, which stimulate the act of eating, and the consequences of eating, which can be positive or negative.

> To cite some examples: 1) The smell of food when you enter a house may trigger salivation and hunger. Eating satisfies the desire created by the smell of food. 2) When you were a child, you may have found that eating relieved feelings of anger or boredom. If so, you would tend to eat again whenever you became angry or bored. 3) You may accept food offered at a party because you don't want to offend the hostess. Eating the food provides you with a reward in the form of the hostess' pleasure and appreciation, as well as a general feeling of social acceptance from the other guests.

Cues to Start and Stop Eating

The following are some of the cues or signals that may cause you to start or stop eating. The goal of this section is to determine which ones are important to you and to help you control them.

Physiological cues include hunger, tension, growling stomach, headache, and the like. These are the stimuli for which eating is an appropriate response. There are two kinds of external cues. The first are what we might call "non-human." They include the sight of food, smells of food, reading, watching television, and others. These types of cues are most easily identified and may be controlled by manipulating the events around us. The other groups of external cues are "human" in origin. They include the presence of friends, social events, coffee breaks, etc. These, too, can be controlled.

Emotional cues such as anger, depression, or boredom can also induce eating. These are often more difficult to control but can be dealt with by changing the rewards and activities to which we respond.

Common Cues to Start Eating with Recommended Responses

Physiologic Cues	Suggested Controls
Growling Stomach Salivation Faintness Uneasy Feeling Headache Hunger Fatigue Tension Suggested Controls	The body produces these sensations when it expects or needs food. They are best controlled by always making it a habit to eat at a specific time. Establish a meal pattern, stick to it regularly, and these sensations eventually will appear only when it is time to eat, as planned. Make a ritual of where and when you eat. Substitute low calorie food; keep prepared carrot sticks crisp and accessible for between meal snacks or appetizers when sensations of "hunger" appear.
Bad taste in mouth (or oral sensations)	Use mouthwash, toothpaste or mouth spray

External Cues (non-human)	Suggested Controls
Thoughts of food	Try to make yourself think of something else. Daydream.
Shopping for food	Do it alone (friends and children increase the tendency to impulse-buy). Always shop from a list. Never shop when hungry.
Cooking	Tell yourself the meal you are preparing is so great you don't want to spoil your appetite by nibbling. Choose low-calorie munchies or sip lemon-flavored water or low-calorie drinks. If you train yourself to sit down to eat, it is harder to eat when cooking.
Smell of food	Use the same controls as for cooking (above). In a shopping center, plan to detour or avoid places emitting tempting odors.

External Cues (non-human)	Suggested Controls
Time of day (includes getting home from work, which may have some emotional cue component as well). Others at table are finished Weekends and holidays	Try to select or prepare low-calorie foods. Utilize built-in delays, as with other activities besides eating. Be the one to help the hostess.
Reading or other associated activities	Do not stand or sit within easy reach of food.

External Cues (human)	Suggested Controls
Others eating at meal times Social events, parties, entertaining, etc.	At a cocktail party, try a drink made of soda and lemon juice; no one can tell it's not a gin & tonic. Avoid alcohol, since even one drink can poison your control.
	Slow eating to match pace of others at table. If you often eat with others, using this cue can really reduce total intake.

External Cues	Suggested Controls
Depression (includes feelings of failure) Frustration Anger Boredom Lonely Guilt Rebellion Feelings of deprivation	These negative emotions are common cues to start eating. Food can provide a temporary distraction or self-soothing. Eating does not resolve the roots of these feelings, however. Attempt to identify emotional eating and substitute other behaviors, which can put these negative feelings to rest. Develop a positive attitude, which can be used in a cheerful, optimistic, and self-motivating way.

There are two groups of cues that signal us to stop eating. The following list identifies some of these, with suggestions for gaining control of the internal and external signals.

Your goal is to develop new responses to strengthen and increase the frequency of cues that are already identified as "stopping" eating, with emphasis on using positive or appropriate types of control rather than negative, inappropriate reactions.

Physiologic Cues	Suggested Controls
Full (satisfied)	If only fullness stops your eating, you can never lose weight. Find or develop other cues to stop. If you don't know how, weigh food, eat to fullness, and then next time take a smaller portion.
Belt feels tight	Try tightening the belt one notch before starting to eat.
Drowsiness	A definite signal to stop eating immediately. You can lose control when you are not fully alert and not concentrating.
Indigestion (discomfort)	A personal sense you must study. Is it pure overeating? Is it certain foods or combinations of foods? Is it when eating occurs in association with something else (certain mood, time of day, person)? First identify when and why discomfort occurs. Then control the other associated factor.

External Cues (human)

Food tastes bad	This is a useful cue to *decrease* eating. Whenever you eat, be conscious of taste. If unpleasant, stop eating that food immediately. Food often begins to taste less good as you become physiologically satisfied.
Plate empty, i.e., food all gone	Very common for most people. Again demonstrates "externality." Can be used very positively to reduce food intake by choosing smaller plates, cooking only

exact serving sizes, eating slowly so that you are not finished before others at table have ended meal. Buying smaller amounts and shopping more often will also help.

Out of time (end of lunch hour)
Something else you have to do — Can be very helpful. Become a calculating clock watcher and plan your activities. Example: At work, delay beginning of lunch-hour meal by leisurely bathroom visit, stop to chat, a quick trip to the bank, etc. Try to schedule other things to be done during problem-eating times. Commit yourself to trying alternate activities until you find one or more that suit you.

The internal cues are physiologic, such as a full stomach and feelings of satiety. Tight clothing and a tight belt are external cues to this same "internal state." When your belt gets tight, it is a clue that you have eaten too much. These are appropriate cues to which we wish you should attend and respond appropriately.

There are also a number of external cues to decrease eating. An empty plate is obvious. It is one of the most common cues and is relatively easy to control. Next time use a smaller plate, smaller portion sizes, and cook only what you can eat at one serving. Use tall glasses rather than short, squat ones—the optical experience of seeing a glass fill quickly helps you think you are getting more. Do not put serving dishes on the table. When you can see more food, it can stimulate your desire for "seconds." Portion-controlled frozen foods can help here, too.

External cues can also come from human beings. These are usually different people or different situations than those that provide cues to start eating. But we can capitalize on these to help us stop eating earlier.

An understanding of these cues and the exercise that follows are designed to:
1) help you analyze your eating behavior and the specific signals that start and stop your eating;
2) control your extraneous, irrelevant, or distorting cues by breaking their association with eating;
3) reinforce or reward new, healthier controls;
4) substitute other behavior for some eating incidents to help you control the frequency of eating;
5) make eating more pleasurable by increasing your awareness of the taste of food; and
6) increase your awareness of physical hunger as a cue to start and stop eating.

Remember these behavioral goals as you begin to identify the things you do when you eat. Also, keep our goal of reducing the intake of "bad fructose" front and center. Conscious awareness and self-observation are the keys to controlling your eating habits. Set short-term goals and stick to them.

I want you to keep a record of what you are doing every time you eat and learn the places that are associated with your eating. This will help you identify those places that habitually cause you to eat.

You need an honest, current pattern of the things you do when you eat so you can see how to control eating. These are for your benefit to help you lose weight. Some changes may occur simply because you become more aware of what you are doing.

The "Where" of Eating

The first thing to do in analyzing your eating behavior involves identifying and keeping a monitor of the places where you eat. This section has been designed to provide the specific techniques you will use to analyze your eating behavior in terms of where, what, when, why, and how you eat so you may develop conscious control over all your eating behaviors.

Using a 3×5-inch card designed like the one shown below, pay attention to where you are every time you have something to eat or drink. Watch for places that stimulate a desire to eat, such as walking past a bakery or a pizza parlor. Making a list may help you gain better control over the kinds of situations that trigger or stimulate your eating.

Bray Plan Monitor	
MONITOR FOR PLACES OF EATING	
Day	
Food Eaten	Place

Figure 2. Monitor for places of eating. You will use this to record the foods you eat and the places where you eat them. You might assign 1 = kitchen, 2 = dining room, 3 = living room, 4 = work/car, 5 = bedroom, 6 = fast-food restaurant.

This Bray Plan Monitor will help you keep a more detailed record of the places where you eat each day. Keep your record for a full week. There are two columns. On the left, you should write down the food you eat every time you put food in your mouth. Every bite of food—a cracker or a drink of anything except water—must be recorded. This means you must carry the Bray Plan Monitor with you at all times. In the next column, write down the place where you ate that food or drank that beverage. Since many people eat most of their food in only a few places, it may be easier to give numbers to the common places—like kitchen, dining room, den, cafeteria, etc.—and then record only the number.

The purpose of this monitor is to help you observe where you eat and become more consciously aware of eating. The more accurate your records, the easier it will be for you to locate some of your problem areas and then make changes in your eating habits. Be honest and be thorough. You have only yourself to help! This is only one of many records you will learn to keep. If you master it, the others will be easy. Use these guidelines to avoid possible pitfalls.

1. Remember to record everything you eat or drink, and do it immediately.
    *   Concentrate on eating and avoid other activities that can distract you.
    *   Tying a string on your finger may help to remind you of the record-keeping.
    *   Involve your spouse or a friend in the recording.

2. Keep your record even when you do not eat at home.
    *   Have your monitor with you at all times; it is designed to fit into your pocket or purse.
    *   If you prefer to make your recording in private, leave the table and record in the privacy of the bathroom.

3. Learn to identify what goes into the food you eat.
    *   Concentrate on the food and examine what you eat. This is part of the goal in becoming more aware of your eating behavior.
    *   At a friend's house, request the recipe; the cook will be flattered.
    *   At restaurants, it is usual for people who are on special diets (such as diabetics) to request information on ingredients. Pretend to be allergic if necessary.

Analyzing Where You Eat

Now that you have recorded what and where you ate or drank for the past week, I will show you how to analyze these records and recognize your patterns of eating. You may find you need to reduce the number of places where you eat.

Take out the monitors you used during the past week and lay them out in front of you. Below is an illustration of a completed analysis for places of eating to show you what the finished result might look like. The blank form printed below is for you to use. Several places where people commonly eat are printed, and several empty lines have been left for your use. First, add the places where you ate that are not listed on the form.

Bray Plan Monitor ANALYSIS FOR PLACES OF EATING																
	1	2	3	4	5	6	7	8	9	10	11	12	13	14	Add'l	Total
Kitchen																
Dining Rm																
Living Rm																
Work/Car																
Bedroom																
Restaurant																
Other																

Figure 3. Analysis form for recording the number of times you have eaten. Place a mark in a box next to each time you have eaten in that place.

Next, blacken a box opposite the first place you ate on day one. For example, if you ate breakfast in the kitchen, lunch in a restaurant, a snack in your office, dinner in the dining room, and a snack in the kitchen, then there should be two blackened squares for kitchen, one blackened square for dining room, one for work and one for restaurant. Continue to fill in the places you ate until all seven days have been transferred to the analysis sheet. Among the most common places for people to eat these days is in their car and in the bedroom, while watching television. Because these can be settings in which control of food intake is problematic, these are the first ones to concentrate on if they are among your common eating places. Here is an example from one of my patients.

Bray Plan Monitor **ANALYSIS FOR PLACES OF EATING**																
	1	2	3	4	5	6	7	8	9	10	11	12	13	14	Add'l	Total
Kitchen	■	■	■	■	■	■	■	■	■	■	■	■				12
Dining Rm																
Living Rm	■	■	■	■	■	■	■									7
Work/Car	■	■	■	■	■	■	■	■	■	■						10
Bedroom	■	■	■	■	■	■	■	■	■	■	■	■	■			13
Restaurant	■	■														2
Other																

Figure 4. Analysis form for places of eating. Several places have been listed at the left, but they can be replaced with places you eat that are not included. The "other" row is also for places you eat that are not listed.

Controlling Where You Eat

- Certain places often become, by habit of long association, direct cues to eat. They may include ball games, movies, or a chair by the television.
- Some people eat everywhere and anywhere. Instead of saying, "I can't eat," tell yourself, "I can eat only in one or two designated places."
- Eliminate the places not directly associated with food first. But be flexible. For example, if you live in an efficiency apartment, it may not be possible to stop eating in the bedroom. But you don't have to eat in bed!

It may be helpful to make a big occasion of each eating incident. Set a place at your own designated eating area, use special dishes, a special place mat, flowers or candles, and the like.

You may want to designate one special place to eat at home (and also one at work) and simply change the habit of where you eat. Eating only at that place may help you gain control.

If you eat in the cafeteria at work, this is an appropriate place. If you eat at your desk or elsewhere, this may be an appropriate or inappropriate place, depending on your work situation. It is one you need to look at carefully. Circle these inappropriate times and places on your analysis sheet and try to stop eating at your desk. Move to the cafeteria or a different part of the office to eat.

Your goal is to reduce the number of places where you eat. You are now ready to repeat the monitoring for another week to see how successful you have been in changing the number of places you eat. Complete a second analysis form in the same way.

Now you are ready for the second monitor.

What You Are Doing When You Eat

This section is designed to help you become aware of the things you do while you are eating. Remember, eating is a behavior that can be initiated by both internal and external cues. The need to eat is inborn, but the culture in which we are raised teaches us to adapt this need in accepted ways. In our culture, rewards are often associated with food. If the rewards are positive, they will tend to reinforce the association between eating behavior and the cues that lead up to eat. If the rewards are negative, they will tend to weaken these associations.

The goal of this Bray Plan Associated Activity Monitor is to help you focus on the problem areas associated with eating and make step-by-step changes to achieve gradual control. Remember, the more accurately you keep your records, the more they will ultimately help you to change your eating patterns.

In Column 1, write down the foods you eat. It is essential to record every bite and every sip you put in your mouth, including low-or non-calorie foods and drinks. Make your record immediately as you eat. If you do not have your monitor with you, it is better not to record that food or meal at all. Never fill in the monitor from memory. Inaccurate records will mislead you.

In the column on the right, record what you are doing when eating. For example, let's say you are going to sit down and have lunch. You are eating at the dining room table at a friend's house and you are talking. You should record food eaten (such as a fruit salad, soup, and coffee) and the fact that you were talking with your friend.

The most common activities associated with eating are watching television, talking, reading, and preparing food. You may want to give these activities numbers (1–4) and only write out the other things you do while eating. Keep your record for a full week.

Bray Plan Monitor **MONITOR FOR ASSOCIATED ACTIVITY**	
Day	
Food Eaten	Associated Activity

Analyzing What You Are Doing When You Eat

Now that you have a week's record of the activities associated with your eating behavior, you are ready to analyze them. Below is an illustration of what a finished one might look like.

Bray Plan Monitor **ANALYSIS FOR ASSOCIATED ACTIVITY**																
	1	2	3	4	5	6	7	8	9	10	11	12	13	14	Add'l	Total
Reading																
Watching TV																
Preparing Meals																
Talking																

Figure 5. Analysis of activities associated with eating. Use of this monitor is similar to the others. You may want to use 1 = reading, 2 = watching TV, 3 = preparing meals, 4 = car.

Begin by assembling the monitor cards you used this past week. Notice on the analysis form that we have listed the four most common activities associated with eating (reading, watching television, preparing food, and driving your car). There are three blank spaces for any other activities you do often while eating. Fill in a square, beginning at the left, for each instance of eating for a given activity. Do this for the entire week, blackening one square for every time you had something to eat.

Use the blank column labeled "additional" (add'l) for any number or events over 14. This can be done by putting extra check marks in this box to indicate each extra instance of eating. Circle the square if that eating instance consisted only of non-caloric food, such as black coffee, tea, or diet soda. If the beverage had sugar or milk in it or if anything else was con-sumed, do not circle it. Here is an example from one of my patients.

Bray Plan Monitor **ANALYSIS FOR ASSOCIATED ACTIVITY**																
	1	2	3	4	5	6	7	8	9	10	11	12	13	14	Add'l	Total
Reading																4
Watching TV																3
Preparing Meals																2
Talking																3
Other (Car)																2

Figure 6. Analysis form for summarizing activities associated with eat-ing. The blank rows are for adding other places you may eat.

When you have gone through the entire week's records, count the number of checks and boxes and put the total number in the last column labeled "total."

How an Awareness of Associated Activities Can Be Used to Control Eating

Associated activities, like places of eating, can become cues for eating. They can also distract you from focusing on eating. You need to become aware of the activities that accompany eating because research has shown that over-weight people eat more when they are distracted. It is easy to overeat when you are watching television or when you are engrossed in a book or a con-versation. When you aren't paying attention to the food you eat, you can-not use your consciousness to control it. When you eat automatically and unconsciously, it is easy to overeat.

The following guidelines can help you:
- Make a conscious effort to turn off the television and avoid reading when you eat. Your goal is to make eating an enjoyable occasion in itself.
- Avoid being distracted. Distracting events may lead you to eat more than you otherwise would.
- I don't advise "no talking when eating," as eating should be a pleas-ant and sociable time and talking is part of it. But take your mind off the conversation every minute or two to concentrate upon your food and your feelings about it. Concentrate on how you eat.
- Chew food slowly and thoroughly, savoring the flavors. Whenever you eat, you should try to do little else.

- Your goal is to reduce the non-eating activities associated with eating, while enjoying your food more fully.

Substitute Alternative Behavior

A number of cues or signals may trigger an automatic habit of eating, but you can change these patterns. Some added suggestions:

1) **Television food commercials**

    Change channels; mute the channel; leave the room (this also increases exercise); use TIVO to record your favorite programs so you can fast-forward through the ads; do a self-rewarding chore or activity (i.e., wash a shelf, change your clothing, brush your teeth). Try to reduce TV time, especially if TV watching is associated with eating.

2) **Sight of food**

    Keep food out of sight; use opaque containers, which reduce both visual and olfactory cues; repackage food as soon as you bring it home from the market; don't put serving containers on the table; put portions directly on plates; remove leftovers immediately and scrape plates into disposal.

3) **Thoughts of food**

    Try not to think about food; put it out of your mind by thinking about something else—your favorite place, for example. This is a substitute activity, replacing one thought for another.

4) **The way you eat**

    Choose low-calorie foods over foods that are high in calories. Focus on limiting "bad fructose" when you eat. Build in delays in the rate of eating. For example, drink water between bites of food or go to the powder room. Help serve or clear the food as a substitute activity.

5) **Emotional cues**

    Eating is not an appropriate response to emotional situations. Develop substitute activities for boredom or depression, such as taking a hot bath, walking, reading, involving yourself with a hobby, or calling a friend. Eating is not an appropriate response to anger or guilt. Physical exercise often helps relieve this kind of tension. Emotions are generally arousing. This means that happy emotions as well as anger and depression can trigger overeating; therefore, it is important to learn appropriate responses to emotions, as well as knowing which cues and activities may trigger your eating.

After completing your analysis of activities associated with eating, you can apply what you have learned by recording these activities for a second week, using some of the controls and behavioral changes we have discussed.

Are You Hungry When You Eat?

The third Bray Plan Monitor is for your personal evaluation of hunger, that is, how hungry you are every time you have something to eat. It will be helpful to ask yourself these questions:

1) What is hunger?
2) How do you experience hunger?

The following are some of the answers we have had from patients over the years. Which ones do you associate with hunger?

salivation	light-headedness	tension
growling	knots in stomach	weakness
depression	nausea	irritability
headache	"climbing the wall"	anxiety

3) How hungry are you right now? Very hungry, not hungry, or somewhat hungry?
4) How often do you eat when you are not really hungry?

When filling out this monitor, we want you to be able to distinguish between the physical sensations of hunger and the desire to eat. There is a difference between the appetite and hunger. Appetite refers to a desire for food, often for a particular food. Hunger indicates a physiological need for food, usually independent of the type of food.

During the coming week, you will use this monitor for evaluating hunger to record your hunger at the beginning of each meal.

Bray Plan Monitor	
MONITOR FOR HUNGER	
Day	
Food Eaten	Degree of Hunger

Figure 7. Monitor for recording hunger sensations. Rate hunger on a scale of 1 to 5 with 1 = not at all hungry, 2 = slightly hungry, 3 = moderately hungry, 4 = very hungry, 5 = extremely hungry.

- Focus on how hungry you are each time you start to eat.
- Note whether it is a full meal or a snack.
- Each time you start to eat a meal or a snack, take a moment to decide how hungry you are. Use a rating scale of 1 to 5 as follows, which is also on the monitor.
  1 = No hunger
  2 = Slightly hungry
  3 = Moderately hungry
  4 = Very hungry
  5 = Extremely hungry

Define hunger as you sense it. Note the different sensations of hunger you have.

Analyzing Your Feelings of Hunger

Now that you have recorded your relative hunger during one week, you are ready to analyze how this relates to your eating behavior. A sample of what a finished analysis form might look like is shown below.

									Number of Times							
Rating	1	2	3	4	5	6	7	8	9	10	11	12	13	14	Add'l	Total
1																
2																
3																
4																
5																

Bray Plan Monitor
ANALYSIS FOR HUNGER

Figure 8. Analysis of hunger. Check the number of times during the week you rated hunger and each level.

The hunger ratings (1 to 5) are printed in the left column. The number of times you recorded each rating for the past week are printed across the top. Fill in the form as you did before.

- Mark a square alongside the appropriate hunger rating for each time you felt that degree of hunger when starting to eat.
- Use check marks for any "additional" ratings at each level.
- Count all boxes plus "additional" checks and write the total number of each rating.
- Circle any non-caloric food.

Here is a completed example from one of my patients.

	Bray Plan Monitor **ANALYSIS FOR HUNGER**															
Rating	Number of Times															Total
	1	2	3	4	5	6	7	8	9	10	11	12	13	14	Add'l	
1																1
2																3
3																5
4																8
5																3

Hunger is an internal tension, which may be perceived as a headache, depression, anxiety, or a growling sensation. Your goal is to become more responsive to your body's signals for "hunger." There are two factors to consider:

1) Are you finding it easier to identify hunger? If not, keep practicing until you can separate sensations of hunger from other environmental cues.

2) When are you hungry? Some people find it easy to identify hunger patterns; others find it hard. It may help to rearrange your meal schedule to eat when you are hungry; when you identify cues other than true hunger, try to do something other than eat. This is where hobbies and other activities you enjoy are particularly important.

You can begin to control your behavior based on responses to hunger while eating. For the coming week, at one meal each day, stop eating as soon as you realize you are no longer hungry. Select and write down at which meal each day you will practice that response. Select the meal most regularly included in your daily pattern.

Your goal is to learn to "tune in" to your body signals. I want you to understand your personal hunger better and to recognize the "cues" that trigger your appetite. These are some of the results you may expect:

1) Your attitude toward your food may change. Leave waste on the plate, not on your waist. When our parents taught us that waste is "sinful," we were being trained to overeat. But eating more than we need is also "waisting" food. A little wasting (or discarding) of food now can be compensated for later as you learn to shop and eat more economically.

2) You may consider not eating dessert. This might mean taking more food than planned as second helpings in order to stop the feeling of hunger and the urge to eat the wrong foods. Remember, sensory-specific satiety[2] can work for you. We always seem to have room for dessert, so don't have dessert in the house.

For the coming week, ask yourself how hungry you are before a meal or snack and try to eliminate as many ratings in the #1 and #2 columns as you can. You don't have to be ravenous (#5), but try to be moderately hungry before eating (#3 and #4). This may mean skipping a meal if you decide you are not really hungry at that time.

Eating and the Taste of Your Food

Taste is a subjective evaluation that elicits different responses from different people. Ask yourself what taste means to you. Is there a good taste? A bad taste? How do you taste food? Some of the factors that determine our sense of taste include flavor, aroma, and texture. You may gain better control over your eating habits by improving your perception of taste. The number of tastes has gone up since we were in school. The classical ones are sour, bitter, sweet, and salty. Two other tastes have been added. One is "umami," produced by things like monosodium glutamate. The other is the taste for fatty acids that was initially identified at the Pennington Center.[1] In addition to these six tastes, we recognize food by the odors they give off that affect our nose.

Try the following tests with some dehydrated apple slices and some flavored crackers:

- Unwrap the package of dried apples very slowly. Is your mouth watering? If it is, you know that external cues (i.e., the thought, smell, and sight of food) are triggering your hunger. This can be a very strong incentive for eating.
- Take a slice of apple, but do not start eating. Look at the apple. Smell it. What sensation do you perceive?
- Take a small bite, but don't swallow. Chew it thoroughly and slowly. How does it taste?
- Continue to chew slowly. Does the taste change? How?
- Now, repeat the steps with the crackers. First, open the package as slowly as you can. Is your mouth watering?
- Take a cracker, but do not start eating. Look at it, smell it. What do you feel?
- Take a small bite, but don't swallow. Chew it slowly and thoroughly. Try to taste it as intensely as you can. How does it taste? Do the taste and the texture change as you continue to chew the cracker?

What does this test really tell you about tasting food?

- You must chew your food thoroughly.
- Decide how good a food tastes by judging how long its flavor lasts.

Flavors change with enzyme action in saliva, but you won't notice that if you gulp down your food. Appearance, smell, and texture influence the sensation of taste. Food chemists know this very well—that's why some food products can claim that if you take the first bite you will eat the whole package. From now on, try to practice really tasting everything you eat, just as you did with the apples and crackers.

For the next week, your record-keeping will focus on the taste of your food. A sample of the Bray Plan Monitor is shown below.

Bray Plan Monitor **MONITOR FOR TASTE**	
Day	
Food Eaten	Taste of Food

Figure 9. Monitor for taste of foods. Use the following numbers to rate your taste of the foods you select to rate: 1 = poor taste or no taste 2 = fair taste, 3 = good taste, 4 = very good taste, 5 = fantastic taste.

Down the left side, you will write down every food you eat and every beverage you drink. As you are putting the food into your mouth, do what you have just done with the dehydrated apples and the crackers—that is, let the food stay in your mouth for a few seconds, and then chew it slowly. Make an evaluation of the taste on a scale of 1 to 5. Use the following rating scale that is also attached to the figure:

> 1 = Poor taste or no taste
> 2 = Fair taste
> 3 = Good taste
> 4 = Very good taste
> 5 = Fantastic taste

Do this with each different food item that you eat. As you go through the meal bite by bite, note how the taste of the food changes. Record this, too. Do you keep eating after the flavor changes? If so, here may be the opportunity for you to make some changes. Keep this record for one week.

Analyzing Eating and the Taste of Food

Now that you have kept a record of how you taste food for a full week, you can begin to analyze how taste affects your eating habits. A sample taste analysis form is reproduced below. You can see it is similar to the other forms we have used before.

On the left side, you will see the taste ratings (1 to 5); across the top are the number of times you recorded each rating during the past week. Count your ratings and fill in the squares as you did when rating hunger. Circle any non-caloric foods.

Your goal with this monitor is to heighten your taste awareness and your enjoyment of food. In the coming week, try to increase the number of ratings in columns #3 and #4 and to reduce the number of ratings in column #1 and #2. Too many #5 ratings can stimulate overeating.

For the next week, repeat the monitoring of the taste of your foods. As you did last week, go through your monitors and record all your taste ratings from everything you ate. Follow the same procedure as you did before, always beginning at the left.

	Bray Plan Monitor **ANALYSIS FOR TASTE**															
	Number of Times															
Rating	1	2	3	4	5	6	7	8	9	10	11	12	13	14	Add'l	Total
1																
2																
3																
4																
5																

Figure 10. Analysis for recording taste preferences. Put your ratings of the foods you selected under the appropriate rating score and total the number of times for each taste level.

Were you able to make changes? What were they? How did you do it? Continue to evaluate the taste of your food when you are hungry and after you are full. Remember, awareness can give you control over eating.

- Any time you realize you are no longer hungry and the food doesn't taste really good, STOP EATING.
- Any time you are not really hungry, don't eat.
- Anything not tasting good (#1, #2) should lead you to ask yourself: "Why am I eating this?"

Let me re-emphasize my message. Your goal is to break the cue-response chains that help you retain bad eating habits. There are several techniques to help you change your habits:

1) Select a specific place to do all your eating.

2) Eat on one special plate of small size, with your own special utensils. Selecting tall, thin drinking glasses may reduce how much you drink at each sitting.

3) Always sit down to eat. This makes it difficult to nibble while preparing food or while doing other activities.

4) Eliminate distracting influences while eating, such as watching television or reading. When the phone rings, however, use it as a chance to interrupt eating and take the call standing up—you spend more energy.

5) Try to internalize and personalize these ideas so they apply to your needs and problems.

6) Do not try to eliminate your most difficult problems first. "Cut down rather than cut out" should be your motto for the early changes.

Here is an example from one of my patients.

Bray Plan Monitor **ANALYSIS FOR TASTE**																
Rating	Number of Times														Add'l	Total
	1	2	3	4	5	6	7	8	9	10	11	12	13	14		
1																1
2																2
3																6
4																10
5																3

How Fast and How Often Do You Eat?

How fast you eat and how often are two important factors affecting your overall eating behavior. Learning about the frequency and rate of eating will help you identify problem areas and change to more positive habits. The monitor we use for this is shown below.

Bray Plan Monitor **MONITOR FOR FREQUENCY & RATE OF EATING**				
Day		Time	Meal	Snack
Food Eaten		Start	Stop	

Figure 11. Monitor for the rate of eating. For each food item you eat in the next week, record the time you start and stop and with a check mark note whether it was a meal or a snack.

In column #1, write down all the foods and beverages you eat, just as you have been doing with the previous monitors for where you eat and for the associated activities. Remember, you must record immediately, each time you eat. Do not rely on memory; carry the monitors with you at all times.

Under the column labeled "Time-Start," write down the exact time (for example, 10:16 P.M. or 12:21 A.M.) when you start eating anything, even one bite. You must have a clock or watch available at all times. Again, write down the time immediately; don't rely on memory. To see why this is important, try to recall how many separate times you ate yesterday. What time did you start to eat? When did you stop? You can see how difficult it is to remember these things even one day later.

In the column labeled "Time-Stop," record the exact time you stopped eating each meal or snack. In the second column labeled "Meal or Snack," put a check mark to note what type of eating even it was. Spend the next seven days recording the frequency and timing of your meals and snacks, using 3×5-inch cards made to look like this Bray Plan Monitor.

Analyze the Rate and Frequency of Eating
Here is the analysis form — a completed sample is shown below.

Bray Plan Monitor ANALYSIS OF FREQUENCY OF EATING									
Time	1	2	3	4	5	6	7	Add'l	Total
6-7 AM									
7-8									
8-9									
9-10									
10-11									
11-12									
12-1 PM									
1-2									
2-3									
3-4									
4-5									
5-6									
6-7									
7-8									
8-9									
9-10									
10-11									
11-12									

Figure 12. Analysis form for frequency of eating. On this form, record the times of day when you eat food in the one-hour intervals.

The left column for "Frequency Analysis" has the day divided into one-hour periods. Across the top is the number of eating incidents. From your monitor cards, count the number of meals and snacks. Each incident should be recorded separately. Fill in the number of squares for that time period. Do one day at a time. Mark the time column when you begin to eat. Circle each non-caloric eating incident (i.e., black coffee, black tea, diet soda, etc.). When all the columns are filled in, use marks in the "additional" column. Put the total number in the "total" column.

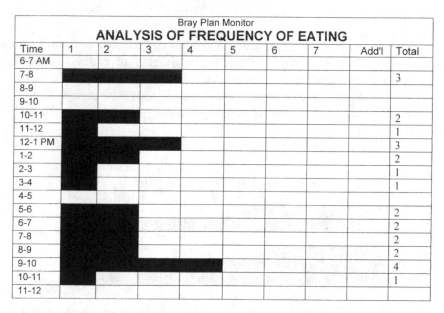

Bray Plan Monitor ANALYSIS OF FREQUENCY OF EATING									
Time	1	2	3	4	5	6	7	Add'l	Total
6-7 AM									
7-8									3
8-9									
9-10									
10-11									2
11-12									1
12-1 PM									3
1-2									2
2-3									1
3-4									1
4-5									
5-6									2
6-7									2
7-8									2
8-9									2
9-10									4
10-11									1
11-12									

Figure 13. Form for recording the frequency during the day at which you eat. For this individual breakfast, lunch and dinner were most common, but there was grazing throughout the evening.

Analyze the Rate of Eating

	Bray Plan Monitor ANALYSIS RATE OF EATING								
MINS	1	2	3	4	5	6	7	Add'l	Total
0-5									
6-10									
10-15									
15-20									
20-25									
>25									

Figure 14. Monitor for time of eating. Record the duration of each eating event.

The left side of the "Rate Eating Analysis" has the number of minutes for each eating incident. Across the top is the number of eating occasions. Count the number of minutes spent on each meal or snack. Fill in the squares for the number of eating occasions beside each time period. Use the "additional" column when the others are filled up. Remember to circle each non-caloric eating incident.

Below is an example from one of my patients.

	Bray Plan Monitor ANALYSIS RATE OF EATING								
MINS	1	2	3	4	5	6	7	Add'l	Total
0-5	■	■	■	■					4
6-10	■	■	■	■	■	■	■	+2	9
10-15		■							1
15-20			■						3
20-25							■		6
>25	■	■	■	■	■	■		+8	15

Figure 15. Analysis form to summarizing the rate at which you eat meals during the day. For this individual, the peak rates were between 6 and 10 minutes and then longer than 25 minutes.

Controlling How Often You Eat

1. If your problem is eating all day long, you can control it by reducing the number of times you eat.
   - Pre-planning and pre-preparing can be a good defense strategy. When you get up in the morning, plan when and where you will eat that day. This will help you control your responses to those food-associated stimuli that can turn you "on" at any particular moment.
   - Eat only when and what you planned.
   - Select a one-hour time period when you will eat nothing. Pick an hour that typically has at least one eating instance in it per week that

is not a meal.

- Try to control the places where you eat and the activities associated with eating. As you change one, other aspects will be affected. The results from the behavior change will be multiplied with every small change.
- Do not attempt to eat a lot of food at meals or at breakfast in order to reduce the number of other instances. Cut out, but do not replace.

2. If your principal problem is eating most of your food at meal times, try other tactics:
   - Use a smaller plate; portions will look larger.
   - Do not put serving dishes on the table; this will make it harder to get second helpings.
   - Eat more slowly. This will give you a chance to feel full earlier. When others at the table are done, STOP, even if there is food left on your plate.
   - Have sparkling water with ice and lemon juice or a diet drink before your meals.
   - Learn to put down your knife and fork between bites. Concentrate on creating delays. Drink water between finishing one bite and taking the next.
   - If you have a three-meal pattern, ask yourself if that includes everything you ate. If it does, your problem may not be the frequency but the quantity being eaten at each meal.

Controlling How Fast You Eat

1. If most meals are eaten in 10 minutes or less, the body's signals for satiety may not have time to tell you to stop. The food may not have had time to signal you that you've had enough by activating internal responses.
   - Aim for 15–25 minutes for each meal.
   - Sit down to eat all meals.
   - Concentrate on enjoying food by having an attractive table setting, using nice dishes, and trying to really taste your food. This requires chewing thoroughly.
   - Do not drink liquid unless your mouth is empty.
   - Plan occasional 1- to 2-minute delays between courses.
   - Do not put serving dishes on the table (to reduce ease of second helpings).
   - Pause between bites. Cut food into smaller pieces. Try to chew more slowly. This will give you a chance to feel fullness.
   - In a restaurant, watch how thin people eat. They often put utensils

down between bites, wipe their mouths, etc.—all of which slows down the eating process.

2. Beverages can be an important control mechanism.
   - They can increase the volume of the stomach, which may help to signal that you've had enough to eat.
   - Drink one or more glasses of water per meal.
   - As noted before, some fast eaters wash unchewed food down. The emphasis should be on changing rapid eating (5 minutes or less) and prolonged eating (over 26 minutes).
   - Try to keep more eating events toward the middle (10–25 minutes). Again, remember to make simple, gradual changes.

Pre-plan Your Meals

1. The goal of this monitor is to bring pre-planning into your life and begin to focus on practical ways to control your eating throughout the day and week.
2. The technique includes an analysis form in which the kinds of activities that were pre-planned and executed can be recorded. It is a tool that prepares you for difficult situations: meals away from home, foods eaten during the weekend, parties, and other social occasions where temptation to overeat may be a problem.

Bray Plan Monitor **MONITOR FOR PREPLANNING**	
Day	
Pre-Planned Activity	Success

Figure 16. Monitor for pre-planning foods and eating events. This monitor provides space for listing the eating activities for the day that you pre-planned and for noting your degree of success: A = very successful, B = moderately successful, C = Okay, D = not very successful.

In the coming week, I want you to pick a time to try out pre-planning. There are three assignments.

For two days, one regular, routine day and one weekend day, pre-plan one part of the day. Choose from the following what you are going to eat, the amounts you think you will eat, the exact time you will eat, and where you will eat it. Do this the evening before or the first thing in the morning on that day. Make sure it is not done at the very last moment. The goal is to enable you to make conscious decisions about what, when, where, and how much you eat. Also, remember that changes in your activities may require you to alter your plans.

On the selected day, record what you actually ate, including the exact time and amount. This gives you a chance to apply awareness of calories and of eating situations and to restructure your plan if the circumstances change.

For example: Friends invite you to a restaurant for dinner. Before going, think about what you will order—maybe even look up the menu online. This gives you insulation against the psychological turn-on most of us experience when presented with a menu and its many choices.

If your plan fails, you can still get useful information from it. Analyze and write down why you were unable to follow the plan. Then, rather than blaming yourself or anyone else, try to develop a plan once again. Think positively and plan positively.

Becoming Better at Pre-planning

During the past week, you have pre-planned one meal and/or one day. How did it go? For how many days did you pre-plan and then record actual intake?

Let me repeat the goals of pre-planning. They are:
- To help you identify difficult situations before they arise.
- To help you make a more conscious approach to these difficult situations.
- To give you the upper hand by planning ahead rather than becoming a victim of fate.

How accurate was your pre-planning? Record your answers to the questions on the form below. For each day or part of a day you pre-planned, record whether you ate or didn't eat what you planned. Also record whether you ate more or less than you planned.

Bray Plan Monitor **ANALYSIS OF PREPLANNING**												
Category	Number of Times											
	1	2	3	4	5	6	7	8	9	10	12	
Food Item Eaten Planned												
Food Planned Not Eaten												
Less Eaten Than Planned												
Eating at time not planned												
Eating at place not planned												
Eating as planned (gold *)												

Figure 17. Analysis form for pre-planning. Fill in as described in the text.
Pre-planning can have several uses:

It can help you with planning weekends, which tend to be less structured than weekdays.

It can be used when dining out. Although you cannot anticipate what the hostess will serve, you CAN plan what to cut down on, how to leave food on your plate, how to praise the dessert but not finish it, and how to win support for your weight goals from others by showing the proper restraint.

Some helpful tips include drinking plenty of water, using the bathroom during the dinner hour to delay the rate of eating, and putting your fork down between each bite. Since alcohol dulls your taste and ability to follow your plan, I urge you to avoid alcoholic drinks. Lemon juice in sparkling water with ice can be quite refreshing, and it has no calories.

The same method can help you in:

- Planning for business luncheons.
- Planning for holidays or trips.
- Planning for days when emotional problems are apt to arise (report cards, end-of-the-month bills, etc.).
- Planning for your shopping trips.

Here is an example of a pre-planning analysis from one on my patients.

Bray Plan Monitor **ANALYSIS OF PREPLANNING**												
Category	Number of Times											
	1	2	3	4	5	6	7	8	9	10	12	
Food Item Eaten Planned	███											
Food Planned Not Eaten	███	███	███	███								
Less Eaten Than Planned	███	███										
Eating at time not planned		███										
Eating at place not planned	███											
Eating as planned (gold *)	███	███	███	███	███	███						

Figure 18. Analysis for summarizing your pre-planned activities.

As you can see from this analysis, this individual is making good progress, just as you can. Good luck!

CHAPTER NINETEEN

Success with Being Active

How Active Are You?
Let's begin by reviewing your energy needs. This is done by referring to the Energy Balance Diagram below. This diagram was discussed earlier in Chapter 7.

Human Energy Balance

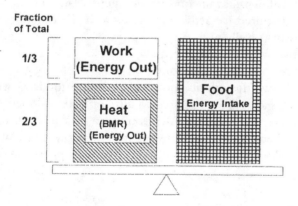

Figure 1. Diagram of energy balance. This figure was presented in Chapter 7. The right-hand bar represents the energy from food intake, which provides all of our energy. The left-hand bars divide energy expenditure into the resting component, which is about 2/3 of the total, and the part we control with our activity, which is about 1/3. There is about 10% that is accounted for in the processes of digestion, absorption, and storage of food (the thermic effect of food).

As you now know, the only source of energy for the body is from the food and beverages you ingest. The energy value of the food and beverages you eat is measured in calories. As your food is digested, the energy it contains enters your body to meet your daily needs or to be stored for later.

Learn the law of energy intake and output, and you will understand that when you steadily eat more calories than your body needs each day, you will gain weight.

There are two important routes for using up energy: your body metabolism and daily activity.

Your basal or resting metabolism accounts for about two-thirds of your total daily energy expenditure. The beating of your heart, the chemical changes that occur in your kidneys, brain, intestines, etc., are major contributors to your resting metabolic needs. If your basal metabolic rate slows down, as it does with every decade of your life, and you fail to reduce food and beverage intake accordingly, the excess calories you consume will be stored as fat.

Your daily activity accounts for less energy than resting metabolic rate. For most of us, it is about one-third of our total energy needs.

The quantity of energy used by your body for activity goes up as body weight increases. Thus an overweight person does more work walking about a room, getting out of a chair, or getting dressed than does a person of the same height, sex, and age who is of normal weight. As a consequence, overweight people tend to perspire more readily and frequently find exercise unpleasant, if not downright uncomfortable and distasteful.

The energy required for activity increases with the duration, intensity, and rate of activity as well.

There are two ways to look at activity:

1. Activity can be related to calories in food.

This table shows the caloric equivalent of some foods as well as the number of minutes of walking required to burn up extra calories. Note that the heavier you are, the fewer minutes you must walk to burn up a given amount of food. Because of the extra weight, however, the insulating effect will make you feel warmer, and this often discourages people from making the effort.

Table 1. Minutes of Walking to Burn the Calories in Various Foods

Minutes to BURN CALORIES

Food	Calories in Food	Walking at 3 mph Body Weight (lb)		
		120	160	200
Apple (1) (2½" diam.)	75	21	17	14
Apple Pie (1/6 of 9" pie)	410	115	93	78
Beer (12 oz)	170	47	38	31
Blueberries (cup)	87	23	19	16
Beef Steak (cubed, 4 oz)	300	83	68	57
Biscuit (1) (2" diameter)	130	36	30	24
Bologna (1 sl)	88	23	19	22
Bread (1 sl)	65	18	15	12
Broccoli (cup)	50	14	12	10
Cola (8 oz) (Coke)	100	28	23	19
Cereal-Cooked (cup)	165	46	38	31
Cheese (1 oz) (Gouda) (Caraway)	100	28	23	19
Chocolate Cake (1 piece) (2"×3"×2") no icing	165	46	38	31
Egg (medium)	78	22	18	15
Flounder (4 oz) (raw)	78	22	18	15
Frankfurter	124	34	28	23
Hamburger & Bun, (1 bun) (3 oz., high-fat meat)	400	111	91	76
Milk (whole) (8 oz)	166	46	38	31
Orange, large (3" diam.)	115	32	27	23
Potato (baked—1) (no skin) (2½" diam.)	100	28	23	19
Salmon (canned) (3½ oz)	200	56	46	38
Strawberries (cup)	54	15	12	10

2. Energy expenditure from activity can be related to various levels of activity as well as to type of activity.

Table 2 is from the Recommended Dietary Allowance[1] of the National Academy of Sciences to show you the energy levels related to various activities. From sleeping to the highest levels of exercise and work, the energy expenditure may go up as much as ten times. Note also, however, that almost no time is spent in high-level activities while nearly 75% of the day is spent in activities with very low levels of energy expenditure. One key difference between overweight and normal-weight people is that overweight people sit about two hours more per day.[2] If you are overweight, plan to stand more during such activities as talking on the phone.

Table 2. Levels of Activity

SCORE	TYPE	EXAMPLES
0	Sleeping:	
1	Reclining:	Watching television, reading quietly.
2	Very Light:	Seated or standing activities such as done by painters, cab and truck drivers, laboratory workers, typists, musicians, stitchers, office workers.
	Men:	Office workers, most professional occupations.
	Women:	Office workers, housewives with mechanical aides such as dishwashers, etc., teachers, and most other professional women.
3	Light:	Walking on level at 2.5–3 mph, tailors, pressers, garage work, electricians, carpentry, restaurant trades, cannery workers, manual clothes washing, shopping with light load, golf, sailing, table tennis, volleyball.
	Men:	Most men in light industry, students, building workers, except for heavy laborers, many farmers.
	Women:	Light industry, housewives without mechanical appliances, department store workers, students.
4	Moderate:	Walking 3.5–4 mph, plasterers, seeding and hoeing, scrubbing floors, stockroom with loading and stacking heavy loads, shopping with a heavy load, bicycling, skiing, tennis, and dancing.
	Men:	Some agricultural workers, unskilled laborers, forestry workers (except lumberjacks), soldiers, miners, steel workers.
	Women:	Some farm workers, dancers, athletes.
5	Heavy:	Walking uphill with a load, lumberjack, pick and shovel work, basketball, swimming, climbing, football.
	Men:	Lumberjacks, blacksmiths, rickshaw-pullers.
	Women:	Construction workers

The Great Calorie Count

For the next week, I want you to learn how much energy you use each day through activity. You will record your activity on a daily basis for the next week on the Bray Plan Activity Monitor below.

Bray Plan Monitor **MONITOR FOR ACTIVITY**		
Day		
Activity	Time	
	Start	Stop

Figure 2. Monitor form to record activity levels for each hour using the levels described in Table 2.

For each day of the week, you will record your activity level for each hour of the day, whether you are awake or asleep. At the end of the hour, figure out the most active thing you did for at least fifteen minutes of that hour. Then use the numbers in Table 2 to record the level (0–5) of that activity. Now that you have finished your week-long log of activity levels on an hour-by-hour basis, let's see how many calories you expended through this activity. Keep in mind that I'm using the word "activity" for both muscular activities and basal or "resting" activity. To analyze the activity you have recorded, we will use the figure below and the two tables that follow.

Bray Plan Monitor **ACTIVITY MONITOR**					
Day					
Hour		Hour		Hour	
12A -1		8-9		4-5	
1-2		9-10		5-6	
2-3		10-11		6-7	
3-4		11-12 P		7-8	
4-5		12-1		8-9	
5-6		1-2		9-10	
6-7		2-3		10-11	
7-8		3-4		11-12	

Figure 3. Analysis of daily activity. To fill in this form, you will use the two tables described below. An example from one patient is shown below to give you an idea of what it should look like.

For the first day, add up the number of hours spent at each of the five levels of activity. Put these totals under Day One of the chart. The total hours for that day and for other days should add up to 24. Repeat for the remainder of the days of the week until you have determined the number of hours spent for the week at each of the levels. Now average the totals for each day to come up with an average daily total at each of the levels.

The next step is to turn to the table for "Basal Energy"(Table 3). This table relates your height, weight, and age to average basal energy expenditure. Identify your half of the chart. The top is for men and the bottom is for women. Find the range of heights that applies to you. Let's say you are a man 5 feet 7 inches (67 inches) tall and 180 pounds. Your group of numbers is in the middle of the first chart. Next, find the weight closest to your own. Finally, read across to the column that includes your age. Let's assume it's 40. Then you would be in the 36-55 category. Your basal energy is approximately 1376. Record that number on the right-hand side of your activity analysis worksheet next to the word "basal."

Table 3. Basal Energy Needs For Men (Top) and Women (Bottom)
Men

Height (in)	Weight (lb)	Age Group (yr)		
		18–35	36–55	56–75
60–65	160	1240	1171	1093
	200	1550	1464	1367
	240	1860	1757	1640
66–71	180	1492	1376	1286
	220	1824	1682	1572
	260	2155	1988	1858
72–78	200	1750	1658	1550
	240	2100	1990	1860
	280	2450	2322	2170

Women

Height (in)	Weight (lb)	Age Group (yr)		
		18–35	36–55	56–75
60–65	120	900	821	772

	160	1200	1094	1030
	200	1500	1367	1288
	240	1800	1640	1545
66-71	140	1108	1000	945
	180	1388	1286	1215
	220	1668	1572	1485
	260	1972	1858	1755
72-78	160	1380	1240	1166
	200	1600	1550	1458
	240	1910	1860	1750
	280	2240	2170	2042

Based on the information in Table 4, you can estimate the number of calories expended through the various activity levels.

Table 4. Energy Expenditure in Relation to Body Weight and Activity Level*

		Body Weight (lb)		
Activity Level	<u>120</u>	<u>160</u>	<u>200</u>	<u>240</u>
		Calories/hr		
1	28	37	46	55
2	32	43	54	65
3	43	58	72	86
4	60	80	100	120
5	92	123	154	184

* Activity level is defined in Table 2.

If you weigh 200 pounds, you spend 46 calories per hour at level 1 of activity. If your weight is 120, 160, or 240 it is also easy to read these numbers and directly place them on the Analysis Monitor in Figure 3. If you weigh 180 pounds, the values are between those under columns you have to do a little more work. If you weigh 180, you use the number halfway between

160 and 200 pounds. Thus at activity level 1, you spend approximately 41 calories per hour; at level 2, approximately 47 calories per hour; at level 3, 65 calories per hour; at level 4, 90 calories per hour; and at level 5, 138 calories per hour. You have to recognize that these are estimates. The numbers are now transferred to the column labeled "calories per hour," which is adjacent to the column labeled "average" on the analysis sheet. Now multiply the average number of hours at each level by the calories per hour for this level and write the number in the column at the far right. A sample from one of our patients is shown below. The number in the total should give a reasonable estimate of the number of calories you have expended during the past week. Since you have recorded an activity level with only fifteen minutes of time spent at that level, this first total is obviously an overestimate. If you want to be more accurate, repeat the same Bray Plan recording monitor and record the level when you spend forty-five minutes or more at a given level. With this additional information, which should be lower than the previous one, you will have a good estimate for the range of energy you need to maintain your own body weight.

Figure 4. Analysis of Daily Activity. A description of the analysis is provided above.

Bray Plan Monitor **ANALYSIS FOR ACTIVITY**											
Level	Days							Average	Calories per hour	Level	Calories
	1	2	3	4	5	6	7				
0 Sleeping	8	9	9	7	8	7	9	8.1	Basal*	Basal	1500*
1 Reclining	13	14	13	15	14	15	12	13.7	46	1	630
2 Very light	1	2	2	1	1	1	2	1.4	54	2	75.6
3 Light	0	0	0	1	1	0	0	0.3	72	3	21.6
4 Moderate	1	0	0	0	0	1	1	0.4	100	4	40
5 Heavy	0	0	0	0	0	0	0	0	154	5	0
										Total	2266

*Basal calories were obtained from Table 3 for a woman aged 20–35 with a height of 60 to 65 inches and a weight of 200 pounds.

§Calories per hour were obtained from Table 4 for an individual weighing 200 pounds. Note that for the Basal Calories, you need an age, height and weight, but for Calories per hour, you need only a weight.

There is a second way to estimate your energy expenditure. This uses the step counter. For the next week, I want you to use the step counter you have to record your daily steps. This can be done with the Bray Step Counter Monitor shown in Figure 5.

Bray Plan Monitor **MONITOR FOR STEP COUNTER**	
Day of the Week	Number of Steps
Monday	
Tuesday	
Wednesday	
Thursday	
Friday	
Saturday	
Sunday	

Figure 5. Step Counter Monitor. Fill in the number of steps you record from your step pedometer each day. Set it at zero each morning and then record the number of steps the next morning before resetting it to zero.

Now that you have completed a week's worth of recording, let's see what you have. The analysis form below allows you to record the number of days during the week you achieved a given number of steps. Blacken the appropriate number of bars along each row. Since there are only seven days in a week, there should only be seven boxes filled. Remember—it takes about 2000 steps for a mile. Note the number of steps you walked each day: 2000 steps is about one mile. Now for the next week, let's repeat this and increase your steps on each day by an average of 1000 or ½ mile. See how it goes. We will then continue this until you are getting 5,000 steps each day. This is equivalent to about 2-1/2 miles and will give you the 30–45 minutes of walking you need each day. You can use the analysis form to keep track of your progress with increasing the number of steps.

Bray Plan Monitor **ANALYSIS FOR NUMBER OF STEPS**								
Steps	1	2	3	4	5	6	7	Total
<1000								
1-2000								
2-3000								
3-4000								
4-5000								
5-6000								
6-7000								
7-8000								
8-9999								
>10000								

Figure 6. Analysis form for step counting. Check off the boxes that correspond to the number of steps you took. There are only seven days in a week, so there should be seven checks.

The other side of the energy-balance equation is the calorie value of the foods you eat. If this value is equal to the energy you expend through daily activities, then your weight will remain stable over time. To carry this idea further, if the calorie value of the foods you eat is less than the amount of energy you burn up, you will lose weight.

An example from a relatively inactive individual is shown below. It shows there is considerable room for improvement. Keep walking!

Bray Plan Monitor
ANALYSIS FOR NUMBER OF STEPS

Steps	1	2	3	4	5	6	7	Total
<1000	█							1
1-2000	█	█	█					3
2-3000	█	█						2
3-4000								
4-5000	█							1
5-6000								
6-7000								
7-8000								
8-9999								
>10000								

Figure 7. Analysis form for summarizing the steps you take each day during the week

Calories You Spend in Various Activities
In contrast to the earlier table, the following table is not divided according to sex or height. The only variable you use is your weight.

Although increased activity may be good for you, any sudden change, particularly if you are older (over 50 years of age) and have been inactive in the past months or years, can cause trouble. Before increasing your activity level by introducing new activities that you are not already doing, you are strongly advised to consult with your physician to obtain his or her clearance to engage in new or more strenuous levels of physical activity.

Activity and You
There are at least two kinds of activities you can perform. The first is called aerobic, and the second is called anaerobic. "Aerobic" means using oxygen; "anaerobic" means not using oxygen.

Aerobic activities involve such things as walking, swimming, bicycling, and jogging—the kinds of activities that get you breathing faster and your heart pumping more blood. Anaerobic activity, on the other hand, tends to involve isometric or muscle-building activity, where changes in heart rate are more variable (Chapter 7).

For most people, aerobic activities are preferable because they increase your metabolism and help you burn fat. Swimming and bicycling are good activities for overweight people because your weight is supported by the water or the bicycle seat.

To give you some feeling about the calorie expenditure during various activities, I prepared Table 5, which shows the calories used per minute above basal level for different activities. Note that for many activities, you expend few calories above basal levels. If you do any of these activities for a long time, however, the effect can be important to you. The values in this table represent the increase over basal energy expenditure associated with each activity. When you calculated your basal energy earlier, you saw that it changes with your age, weight, and height. The values in the table are corrected by subtracting the energy you would spend at basal level from the total associated with each activity. For most people, basal energy is just below 1 calorie per minute. Lying down adds only a little to the extra energy, but standing can increase it to about 1.2 calories per minute—a 20% increase above basal, depending on how heavy you are. Your motto should be "keep moving, no matter how slowly."

Table 5. Energy Expenditure Above Basal Levels Related to Body Weight and Activity

| | Body Weight | | |
| | 120 | 160 | 200 |
Activity		Cal/min	
Lying down	0.10	0.12	0.15
Sitting	0.38	0.50	0.62
Standing	0.45	0.61	0.77
Ironing	0.90	1.22	1.54
Walking (3 mph)	1.80	2.41	3.03
Carpentry	2.10	2.80	3.50
Bicycling	2.30	3.05	3.80
Calisthenics	2.50	3.35	4.20
Dancing	2.70	3.65	4.60
Walking (4 mph)	3.12	4.12	5.13
Skating	3.20	4.26	5.33
Swimming (2 mph)	7.10	10.05	12.00
Running (10 mph)	12.83	17.06	21.28

We know that activity and movement can be helpful when trying to manage your weight. For many overweight people, walking is most desirable, since it can be done anywhere at almost any time of year and is a form of activity we all do. And remember, in snowy or rainy weather, you can always walk in a mall and window-shop at the same time. Walking is helpful in maintaining weight loss (Chapter 7)—once you have lost it. While activity alone is unlikely to bring about a major loss of weight, it can help enormously when combined with careful control of food intake.

For example, if you increase your energy expenditure by as much as 10 to 15% through walking or other activity, your calorie intake can move up some without gaining weight. And if your activity program is followed faithfully, you will be able to afford more calories, thus more food each day, without regaining weight.

Even a small amount of walking or other activity each day can make a difference in your caloric expenditure. Pursuing this activity over the course of a year will produce a significant weight loss. On the other hand, if you cut down on your activity, you will gain weight, unless you also cut down on your food. It is a trade-off.

Being active implies a number of things. It is the way you move and the way you breathe, as well as the way you walk. It is not something to be done just when you feel like it. Ideally, walking or other activity should be regular and consistent, according to your age and sex.

Warming Up
Warming up before you start is important.

Here are some simple warm-ups for you:

1. Relax your arms, let your hands hang limp, and then shake your hands.

2. Rotate your arms, leading with the elbows.

3. Rotate your head, permitting the jaw to hang slack. Close your eyes while doing this exercise.

4. Rotate just the shoulders, first together and then separately.

Getting into Shape
In order to become more active, your body may need conditioning. First, you need to get into shape.

Increasing your activity can get you into shape, keep you supple and limber, improve your muscle tone, and relax you all at the same time. It may even help correct your posture and, above all, reduce your weight.

Think of your body as a machine. To keep a machine in good working order, you would not permit it to sit idle, would you? In the same way, your body functions better when it is kept in good working order. And your body—because of nature's wonderful powers—will respond positively and become stronger when used properly. If you plan to increase your walking, do it gradually.

Three Keys to Becoming More Active

Before you begin any activity, consider the three things you will always be doing, whether exercising or not: thinking positively, breathing correctly, and keeping a good posture. Let's make sure you do them correctly and you have your doctor's approval before beginning any major departure from your usual habits of activity.

1. Thinking Positively

Walking should become part of your life. When you embark on this program, it should be important not only to want to feel better now, but to want to continue feeling better. Form a mental picture of what you would like to look like and how you would like to feel. Place it alongside the image of what you look like now and how you feel now. This should help motivate you every day.

2. Breathing Effectively

People use only ⅛ of their total lung capacity when breathing normally. Poor breathing habits can further decrease your capacity to walk or do anything else. It is wise to adopt good breathing habits because you will find walking or other activity much easier if you breathe properly.

When you breathe, you take oxygen into your lungs and you exhale carbon dioxide. A normal person takes about 16 to 20 breaths per minute, or some 23,000 breaths a day. Our breathing tends to become more shallow as we get older and heavier. Breathing is, of course, vital to your entire body. The more efficiently you breathe, the more effectively your body will function. There are two methods of deep breathing: 1) breathing through your mouth, drawing in the air in gasps, and 2) closing your mouth and breathing deeply through your nose. With either method, stand "large," spreading your ribs to the side.

Here are some exercises to increase your lung capacity, strengthen your diaphragm, and help you develop good breathing habits:

- Take a deep breath, fill your lungs full, and see how long you can hold that breath. Then, with teeth closed, expel it with a hissing noise. Do this as slowly as possible and finish with one last, forceful hiss. This will help clear your lungs. Repeat this exercise several times or whenever you think of it.

- Take a deep breath and enjoy it. Count to 20 as you exhale. As singers and swimmers know, the amount of air you can hold in your lungs is extremely important.

- Light a candle and hold it about 10 inches from your mouth. Take a deep breath and fill your lungs. Expel the air slowly in such a way as to keep the candle burning. It will waver but should not be blown out.

3. Correct Posture

In order to breathe properly, you must sit and stand straight. Obviously, you cannot fill your lungs if they are distorted by your posture. Picture your lungs as two balloons you must fill, one on either side of your chest.

Whether you are sitting or standing, your back should be upright, shoulders back and relaxed, chest and head up. One of the easiest ways of picturing this position is to imagine a string tied to the top of your head and to your chest, puppet fashion. When the string is pulled taut, everything falls into place without much effort.

This position can also be practiced by backing up to a wall. Make an effort to touch the small of your back, your calves, and the back of your head (in chin-down position) to the wall. Stay in this position and try the deep-breathing exercises. The very few minutes spent on them can benefit you tremendously. In addition, these breathing exercises are necessary for forming a firm foundation for your activity program and can be sandwiched into your day easily and frequently.

Begin Slowly and Keep Going

Now you are ready to begin moving your entire body. The important thing to remember is that it is far better to begin slowly than to start off with a bang and then not be able to keep it up. Even a limited program can help you feel much better.

Some of you may do no more than what has already been mentioned— the basic warm-ups, breathing, and posturing and all with a good mental attitude.

You should also respect your fatigue point. When walking, if you feel pain in any part of your body, stop immediately. Never push yourself to continue under these circumstances. Consult with your physician before you make a significant increase in your activity, particularly if you are over 50 years of age or have had any evidence of early heart disease in your family or yourself.

Your fatigue point is not stationary, however, and with activity you can usually gradually increase the amount of walking.

There is nothing magical about any program for activity. Yours should include some form of aerobic activity. Walking is the most suitable activity for all of us. Learn to think in terms of energy exchange and you need never be overweight again.

To emphasize the importance of energy expenditure in your everyday life, we want you to maintain a regular record of the activity you do each and every day. Using a monitor like the one below, record each time you do activities outside of your regular job. Remember, the more you move, the more energy your body can use without gaining weight. Walking is certainly the easiest activity for most people, and it is the one we can do every day. Other activities you normally engage in should also be noted. Remember that if you have no activity above your daily job requirements, then the day should have a "0" (zero) for extra energy expenditure. As you become more conscious of your activities, the number of days with "0" should fall as the number of days with extra activity increases.

Bray Plan Monitor **MONITOR FOR ACTIVITY**			
Day			
Activity		Time	
		Start	Stop

Figure 8. Monitor for Activity. For one week, record the activities you do each of the day such as walking, playing golf, and riding a bicycle, along with the time when you start and stop the activity.

A Bray Plan analysis form to record the number of times you perform various activities is shown below. Record each time you spent more than the listed time at an activity, and following that as an example of the recording from a patient of mine. Walking > 30 minutes.

Bray Plan Monitor **ANALYSIS FOR ACTIVITIES** Number of times																
	1	2	3	4	5	6	7	8	9	10	11	12	13	14	Add'l	Total
Waling > 30 minutes																
Walking down stairs																
Walking up stairs																
Cycling > 15 minutes																
Swimming > 15 mins																
Jogging > 15 minutes																
Other																

Figure 9. Analysis for activities. Record the number of times you did specific activities in the blank spaces. You can now follow changing activity patterns in the future.

The example below was from a relatively sedentary individual who had lots of room to increase activity in her life.

Bray Plan Monitor **ANALYSIS FOR ACTIVITIES** Number of times																
	1	2	3	4	5	6	7	8	9	10	11	12	13	14	Add'l	Total
Walking > 30 minutes																3
Walking down stairs																10
Walking up stairs																1
Cycling > 15 minutes																
Swimming > 15 mins																
Jogging > 15 minutes																
Other																

Figure 10. Analysis form for summarizing the number of times you do some activities. You can substitute some of the activities on this form on the one you use to get the activities you do recorded.

Remember, to reach and maintain your weight goal, you need to substitute activities, such as walking, for times you might eat. It is harder to eat on the move than when standing still. Two large studies in which the Pennington

Center participates have tested two levels of exercise. One has a goal of 150 minutes of exercise per week, the other 225 minutes per week. Weight loss was, as might be expected, slightly higher in the study with the higher level of physical activity per week, but both levels were effective for weight loss. So keep moving!

CHAPTER TWENTY

Buyer Beware

The Economics of the Obesity Epidemic

Foods on "Sale"

We are all influenced by the prices of the goods we buy. When a sale occurs, we tend to "stock up" with things, even when we don't need them. When we do this with food, we are at risk of putting "the waste on the waist." With the reduction in some food prices over the past thirty years, there has been a shift in the commercially profitable products that result from federal subsidies of corn, sugar, and rice. The food industry has been able to produce cheap, good-tasting, energy-dense foods—"bad fructose" (HFCS/sucrose), high-fat foods[1,2]—and to sell them to you cheaply and in large portion sizes. In contrast, foods like fruits and vegetables with "good fructose" are not subsidized and are more expensive; thus you tend to buy less of these foods, particularly when you are on a tight budget. Some experts recommend that we spend our money for the good foods and leave the bad ones alone.[3]

Costs of Food

Let me give you some examples of the changes in food prices for subsidized and non-subsidized categories. Between 1985 and 2000, the prices of fresh fruits and vegetables rose 118%, the price of fish rose 77%, and the prices of dairy products (which are subsidized) increased by 56%. Compare this with the smaller rise in prices for foods made from federally subsidized items that often include "bad fructose" and fat. Sugar and sweets rose only 46%, fats and oils only increased 35%, and carbonated beverages, a prime source of "bad fructose," only rose by 20%.[4] Is it any wonder that people with limited incomes eat more foods that are high in sugar and fat?

Providing more "healthy" food alternatives is one alternative to helping fight the obesity epidemic. Healthy foods are usually "engineered" and will almost certainly cost more. What is healthier than fresh fruits and vegetables, low-fat or skim milk, and fish, poultry, and nuts? Since our food choices are often based largely on price, healthy food choices may not be economically healthy. Moreover, I doubt these healthy new items will alter consumer choices as long as good tasting, energy-dense, high-fructose/high-fat foods of the kinds you get at fast-food restaurants remain cheap.

Economic factors may have a lot to do with the small numbers of "excess calories" people eat that, over time, lead to weight gain. What we consume is influenced by the price we have to pay for it. As noted above, the prices for different types of food have risen at different rates over the past thirty years. Since the beginning of the 1970s, the prices of foods that have a high energy density, such as those rich in fat and sugar, have fallen relative to other items. The Consumer Price Index (CPI) has risen at the rate of 3.8% per year from 1980 to 2000 while food prices have gone up at only 3.4% per year. In the period from 1960 to 1980, when there was only a small increase in the prevalence of overweight people, food prices rose at a rate of 5.5% per year—slightly faster than the CPI, which grew at a rate of 5.3% per year. Is it any wonder that people with limited income eat more "bad fructose" (HFCS/sucrose)- and fat-containing foods? At the present time, it costs between $0.30 and $1.50 for 1,000 calories of fats/oils, sugars, and grains, and between $1.00 and $90.00 for 1,000 calories of meat, fish, dairy products, and fruits or vegetables.[5] Is it any wonder that cheap, good-tasting, energy-dense foods with lots of "bad fructose" and fat are widely consumed?

Eating more food energy over time than we need for our daily energy requirement produces extra fat, and we gain weight. In the current obesity epidemic, the average increase in body weight is 1 to 2 pounds per year. You can calculate the amount of net energy storage required by an adult to produce 1 pound of added body weight, 75% of which is fat, by using a few assumptions. One pound of adipose tissue contains about 3,500 calories of energy. If the efficiency of energy storage were 50% (with the other 50% being used by the synthetic and storage processes), we would need to ingest 14,000 calories per year of food energy to gain 1 to 2 pounds per year. Since there are 365 days in the year, it would only take an extra 40 calories per day (40 kcal/d × 365 d/year = 14,600 calories) to produce the current epidemic! For simplicity we can round this to 50 calories per day or the equivalent of 10 teaspoons of sugar or 6 oz of a soda with "bad fructose." Any wonder the Low-Fructose Approach to Weight Management came into existence?

Has our intake of food energy increased? From information collected by the U.S. Department of Agriculture on food use, we can now answer this question. The number of calories the average person ate per day was relatively stable during the first eighty years of the twentieth century. During the last twenty years (from 1980 to 2000), however, there was a clear rise in energy intake, from about 2,300 calories a day to about 2600 calories a day, an increase of 300 calories eaten each day.[6] As we calculated above, it would only take an additional 50 calories a day to produce a two-pound weight gain in a year. No wonder we're in an epidemic of weight gain.

We know that our pattern of energy intake changes during our lifetime. Right after birth, our need for food goes up rapidly as we grow from infancy to adulthood. There is thus a rapid increase in food intake for both boys and girls during the first decade of life. As puberty begins and both boys and girls go into their last growth spurt, the energy intake also goes into a "spurt," particularly for males but also in females, reaching a peak during adolescence for both sexes. From age 20 onward, there is a slow decrease of food intake by both sexes, but again males remain higher on average than females throughout lives.[7] This is because males have more muscle tissue in their bodies than do females (see Chapter 1).

Portion sizes and the number of foods that come in large portion sizes have dramatically increased in the past forty years.[8] We need to reduce them if we are to combat the epidemic of overweight successfully. One consequence of the larger portion sizes is that we eat more food and thus get more calories.[9] The USDA estimates that between 1984 and 1994, daily calorie intake increased by 340 calories a day, or 14.7%. Refined grains provided 6.2% of this increase, fats and oils 3.4%, but fruits and vegetables only 1.4%, and meats and dairy products only 0.3%. Beverages sweetened with high-fructose corn syrup contain about 5% "bad fructose" made from these grain products. These beverages are available in containers of 12, 20, or 32 ounces, which provide 150, 250, or 400 calories if all of it is drunk. Many foods list the calories per serving, but the package often contains more than 1 serving, thus making it difficult for consumers to readily measure calorie intake. In 1954 the hamburger served by Burger King weighed 2.8 oz and had 202 calories. By 2004 it had grown to 4.3 oz, with 310 calories. In 1955 McDonald's served French fries weighing 2.4 oz and having 210 calories. By 2004 this had increased to 7 oz and 610 calories. Popcorn served at movie theaters has also grown up, going from 3 cups containing 174 calories in 1950 to 21 cups with 1700 calories in 2004. The increased energy available and consumed by Americans is certainly related to these larger portions.[7] And this "super-sizing" is found in essentially all the items that are on your grocery shelves. Guidance for intake of beverages suggests we drink more water, tea, coffee, and low-fat dairy products with less consumption of beverages that contain primarily water and caloric sweeteners (sugar or

HFCS).[10] The importance of drinking water as an alternative to consuming calories was shown in a recent study. In this study, the more water you drank, the fewer the number of calories you got from solid foods. The scientists measured all the water a person consumed, both from food and drinks, as well as the total energy intake. They then compared the amount of water a person drank to the amount of food and non-water beverages combined. When the total water intake averaged less than 20 grams for each gram of food and non-water beverage, energy intake was 2,485 calories. In people whose water intake was in the top 25% (above 90 grams per gram of food + beverage), energy intake was nearly 30% lower, at 1,791 calories.[11] Thus drinking water may be one strategy for lowering overall energy intake.

Portion size influences what we eat, both in the laboratory and when we dine in such places as cafeterias.[9] Using a laboratory setting, both normal and overweight men and women were given different amounts of a good-tasting pasta entrée and told to eat as much as they liked for 30 minutes. When they were offered the largest size, they ate 30% more than when offered half the amount. The same thing happened when different-size packages of potato chips were offered. Women ate 18% more and men 37% more when the package size was doubled. **Tip:** Select smaller-size packages, smaller serving dishes, and tall, thin glasses rather than shorter, squat ones.

CHAPTER TWENTY-ONE

Supplements Used in Weight Management

Many dietary supplements are marketed to help manage your weight. We have worked on some of these at the Pennington Center. Do they work? Are they safe? I will briefly summarize the evidence showing how safe and effective various weight loss supplements are. To help walk you through the many available products, I have prepared Table 1 with three categories of supplements. They include minerals and metabolites, herbal preparations, and dietary fiber.

Minerals and Metabolites
1. Chromium picolinate: Chromium is a trace mineral and a co-factor that is involved in the action of insulin. It has been claimed that chromium can cause weight loss and fat loss while increasing lean body mass in animals. In 10 human studies, there were small weight losses of 2.4 to 12.8 lb. There were no complications of treatment. These data must be interpreted cautiously, since they rely heavily on one robust study. Chromium picolinate may have a significant effect in preventing weight regain.[1] If this holds up under further study, it might be a beneficial supplement. Thus at this point, there is little evidence of benefit but also few or no adverse events.[2,3]

2. Hydroxymethyl butyrate: -hydroxy--methylbutyrate is formed from an essential amino acid, leucine. A reduction in fat mass and the possibility of an increase in lean body mass have been found in animals. These results indicate that further studies are warranted.[2,3]

3. Pyruvate: Pyruvate is a middle-man in the metabolism of glucose and can serve as a shuttle in the blood stream between liver and muscle. It has been suggested to improve exercise performance and body composition. Two human studies showed no significant effects on body weight compared to placebo. Thus there is little current value in pyruvate.[2,3]

4. Conjugated linoleic acid: The word "conjugated" in linoleic acid refers to chemical structure of an essential fatty acid. There are several different CLA molecules due to this chemical change, and they have different activities. There is little evidence that conjugated linoleic acid produces weight loss in human beings. There is also concern about liver toxicity from the *trans*-10, *cis*-12 isomer. Thus there is little evidence of benefit and concern about harm.[2,3,4]

5. Calcium: This is clearly one of the most interesting and yet most confusing minerals to evaluate. For nearly twenty years, we have known that people with a higher body mass index had a lower intake of dietary calcium. Can calcium by mouth help you lose weight? Some information suggests that high intake of calcium or high-dairy diets may play a part in battling the current epidemic of weight problems.

Our understanding of the relationship between calcium and body weight is particularly confusing to understand. One of the biggest proponents of the effects of calcium also holds a patent for the effects of dairy products for producing weight loss. Such a relationship, where monetary gain is associated with publication of positive studies, raises concerns about the published studies. Moreover, there is inconsistency in both the animal and human studies.

Small clinical trials have been used to claim that calcium supplements or dairy supplements produce weight loss. Larger studies have not supported the value of calcium on weight loss or body composition, leaving the issue in limbo.[5] I would conclude that the evidence of benefit is equivocal and limited to small studies, but there are no major safety concerns.[6]

Herbal Dietary Supplements
A number of herbal products have been proposed as aids in weight loss. The data are generally limited, and because of current federal laws, there is no requirement to show that herbal preparations are effective. Thus buyer beware. To help you understand the field, I have summarized some of these below.

1. Ephedra sinica: *Ephedra sinica* is an evergreen that grows in central Asia, and its principal ingredient is ephedrine. Ephedrine combined with caffeine has been shown to produce weight loss in randomized, placebo-controlled clinical trials conducted in Europe. Two randomized placebo-controlled clinical trials with the ephedra alkaloids contained in Ma Huang have been published. One trial lasted 3 months and the other 6 months. They both showed significantly greater weight loss in the people receiving ephedra and caffeine than with the placebo pill. The ephedra-containing herbal preparations were removed from the U.S. market by the U.S. Food and Drug Administration in April 2004 because of alleged harmful cardiovascular side-effects.[7] This action has recently been reversed by Federal Courts, and ephedra-containing herbals are again available. These are the most widely used supplements for weight loss.

2. Garcinia cambogia: *Garcinia cambogia* contains hydroxycitric acid, which is an inhibitor of a key step in the way the body makes fat. Hydroxycitrate was studied by a major drug company in the 1970s and was shown to reduce food intake and cause weight loss in rodents. Although there have been reports of successful weight loss with small studies in humans, some of which were combined with other herbs, the largest and best designed placebo-controlled study demonstrated no difference in weight loss compared to a placebo.[8] Thus there is currently no evidence to suggest that *Garcinia cambogia* and its herbal components are effective weight-loss agents.[2,3]

3. Yohimbine from Pausinystalia yohimbe: Yohimbine is isolated from *Pausinystalia yohimbe* and acts on specific "lock and key" receptors in the body. The three randomized clinical trials of this herbal preparation yielded conflicting results as to whether there is significant weight loss with this plant extract compared to placebo. More information is needed, and it cannot be recommended at this time.[2,3]

4. Hoodia: *Hoodia gordonii* is a cactus that grows in Africa. It has been eaten by Bushmen to decrease appetite and thirst on long treks across the desert. The active ingredient is called P57AS3 or just P57. P57 decreases food intake in animals according to the Phytopharm website (*http://www.phytopharm.co.uk*). Phytopharm is developing P57 in partnership with a major company. A study with 19 overweight males tested P57. Food intake and body weight fell, and there was no reported illness. Since *Hoodia* is a rare cactus in the wild and cultivation is difficult, it is not clear what the dietary herbal supplements claiming to contain *Hoodia* actually contain or if they are effective in causing weight loss.

5. Citrus aurantium (Bitter Orange): When ephedra was withdrawn from the market by the U.S. FDA, manufacturers of dietary herbal supplements for weight loss turned to *Citrus aurantium*, which contains phenylephrine, which can raise blood pressure and increase energy expenditure. A recent systematic review found only one randomized, placebo-controlled trial involving 20 subjects treated with *Citrus aurantium* for 6 weeks. This trial demonstrated no statistically significant benefit for weight loss.[9] There have been reports of abnormal heart problems when *Citrus aurantium* is used. There is no evidence that *Citrus aurantium* is effective in the treatment of overweight, but there are concerns about its safety.[2,3] Buyer beware.

Fiber
Fiber-containing products are often touted for their ability to help you control your weight. One rationale for these products is that people who eat more fiber tend to weigh less than people who eat less fiber. In a well-known study called the Seven Countries Studies,[10] the men in countries where the fiber intake was higher tended to weigh less than men in countries where less fiber was consumed. Here are some of the "fiber" preparations and what we know about them.

1. Guar Gum: Guar gum is an extract from *Cyamopsis tetragonolobus.* It is the most widely studied of the fiber compounds in this group, with 20 randomized placebo-controlled studies. The data, however, does not show that guar gum works any better than a placebo.[2,3]

2. Chitosan: Chitosan is an acetylated chitin derived from shellfish (crustaceans). It has been widely touted as a weight-loss agent. Chitosan has been studied in 14 randomized clinical trials, with over 1,000 subjects. An analysis of all these studies found that people taking chitosan lost 3.7 lb more, on average.[2,3] It did make a difference but not something to write home about. Another analysis concluded that there is little evidence that chitosan helps people.[6]

3. Glucomannan: Glucomannan is another fiber from the root of the *Amorphophallus konjac* plant. Its chemical structure is similar to that of galactomannan in guar gum. They are both polysaccharide chains of glucose and mannose and serve as water-soluble fibers. In one randomized controlled trial, overweight subjects given glucomannan lost more weight than those given a placebo. But again, the difference was small.[2,3]

4. Plantago psyllium: The psyllium extract from the seeds of this plant is a water-soluble fiber. In one randomized placebo-controlled trial[3], the gold standard for comparisons, there was no significant change in body weight in either the treatment or placebo group.

Conclusion
There are several herbal preparations that may have demonstrated some effect. They are ephedrine-containing, yohimbine-containing, and phenyle-

phrine-containing herbals that are demonstrated to be associated with weight loss. The problem with these products is the potential harm to the heart that could result, particularly when there are no strict controls on dosage. The herbals that seem most promising are, unfortunately, the ones we know least about. Hoodia deserves careful assessment. We need to understand their active ingredients and to carefully assess their safety and effectiveness before our interest is replaced by enthusiasm.

Table 1. Supplements Used in Weight Loss

	Safety Concerns	Weight loss efficacy	Evidence
Minerals and Metabolites			
Chromium	None known	Small weight loss, not clinically important; may prevent weight gain	10 RCTs
β-hydroxy-β-methylbutyrate	None known	? Fat mass reduction	2 RCTs
Pyruvate	None known	No	2 RCTs
Conjugated linoleic acid	Liver toxicity	No	13 RCTs
Calcium	None	No, not in large trials	Epidemiologic association positive; large RCTs negative
Herbal Supplements			
E. sinica – Ma huang	Cardiostimulatory properties, dose-related	Yes – ephedrine effect	2 RCTs
Garcinia cambobia (hydroxycitric acid)	None known	No	1 RCT
Pausinystalia	None known	Conflicting results	3 RCTs

RCT: randomized clinical trial

NOTES AND REFERENCES

Preface
1. Yudkin J. *Pure, White, and Deadly*. London: Penguin Books, 1986.
2. Bray GA, Nielsen SJ, Popkin BM. "High-Fructose Corn Syrup and the Epidemic of Obesity." *Am J Clin Nutr* 2004;79:537–544.
3. Bray GA. *The Physicians Diet Plan*. Unpublished manuscript, Copyright 1982, pp 1–249.

Introduction
1. Bray GA. *The Obese Patient*. Major Problems in Internal Medicine, Vol 9, Philadelphia, Pa.: WB Saunders Company, 1976, pp. 1–450.
2. Ogden CL, Yanovski SZ, Carroll MD, Flegal KM. "The Epidemiology of Obesity." *Gastroenterology* 2007;132:2087–2102.
3. "Obesity: Preventing and Managing the Global Epidemic." Report of a WHO consultation. *World Health Organ Tech Rep Ser* 2000;894:i–xii, 1–253.
4. NHLBI Obesity Education Initiative Expert Panel on the Identification, Evaluation, and Treatment of Overweight and Obesity in Adults. "Clinical Guidelines on the Identification, Evaluation, and Treatment of Overweight and Obesity in Adults—The Evidence Report." *Obes Res* 1998;6:51S–63S.
5. Bray GA. *The Metabolic Syndrome and Obesity*. Totawa NJ: Humana Press, 2007.
6. Bray GA. *The Physicians Diet Plan*. Unpublished manuscript, Copyright 1982, pp 1–249.
7. Ravelli AC, van Der Meulen JH, Osmond C, Barker DJ, Bleker OP. "Obesity at the Age of 50 in Men and Women Exposed to Famine Prenatally." *Am J Clin Nutr* 1999;70:811–816.
8. Franco M, Orduñez P, Caballero B, Tapia Granados JA, Lazo M, Bernal

JL, Guallar E, Cooper RS. "Impact of Energy Intake, Physical Activity, and Population-Wide Weight Loss on Cardiovascular Disease and Diabetes Mortality in Cuba, 1980–2005." *Am J Epidemiol* 2007;166:1374–1380.

9. Bray GA, Nielsen SJ, Popkin BM. "High-Fructose Corn Syrup and the Epidemic of Obesity." *Am J Clin Nutr* 2004;79:537–544.

10. Vartanian LR, Schwartz MB, Brownell KD. "Effects of Soft Drink Consumption on Nutrition and Health: A Systematic Review and Meta-Analysis." *Am J Public Health* 2007;97:667–675.

11. Winett RA, Tate DF, Anderson ES, Wojcik JR, Winett SG. "Long-term Weight Gain Prevention: A Theoretically Based Internet Approach." *Prev Med* 2005;41:629–641.

12. Worthington LS. *De l'Obésité. Étiologie, Thérapeutique et Hygiene.* Paris: E Martinet, 1875.

13. Bray GA. *The Battle of the Bulge.* Pittsburgh: Dorrance Publishing Co., Inc., 2007.

14. Short T. *A Discourse Concerning the Causes and Effects of Corpulency Together with the Method for Its Prevention and Cure.* London: J Roberts, 1727.

15. Flemyng M. *A Discourse on the Nature, Causes, and Cure of Corpulency. Illustrated by a Remarkable Case.* Read before the Royal Society November 1757. London: L Davis and C Reymers, 1760.

16. Rony HR. *Obesity and Leanness.* Philadelphia: Lea and Febiger, 1940.

17. Lavoisier AL. *Traité Elémentaire de Chimie, Présenté dans un Ordre Nouveau et d'après les Découvertes Modernes...; avec figures.* Paris: Chez Cuchet, 1789.

18. Boyle R. *The Works of the Honourable Robert Boyle.* London: A. Millar, 1764.

19. Von Helmholtz H. *Über die Erhaltung der Kraft, eine physikalische Abhandlung: vorgetragen in der Sitzung der physikalischen Gesellschaft zu Berlin am 23sten Juli 1847.* Berlin: G Reimer, 1847.

20. Von Mayer JR. Bemerkungen uber die Krafte der unbelebten Natur. *Ann Chem Pharm (Lemgo)* 1842;42:233–240.

21. Atwater WO, Rosa EB. *Description of a New Respiration Calorimeter and Experiments on the Conservation of Energy in the Human Body.* U.S. Department of *Agriculture*: 63, 1899.

22. Banting W. *Letter on Corpulence Addressed to the Public.* London: Harrison, 3rd ed, 1864.

23. Harvey W. *On Corpulence in Relation to Disease: With Some Remarks on Diet.* London: Henry Renshaw, 1872.

24. Frohlich A. Ein Fall von Tumor der hypophysis ceribri ohne Akromegalie. *Wien Klin Rdsch* 1901;15:883–886.

25. Babinski MJ. Tumeur du corps pituitaire sans acromégalie et avec de

développement des organes génitaux. *Revue Neurologique* 1900;8:531–533.

26. Cushing HW. *The Pituitary Body and its Disorders. Clinical States Produced by the Disorders of the Hypophysis Cerebri.* Philadelphia: JB Lippincott, 1912.

27. The Association of Life Insurance Medical Directors and The Actuarial Society of America. *MedicoActuarial Mortality Investigation.* New York: The Association of Life Insurance Medical Directors and The Actuarial Society of America; 1913.

28. Adams TD, Gress RE, Smith SC, Halverson RC, Simper SC, Rosamond WD, Lamonte MJ, Stroup AM, Hunt SC. "Long-term Mortality after Gastric Bypass Surgery." *N Engl J Med* 2007;357:753–761.

29. Sjöström L, Narbro K, Sjöström CD, Karason K, Larsson B, Wedel H, Lystig T, Sullivan M, Bouchard C, Carlsson B, Bengtsson C, Dahlgren S, Gummesson A, Jacobson P, Karlsson J, Lindroos AK, Lönroth H, Näslund I, Olbers T, Stenlöf K, Torgerson J, Agren G, Carlsson LM; Swedish Obese Subjects Study. "Effect of Bariatric Surgery on Mortality in Swedish Obese Subjects." *N Engl J Med* 2007;357:741–772.

30. Adams TD, Gress RE, Smith SC, Halverson RC, Simper SC, Rosamond WD, Lamonte MJ, Stroup AM, Hunt SC. "Long-term Mortality after Gastric Bypass Surgery." *N Engl J Med* 2007;357:753–761.

31. Bray GA (Ed). *Obesity in Perspective.* Fogarty International Center Series on Preventive Med. Vol 2, parts 1 and 2, Washington, D.C.: U.S. Govt Printing Office, DHEW Publication #75–708, 1976.

32. Howard AN (ed). *Recent Advances in Obesity Research: I. Proceedings of the 1st International Congress on Obesity* 8–11 October 1974 held at the Royal College of Physicians, London. London: Newman Publishing Ltd, 1975.

33. Zhang Y, Proenca R, Maffei M, Barone M, Leopold L, Friedman JM. "Positional Cloning of the Mouse Obese Gene and Its Human Homologue." *Nature* 1994;372:425–432.

34. Farooqi IS, O'Rahilly S. "Genetic Factors in Human Obesity." *Obes Rev* 2007;8 Suppl 1:37–40.

35. Stuart RB, Davis B. *Slim Chance in a Fat World: Behavioral Control of Obesity.* Champaign, IL: Research Press Company, 1972.

36. Flier J. "Obesity Wars: Molecular Progress Confronts and Expanding Epidemic." *Cell* 2004;116:337–350.

37. Larsson B, Svärdsudd K, Welin L, Wilhelmsen L, Björntorp P, Tibblin G. "Abdominal Adipose Tissue Distribution, Obesity and Risk of Cardiovascular Disease and death: Thirteen-Year Follow-up of Participants in the Study of 792 Men Born in 1913." *Br Med J* 1984;288:1401–1404.

38. Appel LJ, Moore TJ, Obarzanek E, Vollmer WM, Svetkey LP, Sacks

FM, Bray GA, Vogt TM, Cutler JA, Windhauser MM, Lin PH, Karanja N. "A Clinical Trial of the Effects of Dietary Patterns on Blood Pressure." *N Engl J Med* 1997;336:1117–124.

39. Sacks FM, Svetkey LP, Vollmer WM, Appel LJ, Bray GA, Harsha D, Obarzanek E, Conlin PR, Miller ER 3rd, Simons-Morton DG, Karanja N, Lin PH; DASH-Sodium Collaborative Research Group. "A Clinical Feeding Trial of the Effects on Blood Pressure of Reduced Dietary Sodium and the DASH Dietary Pattern" (The DASH-Sodium Trial). *N Engl J Med* 2001;344:3–10.

40. The DPP Research Group. "Reduction in the Incidence of Type-2 Diabetes with Lifestyle Intervention or Metformin." *N Engl J Med* 2002;346:393–403.

Chapter 1

1. Adams TD, Gress RE, Smith SC, Halverson RC, Simper SC, Rosamond WD, Lamonte MJ, Stroup AM, Hunt SC. "Long-term Mortality after Gastric Bypass Surgery." *N Engl J Med* 2007 23;357:753–761.

2. Sjöström L, Narbro K, Sjöström CD, Karason K, Larsson B, Wedel H, Lystig T, Sullivan M, Bouchard C, Carlsson B, Bengtsson C, Dahlgren S, Gummesson A, Jacobson P, Karlsson J, Lindroos AK, Lönroth H, Näslund I, Olbers T, Stenlöf K, Torgerson J, Agren G, Carlsson LM; Swedish Obese Subjects Study. "Effects of Bariatric Surgery on Mortality in Swedish Obese Subjects." *N Engl J Med* 2007;357:741–752.

3. Christakis NA, Fowler JH. "The Spread of Obesity in a Large Social Network over 32 Years." *N Engl J Med* 2007;357:370–379.

4. The Association of Life Insurance Medical Directors and The Actuarial Society of America. *Medico Actuarial Mortality Investigation.* New York: The Association of Life Insurance Medical Directors and The Actuarial Society of America, 1913.

5. Society of Actuaries. Build Study. Chicago: Metropolitan Life Insurance Table, 1979.

6. Quetelet LJA. *Sur l'Homme et le Developpement de ses Facultes, ou Essai de Physique Sociale.* Paris: Bachelier, 1835.

7. "Obesity: Preventing and Managing the Global Epidemic." Report of a WHO consultation. *World Health Organ Tech Rep Ser* 2000;894:i–xii, 1–253.

8. NHLBI Obesity Education Initiative Expert Panel on the Identification, Evaluation, and Treatment of Overweight and Obesity in Adults. "Clinical Guidelines on the Identification, Evaluation, and Treatment of Overweight and Obesity in Adults—The Evidence Report." *Obes Res* 1998;6:51S–63S.

9. Ogden CL, Carroll MD, Curtin LR, McDowell MA, Tabak CJ, Flegal

KM. "Prevalence of Overweight and Obesity in the United States, 1999–2004." *JAMA* 2006;295:1549–1555.

Chapter 2

1. Ogden CL, Carroll MD, Curtin LR, McDowell MA, Tabak CJ, Flegal KM. "Prevalence of Overweight and Obesity in the United States, 1999–2004." JAMA 2006;295:1549–1555.
2. Christakis NA, Fowler JH. "The Spread of Obesity in a Large Social Network over 32 Years." *N Engl J Med* 2007;357:370–379.
3. Wing RR, Tate DF, Gorin AA, Raynor HA, Fava JL, Machan J. "STOP Regain: Are There Negative Effects of Daily Weighing?" *J Consult Clin Psychol* 2007;75:652–656.
4. Bray GA, Popkin BM. "Dietary Fat Intake Does Affect Obesity!" *Am J Clin Nutr* 1998;68:1157–1173.
5. Smith SR, de Jonge L, Zachwieja JJ, Roy H, Nguyen T, Rood JC, Windhauser MM, Bray GA. "Fat and Carbohydrate Balances during Adaptation to a High-Fat Diet." *Am J Clin Nutr* 2000;71:450–457.
6. Smith SR, de Jonge L, Zachwieja JJ, Roy H, Nguyen T, Rood J, Windhauser M, Volaufova J, Bray GA. "Concurrent Physical Activity Increases Fat Oxidation during the Shift to a High-Fat Diet." *Am J Clin Nutr* 2000;72:131–138.
7. Ludwig DS. "The Glycemic Index: Physiological Mechanisms Relating to Obesity, Diabetes, and Cardiovascular Disease." *JAMA* 2002;287:2414–2423.
8. Leibel RL. "Molecular Physiology of Weight Regulation in Mice and Humans." *Int J Obes* 2008;32(Suppl): Suppl. 7:S98-S108
9. Pi-Sunyer FX, Aronne LJ, Heshmati HM, Devin J, Rosenstock J; RIO-North America Study Group. "Effect of Rimonabant, a Cannabinoid-1 Receptor Blocker, on Weight and Cardiometabolic Risk Factors in Overweight or Obese Patients: RIO-North America: A Randomized Controlled Trial." *JAMA* 2006;295:761–775.
10. Garrow JS. *Treat Obesity, Seriously.* Edinburgh: Churchill Livingstone, 1982.
11. Garrow JS, Gardiner GT. "Maintenance of Weight Loss in Obese Patients after Jaw Wiring." *Br Med J* 1981;282:858–860.
12. Nedergaard J, Dicker A, Cannon B. "The Interaction between Thyroid and Brown-Fat Thermogenesis. Central or Peripheral Effects?" *Ann NY Acad Sci* 1997;813:712–717.
13. Redman LM, de Jonge L, Fang X, Gamlin B, Recker D, Greenway FL, Smith SR, Ravussin E. "Lack of an Effect of a Novel Beta3-Adrenoceptor Agonist, TAK-677, on Energy Metabolism in Obese Individuals: A Double-Blind, Placebo-Controlled Randomized Study." *J Clin Endocrinol Metab* 2007;92:527–531.

14. Shaw GB. *Misalliance*. IN: *Complete Plays and Prefaces, Volumes I-VI.* New York: Dodd, Mead & Company, 1963.

15. Chua S Jr, Lomax KG, Leibel RL. "Molecular Genetics of Rodent and Human Single Gene mutations Affecting Body Composition." IN: *Handbook of Obesity: Etiology and Physiology.* GA Bray and C Bouchard (eds). New York: M Dekker, Inc, 2004;201–254.

16. Farooqi IS, O'Rahilly S. "Monogenic Obesity in Humans." *Annu Rev Med* 2005;56:443–458.

17. Stunkard AJ, Sørensen TI, Hanis C, Teasdale TW, Chakraborty R, Schull WJ, Schulsinger F. "An Adoption Study of Human Obesity." *N Engl J Med* 1986;314:193–198.

18. Stunkard AJ, Harris JR, Pedersen NL, McClearn GE. "The Body Mass Index of Twins Who Have Been Reared Apart." *N Engl J Med* 1990;322:1483–1487.

19. Bouchard C, Pérusse L, Leblanc C, Tremblay A, Thériault G. Inheritance of the Amount and Distribution of Human Body Fat." *Int J Obes* 1988;12:205–212.

20. Frayling TM, Timpson NJ, Weedon MN, Zeggini E, Freathy RM, Lindgren CM, Perry JR, Elliott KS, Lango H, Rayner NW, Shields B, Harries LW, Barrett JC, Ellard S, Groves CJ, Knight B, Patch AM, Ness AR, Ebrahim S, Lawlor DA, Ring SM, Ben-Shlomo Y, Jarvelin MR, Sovio U, Bennett AJ, Melzer D, Ferrucci L, Loos RJ, Barroso I, Wareham NJ, Karpe F, Owen KR, Cardon LR, Walker M, Hitman GA, Palmer CN, Doney AS, Morris AD, Smith GD, Hattersley AT, McCarthy MI. "A Common variant of the FTO Gene Is Associated with Body Mass Index and Predisposes to Childhood and Adult Obesity." *Science* 2007;316:889–894.

21. Armstrong PJ, Lund EM. "Changes in Body Composition and Energy Balance with Aging." *Vet Clin Nutr* 1996;3:83–87.

22. Bray GA. *Metabolic Syndrome and Obesity.* Totawa, NJ: Humana Press, 2007.

23. Dunaif A. "Polycystic Ovary Syndrome." *Health News* 1998;4:4.

24. Srinivasan S, Ogle GD, Garnett SP, Briody JN, Lee JW, Cowell CT. "Features of the Metabolic Syndrome after Childhood Craniopharyngioma." *J Clin Endocrinol Metab* 2004;89:81–86.

25. Champagne CM, Bray GA, Kurtz AA, Monteiro JB, Tucker E, Volaufova J, Delany JP. "Energy Intake and Energy Expenditure: A Controlled Study Comparing Dietitians and Non-Dietitians." *J Am Dietetic Assoc* 2002;102:1428–1432.

26. Knittle JL, Timmers K, Ginsberg-Fellner F, Brown RE, Katz DP. "The Growth of Adipose Tissue in Children and Adolescents. Cross-Sectional and Longitudinal Studies of Adipose Cell Number and Size." *J Clin Invest* 1979;63:239–246.

27. Spalding KL, Arner E, Westermark PO, Bernard S, Buchholz BA, Bergmann O, Blomqvist L, Hoffstedt J, Näslund E, Britton T, Concha H, Hassan M, Rydén M, Frisén J, Arner P. "Dynamics of Fat Cell Turnover in Humans." *Nature* 2008;453:783–787.

28. O'Hara P, Connett JE, Lee WW, Nides M, Murray R, Wise R. "Early and Late Weight Gain Following Smoking Cessation in the Lung Health Study." *Am J Epidemiol* 1998;148:821–830.

29. Kramer FM, Stunkard AJ, Marshall KA, McKinney S, Liebschutz J. "Breast-feeding Reduces Maternal Lower-Body Fat." *J Am Diet Assoc* 1993;93:429–433.

30. Ludwig DS. "The Glycemic Index: Physiological Mechanisms Relating to Obesity, Diabetes, and Cardiovascular Disease." *JAMA* 2002;287:2414–2423.

31. Nakagawa T, Hu H, Zharikov S, Tuttle KR, Short RA, Glushakova O, Ouyang X, Feig DI, Block ER, Herrera-Acosta J, Patel JM, Johnson RJ." A Causal Role for Uric Acid in Fructose-Induced Metabolic Syndrome." *Am J Physiol Renal Physiol* 2006;290:F625–F631.

32. Yudkin J. *Pure, White, and Deadly.* London: Penguin Books, 1986.

33. Keys A, Brozek J, Henschel A, Mickelsen O, Taylor HL. *The Biology of Human Starvation,* vols. 1 and 2. Minneapolis, University of Minnesota Press, 1950.

34. Klein S, Burke LE, Bray GA, Blair S, Allison DB, Pi-Sunyer X, Hong Y, Eckel RH, American Heart Association Council on Nutrition, Physical Activity, and Metabolism: American College of Cardiology Foundation. "Clinical Implications of Obesity with Specific Focus on Cardiovascular Disease: A Statement for Professionals from the American Heart Association Council on Nutrition, Physical Activity, and Metabolism: Endorsed by the American College of Cardiology Foundation." *Circulation* 2004;110:2952–2967.

35. Poirier P, Giles TD, Bray GA, Hong Y, Stern JS, Pi-Sunyer FX, Eckel RH; American Heart Association; Obesity Committee of the Council on Nutrition, Physical Activity, and Metabolism. "Obesity and Cardiovascular Disease: Pathophysiology, Evaluation, and Effect of Weight Loss: An Update of the 1997 American Heart Association Scientific Statement on Obesity and Heart Disease from the Obesity Committee of the Council on Nutrition, Physical Activity, and Metabolism." *Circulation* 2006;113:898–918.

36. Dhingra R, Sullivan L, Jacques PF, Wang TJ, Fox CS, Meigs JB, D'Agostino RB, Gaziano JM, Vasan RS. "Soft Drink Consumption and Risk of Developing Cardiometabolic Risk Factors and the Metabolic Syndrome in Middle-Aged Adults in the Community." *Circulation* 2007;116:480–488.

37. Aeberli I, Zimmermann MB, Molinari L, Lehmann R, l'Allemand D,

Spinas GA, Berneis K. "Fructose Intake Is a Predictor of LDL Particle Size in Overweight Schoolchildren." *Am J Clin Nutr* 2007;86:1174–1178.

38. Choi HK, Curran G. "Soft Drinks, Fructose Consumption and the Risk of Gout in Men: Prospective Cohort Study." *BMJ* 2008;336:309–312.

39. Weiss EC, Galuska DA, Khan LK, Serdula MK. "Weight-Control Practices among U.S. Adults, 2001–2002." *Am J Prev Med* 2006;31:18–24.

40. "Weight Cycling. National Task Force on the Prevention and Treatment of Obesity." *JAMA* 1994;272:1196–202.

41. Knowler WC, Barrett-Connor E, Fowler SE, Hamman RF, Lachin JM, Walker EA, Nathan DM; Diabetes Prevention Program Research Group. "Reduction in the Incidence of Type-2 Diabetes with Lifestyle Intervention or Metformin." *N Engl J Med* 2002;346:393–403.

42. Sjöström L, Narbro K, Sjöström CD, Karason K, Larsson B, Wedel H, Lystig T, Sullivan M, Bouchard C, Carlsson B, Bengtsson C, Dahlgren S, Gummesson A, Jacobson P, Karlsson J, Lindroos AK, Lönroth H, Näslund I, Olbers T, Stenlöf K, Torgerson J, Agren G, Carlsson LM; Swedish Obese Subjects Study. "Effects of Bariatric Surgery on Mortality in Swedish Obese Subjects." *N Engl J Med* 2007;357:741–752.

43. Adams TD, Gress RE, Smith SC, Halverson RC, Simper SC, Rosamond WD, Lamonte MJ, Stroup AM, Hunt SC. "Long-term Mortality after Gastric Bypass Surgery." N Engl J Med 2007;357:753–761.

Chapter 3

1. Lindner PL. *It's Your Right to Be Thin*. South Gate, CA: The Linder Clinic, 1977.

2. Smith, NJ. *When I Say No, I Feel Guilty*. New York: Bantam Books, 1975.

Chapter 4

1. Christakis NA, Fowler JH. "The Spread of Obesity in a Large Social Network over 32 Years." *N Engl J Med* 2007;357:370–379.

2. Precope J. *Hippocrates on Diet and Hygiene*. London: Zeno, 1952.

3. Pauling L. *Vitamin C, the Common Cold, and the Flu*. San Francisco: WH Freeman, 1970.

4. Fuchs L. *De Historia Stirpium Comentarii Insignes, maximis Impensis et Vigiliis elaborate, adiectis earundem vivis, plusquam quingentis imaginibus, nunquam antea ad naturae imitationem artificiolius effictis & expresis*. Basileae: In officina Isingriniana, 1562.

5. Pollan M. *In Defense of Food. An Eater's Manifesto*. New York: The Penguin Group, 2008.

6. Davis C, Saltos E. "Dietary Recommendations and How They Have Changed over Time." IN: *America's Eating Habits. Changes and Consequences.* U.S. Department of Agriculture, Economic Research Service, Food and Rural Economics Division. Agriculture Information Bulletin No 750. 1999;33–50.

7. U.S. Food & Drug Administration. *Food Guide Pyramid.* Washington, D.C. U.S. Government Printing Office, 1992.

8. *Dietary Guidelines for Americans 2005.* Washington, D.C.: U.S. Department of Health and Human Services; U.S. Department of Agriculture HHS Publication No HHS-ODPHP-2005-01-DGAA, 2005.

9. U.S. Department of Health and Human Services. *Physical Activity and Health: A Report of the Surgeon General.* Atlanta, GA: U.S. Department of Health and Human Services, Centers for Disease Control and Prevention, National Center for Chronic Disease Prevention and Health Promotion, 1996.

10. National Research Council. *Diet and Health, Implications for Reducing Chronic Disease Risk*, National Research Council. Washington, D.C.: National Academy Press, 1989.

11. *Diet, Nutrition and the Prevention of Chronic Diseases.* Report of a Joint WHO/FAO Expert Consultation. WHO Technical Report Series 916. Geneva: World Health Organization, 2003.

12. Appel LJ, Moore TJ, Obarzanek E, Vollmer WM, Svetkey LP, Sacks FM, Bray GA, Vogt TM, Cutler JA, Windhauser MM, Lin PH, Karanja N. "A Clinical Trial of the Effects of Dietary Patterns on Blood Pressure." *N Engl J Med* 1997;336:1117–1124.

13. Sacks FM, Svetkey LP, Vollmer WM, Appel LJ, Bray GA, Harsha D, Obarzanek E, Conlin PR, Miller ER 3rd, Simons-Morton DG, Karanja N, Lin PH; DASH-Sodium Collaborative Research Group." A Clinical Feeding Trial of the Effects on Blood Pressure of Reduced Dietary Sodium and the DASH Dietary Pattern "(The DASH-Sodium Trial). *N Engl J Med* 2001;344:3–10.

14. Bazzano LA, Song Y, Bubes V, Good CK, Manson JE, Liu S. "Dietary Intake of Whole and Refined Grain Breakfast Cereals and Weight Gain in Men." *Obes Res* 2005;13:1952–1960.

15. Barton BA, Eldridge AL, Thompson D, Affenito SG, Striegel-Moore RH, Franko DL, Albertson AM, Crockett SJ. "The Relationship of Breakfast and Cereal Consumption to Nutrient Intake and Body Mass Index: The National Heart, Lung, and Blood Institute Growth and Health Study." *J Am Diet Assoc* 2005;105:1383–1389.

16. Lindner PL. *Test Your Knowledge. What's Your Weight Nutriton I.Q.?* South Gate CA: Peter Lindner, 1974.

17. Wolf A, Bray GA, Popkin BM. "A Short History of Beverages and How

Our Body Treats Them." *Obes Rev* 2008;9:151–164.

18. Funk C. *Die vitamine ihre bedeutung fur die Physiologie und Pathologie mit besonderer Berucksichtgung der Avitaminosen: (Beriberi, skorbut, pellagra, rachitis).* Wiesbaden: J.F. Bergmann, 1914.

19. Ludwig DS. "The Glycemic Index: Physiological Mechanisms Relating to Obesity, Diabetes, and Cardiovascular Disease." *JAMA* 2002;287:2414–2423.

20. Ebbeling CB, Leidig MM, Feldman HA, Lovesky MM, Ludwig DS. "Effects of a Low-Glycemic Load vs Low-fat Diet in Obese Young Adults: A Randomized Trial." *JAMA* 2007;297:2092–2102.

21. Malik R. "Vitamin D and Secondary Hyperparathyroidism in the Institutionalized Elderly: A Literature Review." *J Nutr Elder* 2007;26:119–138.

22. Holub DJ, Holub BJ. "Omega-3 Fatty Acids from Fish Oils and Cardiovascular Disease." *Mol Cell Biochem* 2004;263:217–225.

23. Mozaffarian D, Willett WC. "Trans Fatty Acids and Cardiovascular Risk: A Unique Cardiometabolic Imprint?" *Curr Atheroscler Rep* 2007;9:486–493.

24. Vartanian LR, Schwartz MB, Brownell KD. "Effects of Soft Drink Consumption on Nutrition and Health: A Systematic Review and Meta-Analysis." *Am J Public Health*, 2007;97:667–675.

Chapter 5

1. Wolf A, Bray GA, Popkin BM. "A Short History of Beverages and How Our Body Treats Them." *Obes Rev* 2008;9:151–164.

2. Havel PJ. "Dietary Fructose: Implications for Dysregulation of Energy Homeostasis and Lipid/Carbohydrate Metabolism." *Nutr Rev* 2005;63:133–157.

3. Aeberli I, Zimmermann MB, Molinari L, Lehmann R, l'Allemand D, Spinas GA, Berneis K. "Fructose Intake Is a Predictor of LDL Particle Size in Overweight Schoolchildren." *Am J Clin Nutr* 2007;86:1174–1178.

4. Dhingra R, Sullivan L, Jacques PF, Wang TJ, Fox CS, Meigs JB, D'Agostino RB, Gaziano JM, Vasan RS. "Soft Drink Consumption and Risk of Developing Cardiometabolic Risk Factors and the Metabolic Syndrome in Middle-Aged Adults in the Community. *Circulation* 2007;116:480–488.

5. *Dietary Reference Intakes.* Washington, D.C. National Academies Press, 1997–2002.

6. Wang ZM, Pierson RN Jr, Heymsfield SB. "The Five-Level Model: A New Approach to Organizing Body-Composition Research." *Am J Clin Nutr* 1992;56:19–28.

7. Goldberger J. *The Present Status of Our Knowledge of the Etiology of*

Pellagra. Delamar Lectures, 1925–26. Baltimore: The Williams & Wilkins Company, 1927.

8. Siri PW, Krauss RM. "Influence of Dietary Carbohydrate and Fat on LDL and HDL Particle Distributions." *Curr Atheroscler Rep* 2005;7:455–459.

9. Fremes R, Sabry Z. *The Rate-Yourself Plan for Better Nutrition: NutriScore*. Toronto: Methuen/Two Continents, 1976.

10. Wing RR, Phelan S. "Long-term Weight Loss Maintenance." *Am J Clin Nutr* 2005;82(1 Suppl):222S–225S.

11. Howard BV, Manson JE, Stefanick ML, Beresford SA, Frank G, Jones B, Rodabough RJ, Snetselaar L, Thomson C, Tinker L, Vitolins M, Prentice R. "Low-fat Dietary Pattern and Weight Change over 7 Years: The Women's Health Initiative Dietary Modification Trial." *JAMA* 2005;295:39–49.

12. Flatt JP, Ravussin E, Acheson KJ, Jéquier E. "Effects of Dietary Fat on Postprandial Substrate Oxidation and on Carbohydrate and Fat Balances." *J Clin Invest* 1985;76:1019–1024.

13. Pauling L. *Vitamin C, the Common Cold, and the Flu*. San Francisco: WH Freeman, 1970.

14. Virtamo J, Rapola JM, Ripatti S, Heinonen OP, Taylor PR, Albanes D, Huttunen JK. "Effect of Vitamin E and Beta Carotene on the Incidence of Primary Nonfatal Myocardial Infarction and Fatal coronary Heart Disease." *Arch Intern Med* 1998;158:668–675.

15. Appel LJ, Moore TJ, Obarzanek E, Vollmer WM, Svetkey LP, Sacks FM, Bray GA, Vogt TM, Cutler JA, Windhauser MM, Lin PH, Karanja N. "A Clinical Trial of the Effects of Dietary Patterns on Blood Pressure." *N Engl J Med* 1997;336:1117–1124.

16. Sacks FM, Svetkey LP, Vollmer WM, Appel LJ, Bray GA, Harsha D, Obarzanek E, Conlin PR, Miller ER 3rd, Simons-Morton DG, Karanja N, Lin PH; DASH-Sodium Collaborative Research Group. "A Clinical Feeding Trial of the Effects on Blood Pressure of Reduced Dietary Sodium and the DASH Dietary Pattern" (The DASH-Sodium Trial). *N Engl J Med* 2001;344:3–10.

Chapter 6

1. Wolf A, Bray GA, Popkin BM. "A Short History of Beverages and How Our Body Treats Them." *Obes Rev* 2008;9:151–164.

2. Nielsen SJ, Popkin BM. "Changes in Beverage Intake between 1977–2001." *Am J Prev Med* 2004;27:205–210.

3. Popkin BM, Armstrong LE, Bray GM, Caballero B, Frei B, Willett WC. "A New Proposed Guidance System for Beverage Consumption in the United States." *Am J Clin Nutr* 83:529–542.

4. Wang ZM, Pierson RN Jr, Heymsfield SB. "The Five-Level Model: A

New Approach to Organizing Body-Composition Research." *Am J Clin Nutr* 1992;56:19–28.

5. National Research Council. *Recommended Dietary Intakes.* Washington, D.C.: National Academies Press, 2002–2005.

6. Stookey JD, Constant F, Gardner CD, Popkin BM. "Replacing Sweetened Caloric Beverages with Drinking Water Is Associated with Lower Energy Intake." *Obesity* 2007;15:3013–302.

7. Salazar-Martinez E, Willett WC, Ascherio A, Manson JE, Leitzmann MF, Stampfer MJ, Hu FB. "Coffee Consumption and Risk for Type-2 Diabetes Mellitus." *Ann Intern Med* 2004;140:1–8.

8. Nawrot P, Jordan S, Eastwood J, Rotstein J, Hugenholtz A, Feeley M. "Effects of Caffeine on Human Health." *Food Addit Contam* 2003;20:1–30.

9. Dulloo AG, Seydoux J, Girardier L, Chantre P, Vandermander J. "Green Tea and Thermogenesis: Interactions between Catechin-Polyphenols, Caffeine and Sympathetic Activity." *Int J Obes Relat Metab Disord* 2000;24:252–258.

10. "Artificial Sweeteners: No Calories...Sweet!" *FDA Consum* 2006;40:27–28.

11. Appel LJ, Moore TJ, Obarzanek E, Vollmer WM, Svetkey LP, Sacks FM, Bray GA, Vogt TM, Cutler JA, Windhauser MM, Lin PH, Karanja N. "A Clinical Trial of the Effects of Dietary Patterns on Blood Pressure." *N Engl J Med* 1997;336:1117–1124.

12. Sacks FM, Svetkey LP, Vollmer WM, Appel LJ, Bray GA, Harsha D, Obarzanek E, Conlin PR, Miller ER 3rd, Simons-Morton DG, Karanja N, Lin PH; DASH-Sodium Collaborative Research Group. "A Clinical Feeding Trial of the Effects on Blood Pressure of Reduced Dietary Sodium and the DASH Dietary Pattern (The DASH-Sodium Trial). *N Engl J Med* 2001;344:3–10.

13. Coombes JS, Hamilton KL. "The Effectiveness of Commercially Available Sports Drinks. *Sports Med* 2000;29:181–209.

14. Yudkin J. *Pure, White, and Deadly.* London: Penguin Books, 1986.

15. Havel PJ. "Dietary Fructose: Implications for Dysregulation of Energy Homeostasis and Lipid/Carbohydrate Metabolism." *Nutr Rev* 2005;63:133–157.

16. Mattes R. "Fluid Calories and Energy Balance: The Good, the Bad, and the Uncertain." *Physiol Behav* 2006;89:66–70.

Chapter 7

1. Klem ML, Wing RR, McGuire MT, Seagle HM, Hill JO. "A Descriptive Study of Individuals Successful at Long-term Maintenance of Substantial Weight Loss." *Am J Clin Nutr* 1997;66:239–246.

2. Crespo CJ, Smit E, Troiano RP, Bartlett SJ, Macera CA, Andersen RE.

"Television Watching, Energy Intake, and Obesity in US Children: Results from the Third National Health and Nutrition Examination Survey, 1988–1994." *Arch Pediatr Adolesc Med* 2001;155:360–365.

3. Epstein LH, Roemmich JN, Paluch RA, Raynor HA. "Influence of Changes in Sedentary Behavior on Energy and Macronutrient Intake in Youth." *Am J Clin Nutr* 2005;81:361–366.

4. *Dietary Reference Intakes for Energy, Carbohydrate, Fiber, Fat, Fatty Acids, Cholesterol, Protein and Amino Acids.* Washington, D.C.: The National Academies Press, 2002–2005.

5. *Dietary Guidelines for Americans 2005.* Washington, D.C.: U.S. Department of Health and Human Services; U.S. Department of Agriculture HHS Publication No HHS-ODPHP-2005-01DGAA.

6. Bailey C. *Fit or Fat?* Boston: Houghton Mifflin Co., 1977.

7. Pavlou KN, Krey S, Steffee WP. "Exercise As an Adjunct to Weight Loss and Maintenance in Moderately Obese Subjects." *Am J Clin Nutr* 1989;49:1115–1123.

8. Bray GA. "The Energetics of Obesity." *Med Sci Sports Exer* 1983;15:32–40.

9. Gibbons RJ, Balady GJ, Bricker JT, Chaitman BR, Fletcher GF, Froelicher VF, Mark DB, McCallister BD, Mooss AN, O'Reilly MG, Winters WL Jr, Gibbons RJ, Antman EM, Alpert JS, Faxon DP, Fuster V, Gregoratos G, Hiratzka LF, Jacobs AK, Russell RO, Smith SC Jr; American College of Cardiology/American Heart Association Task Force on Practice Guidelines (Committee to Update the 1997 Exercise Testing Guidelines). "ACC/AHA 2002 Guideline Update for Exercise Testing: Summary Article: A Report of the American College of Cardiology/American Heart Association Task Force on Practice Guidelines" (Committee to Update the 1997 Exercise Testing Guidelines). *Circulation* 2002; 106:1883–1892.

Chapter 8

1. Polivy J, Herman CP." If at First You Don't Succeed. False Hopes of Self-Change." *Am Psychol* 2002;57:677–689.

2. Levine JA, McCrady SK, Lanningham-Foster LM, Kane PH, Foster RC, Manohar CU. "The Role of Free-Living Daily Walking in Human Weight Gain and Obesity." *Diabetes* 2008;57:548–554.

3. Stuart RB. "Behavioral Control of Overeating." *Behav Res Ther* 1967;5:357–365.

4. Brownell K. *The LEARN Program for Weight Control: Lifestyle, Exercise, Attitudes, Relationships, Nutrition.* Dallas: American Health Pub, 1991.

5. Ferguson JM. *Habits, Not Diets. The Real Way to Weight Control.* Palo Alto, CA: Bull Publishing Co., 1976.

6. Skinner BF. "The Operant Side of Behavior Therapy." *J Behav Ther Exp*

Psychiatry 1988;19:171.

7. Pavlov IP. *Conditioned Reflexes: An Investigation of the Physiological Activity of the Cerebral Cortex.* London: Oxford University Press, 1927.

8. Christakis NA, Fowler JH. "The Spread of Obesity in a Large Social Network over 32 Years." *N Engl J Med* 2007;357:370–379.

9. Tillotson JE. "Pandemic Obesity: What Is the Solution?" *Nutr Today* 2004;39:6–9.

10. Mattes R. "Fluid Calories and Energy Balance: The Good, the Bad, and the Uncertain." *Physiol Behav* 2006;89:66–70.

11. Epstein LH, Roemmich JN, Paluch RA, Raynor HA. "Influence of Changes in Sedentary Behavior on Energy and Macronutrient Intake in Youth." *Am J Clin Nutr* 2005;81:361–366.

12. Kissileff HR. "Ingestive Behavior Microstructure, Basic Mechanisms and Clinical Applications. *Neurosci Biobehav Rev* 2000;24:171–172.

13. Blaxter K. "Measurement of the Upper and Lower Segment of Women from 1600 to the Present Showed a Gradual Elongation of the Lower Segment Relative to the Upper One" (Personal Communication).

14. Byrd-Bredbenner C, Murray J, Schlussel YR. "Temporal Changes in Anthropometric Measurements of Idealized Females and Young Women in General." *Women Health* 2005;41:13–30.

Chapter 9.

1. Edney ATB, Smith PM. "Study of Obesity in Dogs Visiting a Veterinary Practices in the United Kingdom." *Vet Rec* 1986;118:391–396; McGreevy PD, Thomson PC, Pride C, Fawcett A, Grassi T, Jones B. "Prevalence of Obesity in Dogs examined by Australian Veterinary Practices and the Risk Factors Involved." *Vet Rec* 2005;156:695–702.

2. Kienzle E, Bergler R, Mandernach A. "A Comparison of the Feeding Behavior and Human-Animal Relationship in Owners of Normal and Obese Dogs. *J Nutr* 1998;128:2779S–2782S.

3. Bray GA, Popkin BM. "Dietary Fat Intake Does Affect Obesity!" *Am J Clin Nutr* 1998;68:1157–1173.

4. Smith SR, de Jonge L, Zachwieja JJ, Roy H, Nguyen T, Rood JC, Windhauser MM, Bray GA. "Fat and Carbohydrate Balances during Adaptation to a High-Fat Diet." *Am J Clin Nutr* 2000;71:450–457.

5. Smith SR, de Jonge L, Zachwieja JJ, Roy H, Nguyen T, Rood J, Windhauser M, Volaufova J, Bray GA. "Concurrent Physical Activity Increases Fat Oxidation during the Shift to a High-Fat Diet." *Am J Clin Nutr* 2000;72:131–138.

6. Hu FB, Cho E, Rexrode KM, Albert CM, Manson JE. "Fish and Long-Chain Omega-3 Fatty Acid Intake and Risk of Coronary Heart Disease and Total Mortality in Diabetic Women." *Circulation* 2003;107:1852–1857.

7. Wing RR, Phelan S. "Long-term Weight Loss Maintenance." *Am J Clin Nutr* 2005;82:222S–225S.

8. Paeratakul S, York-Crowe EE, Williamson DA, Ryan DH, Bray GA. "Americans on Diets: Results from the 1994–1996 Continuing Survey of Food Intakes by Individuals" (CSFII 1994–1996). *J Am Dietetic Assoc* 2002;102:1247–1251.

9. Howard BV, Manson JE, Stefanick ML, Beresford SA, Frank G, Jones B, Rodabough RJ, Snetselaar L, Thomson C, Tinker L, Vitolins M, Prentice R. "Low-fat Dietary Pattern and Weight Change over 7 Years: The Women's Health Initiative Dietary Modification Trial." *JAMA* 2006;295:39–49.

10. Astrup A, Grunwald GK, Melanson EL, Saris WH, Hill JO. "The Role of Low-fat Diets in Body Weight Control: A Meta-Analysis of Ad Libitum Dietary Intervention Studies." *Int J Obes Relat Metab Disord* 2000;24:1545–1552.

11. Bray GA, Flatt JP, Volaufova J, Champagne CM, DeLany JP. "Corrective Responses in Human Food Intake Identified from an Analysis of 7-Day Food-Intake Records." *Am Clin Nutr In Press.* 2008; 88:1504-1510

12. Taubes G. *Good Calories, Bad Calories.* New York: AA Knopf, 2007.

13. Flatt JP, Ravussin E, Acheson KJ, Jéquier E. "Effects of Dietary Fat on Postprandial Substrate Oxidation and on Carbohydrate and Fat Balances." *J Clin Invest* 1985;76:1019–1024.

14. Sparti A, Windhauser MM, Champagne CM, Bray GA. "Effect of an Acute Reduction in Carbohydrate Intake on Subsequent Food Intake in Healthy Men." *Am J Clin Nutr* 1997;66:1144–1150.

15. Roth H. *Harriet Roth's Fat Counter,* 3rd revised edition. New York: The Penguin Group, 2007.

16. Natow AB, Heslin JA. *The Calorie Counter.* New York: Pocket Books, 2007.

Chapter 10.

1. Farshchi HR, Taylor MA, Macdonald IA. "Beneficial Metabolic Effects of Regular Meal Frequency on Dietary Thermogenesis, Insulin Sensitivity, and Fasting Lipid Profiles in Healthy Obese women." *Am J Clin Nutr* 2005;81:16–24.

2. *Recommended Dietary Allowances,* 10th edition. Washington, D.C: National Academy Press, 1989.

3. Pitts GC, Bullard TR. "Some Interspecific Aspects of Body Composition in Mammals." IN: Body Composition in Animals and Man. Proceedings of a Symposium held May 4, 5, and 6, 1967 at the University of Missouri, Columbia, Washington, D.C., National Academy of Sciences, 1968;45-70 Publication No 1598; 1968.

4. Bray GA. *The Obese Patient.* Philadelphia: WB Saunders Co, 1976.
5. Department of Agriculture Handbook No. 8, Composition of Foods: Raw, Processed, Prepared, and its updates, for example: *http://www.nal.usda.gov/fnic/foodcomp/search/*.
6. Pennington JAT, Douglass JS. *Bowes and Church's Food Values of Portions Commonly Used* 18th edition. Philadelphia: Lippincott, Williams and Wilkins Co., 2004.
7. Kraus B, Reilly-Pardo M. *Calories and Carbohydrates.* New York: New American Library, A Division of Penguin Group, Inc., 2003.
8. Bray GA, Flatt JP, Volaufova J, Champagne CM, DeLany JP. "Corrective Responses in Human Food Intake Identified from an Analysis of 7-Day Food Intake Records." *Am J Clin Nutr* 2008 in press.
9. Wansink B, van Ittersum K. "Portion Size Me: Downsizing Our Consumption Norms." *J Am Diet Assn* 2007;107:1103–1106.

Chapter 11.

1. Appel LJ, Moore TJ, Obarzanek E, Vollmer WM, Svetkey LP, Sacks FM, Bray GA, Vogt TM, Cutler JA, Windhauser MM, Lin PH, Karanja N. "A Clinical Trial of the Effects of Dietary Patterns on Blood Pressure." *N Engl J Med* 1997;336:1117–1124.
2. Sacks FM, Svetkey LP, Vollmer WM, Appel LJ, Bray GA, Harsha D, Obarzanek E, Conlin PR, Miller ER 3rd, Simons-Morton DG, Karanja N, Lin PH; DASH-Sodium Collaborative Research Group. "A Clinical Feeding Trial of the Effects on Blood Pressure of Reduced Dietary Sodium and the DASH Dietary Pattern" (The DASH-Sodium Trial). *N Engl J Med* 2001;344:3–10.
3. Vartanian LR, Schwartz MB, Brownell KD. "Effects of Soft Drink Consumption on Nutrition and Health: A Systematic Review and Meta-Analysis." *Am J Public Health* 2007;97:667–675.

Chapter 12

1. Yudkin J. *Pure, White, and Deadly.* London: Penguin Books, 1986. *www. illovosugar.com/sordofsugar.*
2. Howard BV, Manson JE, Stefanick ML, Beresford SA, Frank G, Jones B, Rodabough RJ, Snetselaar L, Thomson C, Tinker L, Vitolins M, Prentice R. "Low-fat Dietary Pattern and Weight Change over 7 Years: The Women's Health Initiative Dietary Modification Trial." *JAMA* 2006;295: 39–49.
3. Rimm EB, Ascherio A, Giovannucci E, Spiegelman D, Stampfer MJ, Willett WC. "Vegetable, Fruit, and Cereal Fiber Intake and Risk of Coronary Heart Disease among Men." *JAMA* 1996;275:447–451.
4. Appel LJ, Moore TJ, Obarzanek E, Vollmer WM, Svetkey LP, Sacks FM, Bray GA, Vogt TM, Cutler JA, Windhauser MM, Lin PH, Karanja

N. "A Clinical Trial of the Effects of Dietary Patterns on Blood Pressure." *N Engl J Med* 1997;338:1117–1124.

5. Cameron E, Pauling L. *Cancer and Vitamin C.* Menlo Park, CA: Linus Pauling Institute of Science and Medicine, 1979.

6. Food and Nutrition Board, Institute of Medicine. *Dietary Reference Intakes for Energy, Carbohydrate, Fiber, Fat, Fatty Acids, Cholesterol, Protein and Amino Acids.* Washington, D.C.: The National Academies Press, 2002/2005.

Chapter 13

1. Bray GA. *The Obese Patient.* Philadelphia: WB Saunders, 1976.

2. *Recommended Dietary Allowances,* 10th edition. Washington, D.C.: National Academy Press, 1989.

3. Davidson MB, Chopra IJ. "Effect of Carbohydrate and Noncarbohydrate Sources of Calories on plasma 3,5,3'-Triiodothyronine Concentrations in man." *J Clin Endocrinol Metab* 1979;48:577–581.

4. Hu FB, Bronner L, Willett WC, Stampfer MJ, Rexrode KM, Albert CM, Hunter D, Manson JE. "Fish and Omega-3 Fatty Acid Intake and Risk of Coronary Heart Disease in Women." *JAMA* 2002;287:1815–1821.

Chapter 14

1. Linn R, Stuart SL. *The Last Chance Diet—When Everything Else Has Failed.* Seacaucus, NJ: Lyle Stuart, Inc., 1976.

2. Sours HE, Frattali VP, Brand CD, Feldman RA, Forbes AL, Swanson RC, Paris AL. "Sudden Death Associated with Very Low Calorie Weight Reduction Regimes." *Am J Clin Nutr* 1981;34:453–461.

3. Howard AN, Grant A, Edwards O, Littlewood ER, McLean Baird I. "The Treatment of Obesity with a Very Low-Calorie Liquid-Formula Diet: An Inpatient/Outpatient Comparison Using Skimmed-Milk Protein As the Chief Protein Source." *Int J Obes* 1978;2:321–332.

4. Wilson FC. *The Cambridge Miracle: A Doctor's Point of View. The Famous Cambridge Diet Explained in Full.* Boca Raton FL: Atlantis Publishing of Palm Beach, 1983.

5. Genuth SM, Castro JH, Vertes V. "Weight Reduction in Obesity by Outpatient Semistarvation." *JAMA* 1974;230:987–991.

6. *Deception and Fraud in the Diet Industry Part I.* Hearing before the Subcommittee on Regulation, Business Opportunities, and Energy of the committee on Small Business House of Representatives, Washington, D.C., March 26, 1990. Washington, D.C.: U.S. Government Printing Office: Serial No. 101–50, 1990.

7. Foster GD, Wadden TA, Peterson FJ, Letizia KA, Bartlett SJ, Conill

AM. "A Controlled Comparison of Three Very Low-Calorie Diets: Effects on Weight, Body Composition, and Symptoms." *Am J Clin Nutr* 1992;55:811–817.

8. Bray GA. "Effect of Caloric Restriction on Energy Expenditure in Obese Patients." *Lancet* 1969;2:397–398.

9. Leibel RL, Rosenbaum M, Hirsch J. "Changes in Energy Expenditure Resulting from Altered Body Weight." *N Engl J Med* 1995;332:621–628.

10. Davidson MB, Chopra IJ. "Effect of Carbohydrate and Noncarbohydrate Sources of Calories on Plasma 3,5,3'-Triiodothyronine Concentrations in Man. *J Clin Endocrinol Metab* 1979;48:577–581.

11. Rosenbaum M, Goldsmith R, Bloomfield D, Magnano A, Weimer L, Heymsfield S, Gallagher D, Mayer L, Murphy E, Leibel RL. "Low-dose Leptin Reverses Skeletal Muscle, Autonomic, and Neuroendocrine Adaptations to Maintenance of Reduced Weight. *J Clin Invest* 2005;115:3579–3586.

12. Flechtner-Mors M, Ditschuneit HH, Johnson TD, Suchard MA, Adler G. "Metabolic and Weight Loss Effects of Long-term Dietary Intervention in Obese Patients: Four-Year Results." *Obes Res* 2000;8:399–402.

13. Look AHEAD Research Group, Pi-Sunyer X, Blackburn G, Brancati FL, Bray GA, Bright R, Clark JM, Curtis JM, Espeland MA, Foreyt JP, Graves K, Haffner SM, Harrison B, Hill JO, Horton ES, Jakicic J, Jeffery RW, Johnson KC, Kahn S, Kelley DE, Kitabchi AE, Knowler WC, Lewis CE, Maschak-Carey BJ, Montgomery B, Nathan DM, Patricio J, Peters A, Redmon JB, Reeves RS, Ryan DH, Safford M, Van Dorsten B, Wadden TA, Wagenknecht L, Wesche-Thobaben J, Wing RR, Yanovski SZ. "Reduction in Weight and Cardiovascular Disease (CVD) Risk Factors in Individuals with Type 2 Diabetes: One Year Results of Look AHEAD Trial." *Diab Care* 2007;30:1374–1383.

Chapter 15

1. Knowler WC, Barrett-Connor E, Fowler SE, Hamman RF, Lachin JM, Walker EA, Nathan DM; Diabetes Prevention Program Research Group. "Reduction in the Incidence of Type-2 Diabetes with Lifestyle Intervention or Metformin." *N Engl J Med* 2002;346:393–403.

2. Hamman RF, Wing RR, Edelstein SL, Lachin JM, Bray GA, Delahanty L, Hoskin M, Kriska AM, Mayer-Davis EJ, Pi-Sunyer X, Regensteiner J, Venditti B, Wylie-Rosett

3. J. "Effect of Weight Loss with Lifestyle Intervention on Risk of Diabetes." *Diabetes Care* 2006;29:2102–2107.

4. Ryan DH, Espeland MA, Foster GD, Haffner SM, Hubbard VS,

Johnson KC, Kahn SE, Knowler WC, Yanovski SZ; Look AHEAD Research Group. Look AHEAD: (Action for Health in Diabetes). "Design and Methods for a Clinical Trial of Weight Loss for the Prevention of Cardiovascular Disease in Type-2 diabetes." *Controlled Clinical Trials* 2003;24:610–628.

5. Look AHEAD Research Group, Pi-Sunyer X, Blackburn G, Brancati FL, Bray GA, Bright R, Clark JM, Curtis JM, Espeland MA, Foreyt JP, Graves K, Haffner SM, Harrison B, Hill JO, Horton ES, Jakicic J, Jeffery RW, Johnson KC, Kahn S, Kelley DE, Kitabchi AE, Knowler WC, Lewis CE, Maschak-Carey BJ, Montgomery B, Nathan DM, Patricio J, Peters A, Redmon JB, Reeves RS, Ryan DH, Safford M, Van Dorsten B, Wadden TA, Wagenknecht L, Wesche-Thobaben J, Wing RR, Yanovski SZ. "Reduction in Weight and Cardiovascular Disease (CVD) Risk Factors in Individuals with Type-2 Diabetes: One Year Results of Look AHEAD Trial." *Diabetes Care* 2007;30:1374–1383.

6. Perri MG, Nezu AM, Viegener BJ. *Improving the Long-term Management of Obesity. Theory, Tesearch and Clinical Guidelines.* New York: John Wiley & Sons, 1992.

7. Wadden TA, Berkowitz RI, Womble LG, Sarwer DB, Phelan S, Cato RK, Hesson LA, Osei SY, Kaplan R, Stunkard AJ. "Randomized Trial of Lifestyle Modification and Pharmacology for Obesity." *N Engl J Med* 2005;353:2111–2120.

8. Stuart RB, Davis B. *Slim Chance in a Fat World.* Champaign, IL: Research Press Co., 1972.

9. Stunkard AJ. "New Therapies for the Eating Disorders: Behavior Modification of Obesity and Anorexia Nervosa." *Arch Gen Psychiatr* 1972;26:391–398.

10. Ferguson JM. *Habits, Not Diets. The Real Way to Weight Control.* Palo Alto, CA: Bull Publishing Company, 1976.

11. Winett RA, Tate DF, Anderson ES, Wojcik JR, Winett SG. "Long-term Weight Gain Prevention: A Theoretically Based Internet Approach." *Prev Med* 2005;41:629–641.

12. Harvey-Berino J, Pintauro S, Buzzell P, Gold EC. "Effect of Internet Support on the Long-term Maintenance of Weight Loss. *Obes Res* 2004;12:320–329.

13. Womble LG, Wadden TA, McGuckin BG, Sargent SL, Rothman RA, Krauthamer-Ewing ES. "A Randomized Controlled Trial of a Commercial Internet Weight Loss Program." *Obes Res* 2004;12:1011–1018.

14. Bray GA. *The Obese Patient.* Philadelphia: WB Saunders, 1976.

15. Nidetch J. *The Story of Weight Watchers.* New York: W/W Twentyfirst Corporation, 1970.

16. Jolliffe N. *Reduce and Stay Reduced on the Prudent Diet.* New York:

Simon and Schuster, Inc., 1963.

17. Stuart RB. *Act Thin, Stay Thin.* New York: WW Norton & Company, Inc., 1978.

18. Tsai AG, Wadden TA. "Systematic Review: An Evaluation of Major Commercial Weight Loss Programs in the United States." *Ann Intern Med* 2005;142:56–66.

19. Heshka S, Anderson JW, Atkinson RL, Greenway FL, Hill JO, Phinney SD, Kolotkin RL, Miller-Kovach K, Pi-Sunyer FX. "Weight Loss with Self-Help Compared with a Structured Commercial Program: A Randomized Trial." *JAMA* 2003;289:1792–1798.

Chapter 16

1. Berland T. *Consumer Guide: Rating the Diets.* Consumer Guide, 1975.
2. *Recommended Dietary Allowances,* 10th edition. Washington, D.C.: National Academy Press, 1989.
3. Kinsell LW, Gunning B, Michaels GD, Richardson J, Cox SE, Leon C. Calories Do Count. *Metabolism* 1964;13:195–204.
4. Freedman MR, King J, Kennedy E. "Popular Diets: A Scientific Review." *Obes Res* 2001;9(Suppl 1):1S–40S.
5. Dansinger ML, Gleason JA, Griffith JL, Selker HP, Schaefer EJ. "Comparison of the Atkins, Ornish, Weight Watchers, and Zone Diets for Weight Loss and Heart Disease Risk Reduction: A Randomized Trial." *JAMA* 2005;293:43–53.
6. Atkins RC. *Dr. Atkins's New Diet Revolution.* New York: Avon, 2002; Atkins R, Gare F. *Dr. Atkins New Diet Cookbook,* New York: M Evans and Co, Inc., 1995.
7. Ornish D. *Eat More, Weigh Less: Dr. Dean Ornish's Life Choice Program for Losing Weight Safely While Eating Abundantly.* New York: HarperCollins, 1993.
8. Sears B, Lawren W. *Enter the Zone: A Dietary Road Map.* New York NY: HarperCollins, 1995; Sears B. *Zone Perfect Meals in Minutes,* New York NY: HarperCollins, 1997.
9. Weight Watchers Publishing Group. *Weight Watchers New Complete Cookbook.* New York: M Evans and Co., Inc., 1995.
10. Gardner CD, Kiazand A, Alhassan S, Kim S, Stafford RS, Balise RR, Kraemer HC, King AC. "Comparison of the Atkins, Zone, Ornish, and LEARN Diets for Change in Weight and Related Risk Factors among Overweight Premenopausal Women: The A TO Z Weight Loss Study: A Randomized Trial." *JAMA* 2007;297:969–977. Erratum in: *JAMA* 2007;298:178.
11. Brownell KD. *The LEARN Manual for Weight Management.* Dallas, TX: American Health Publishing Co., 2000.
12. Sacks FM, Bray GA, Carey V, Smith SR, Ryan DH, Anton S, McMnus

K, Champagne CM, Bishop L, Laranjo N, Leboff, M, Roos J, Levitan L, Loria CM, Obaarzanek E, Williamson D. "Randomized Trial Comparing Fat, Protein and Carbohydrate Composition of Diets for Weight Loss." *N Engl J Med* 2008 in press.

13. Bray GA. Book Review: *Good Calories Bad Calories* by Gary Taubes, New York A.A. Knopf. *Obes Rev* 2008;9:251–263.

14. Bray GA. *The Obese Patient.* Philadelphia: WB Saunders, 1976.

Chapter 17

1. Ronsard N. *Cellulite: Those Lumps, Bumps, and Bulges You Couldn't Lose Before.* New York: Beauty and Health Publishing Co., 1973.

2. Greenway FL, Bray GA. "Regional Fat Loss from the Thigh in Obese Women after Adrenergic Modulation." *Clin Ther* 1987;9:663–669.

3. Caruso MK, Pekarovic S, Raum WJ, Greenway F. "Topical Fat Reduction from the Waist." *Diabetes Obes Metab* 2007;9:300–303.

4. Hamilton EC, Greenway FL, Bray GA. "Regional Fat Loss from the Thigh in Women Using Topical 2% Aminophylline Cream." *Obes Res* 1993;1(Suppl 2):95S.

5. Greenway FL, Bray GA, Heber D. "Topical Fat Reduction." *Obes Res* 1995;3(Suppl 4):561S–568S.

Chapter 18

1. Gilbertson TA. "Gustatory Mechanisms for the Detection of Fat." *Curr Opin Neurobiol* 1998;8:447–452.

2. Rolls ET, Rolls BJ, Rowe EA. "Sensory-Specific and Motivation-Specific Satiety for the Sight and Taste of Food and Water in Man." *Physiol Behav* 1983;30:185–192.

Chapter 19

1. *Recommended Dietary Allowances*, 10th edition. Washington, D.C.: National Academy Press, 1989.

2. Levine JA, Lanningham-Foster LM, McCrady SK, Krizan AC, Olson LR, Kane PH, Jensen MD, Clark MM. "Interindividual Variation in Posture Allocation: Possible Role in Human Obesity. *Science* 2005;307:584-586.

3. Hill JO, Peters JC, Jortberg BT. *The Step Diet. Count Steps Not Calories to Lose Weight and Keep It Off Forever.* New York: Workman Publishing, 2004.

Chapter 20

1. Critser G. *Fat Land: How Americans Became the Fattest People in the World.* New York: Mariner Books, 2004.

2. Tillotson JE. "Pandemic Obesity: What Is the Solution?" *Nutr Today*

2004;39:6–9.

3. Pollan M. *The Omnivore's Dilemma: A Natural History of Four Meals.* New York: The Penguin Group, 2006.

4. Finkelstein EA, Ruhm CJ, Kosa KM. "Economic Causes and Consequences of Obesity." *Annu Rev Public Health* 2005;26:239–257.

5. Drewnowski A, Specter SE. "Poverty and Obesity: The Role of Energy Density and Energy Costs." *Am J Clin Nutr* 2004;79:6–16.

6. USDA ERS *Food Rev* 2002;25:2–15.

7. Bray GA. *Metabolic Syndrome and Obesity.* Totawa NJ: Humana Publishers, 2007.

8. Nestle M. Increasing Portion Sizes in American Diets: More Calories, More Obesity." *J Am Diet Assoc* 2003;103:39–40.

9. Rolls BJ, Morris EL, Roe LS. "Portion Size of Food Affects Energy Intake in Normal-Weight and Overweight Men and Women." *Am J Clin Nutr* 2002;76:1207–1213.

10. Popkin BM, Armstrong LE, Bray GM, Caballero B, Frei B, Willett WC. "A New Proposed Guidance System for Beverage Consumption in the United States." *Am J Clin Nutr* 2007;83:529–542.

11. Stookey JD, Constant F, Gardner CD, Popkin BM. "Replacing Sweetened Caloric Beverages with Drinking Water Is Associated with Lower Energy Intake." *Obesity* 2007;15:3013–3022.

12. Rolls BJ, Roe LS, Kral TV, Meengs JS, Wall DE. "Increasing the Portion Size of a Packaged Snack Increases Energy Intake in Men and Women." *Appetite* 2004;42:63–69.

Chapter 21

1. Cefalu WT, Wang ZQ, Zhang XH, Baldor LC, Russell JC. "Oral Chromium Picolinate Improves Carbohydrate and Lipid Metabolism and Enhances Skeletal Muscle Glut-4 Translocation in Obese, Hyperinsulinemic (JCR-LA Corpulent) Rats." *J Nutr* 2002;132:1107–1114.

2. Pittler MH, Ernst E. "Dietary Supplements for Body-Weight Reduction: A Systematic Review." *Am J Clin Nutr* 2004;79:529–536.

3. Pittler MH, Ernst E. "Complementary Therapies for Reducing Body Weight: A Systematic Review." *Int J Obes (Lond)* 2005;29:1030–1038.

4. Larsen TM, Toubro S, Astrup A. "Efficacy and Safety of Dietary Supplements Containing CLA for the Treatment of Obesity: Evidence from Animal and Human Studies." *J Lipid Res* 2003;44:2234–2241.

5. Reid IR, Horne A, Mason B, Ames R, Bava U, Gamble GD. "Effects of Calcium Supplementation on Body Weight and Blood Pressure in Normal Older Women: A Randomized Controlled Trial. *J Clin Endocrinol Metab* 2005;90:3824–3829.

6. Dwyer JT, Allison DB, Coates PM. "Dietary Supplements in Weight

Reduction." *J Am Diet Assoc* 2005;105(5 Suppl 1):S80–86.

7. Shekelle PG, Hardy ML, Morton SC, Maglione M, Mojica WA, Suttorp MJ, Rhodes SL, Jungvig L, Gagné J. "Efficacy and Safety of Ephedra and Ephedrine for Weight Loss and Athletic Performance: A Meta-Analysis." *JAMA* 2003;289:1537–1545.

8. Heymsfield SB, Allison DB, Vasselli JR, Pietrobelli A, Greenfield D, Nunez C. "Garcinia Cambogia (Hydroxycitric Acid) As a Potential Antiobesity Agent: A Randomized Controlled Trial." *JAMA* 1998;280:1596–1600.

9. Bent S, Padula A, Neuhaus J. "Safety and Efficacy of Citrus Aurantium for Weight Loss." *Am J Cardiol* 2004;94:1359–1361.

10. Kromhout D, Bloemberg B, Seidell JC, Nissinen A, Menotti A. "Physical Activity and Dietary Fiber Determine Population Body Fat Levels: The Seven Countries Study." *Int J Obes Relat Metab Disord* 2001;25:301–306.

APPENDIX 1

Bray Diet Plan

A Guide to the Calorie Values of Foods

Counting calories is one way to help control intake of foods. This abbreviated list of foods with their caloric content is designed to help you. It has been prepared from several sources, but not all foods have been included. The list is arranged into the following groups:

Beverages
Breads and bread products
Cereals and cereal products
Crackers, pretzels, and wafers
Desserts
Eggs
Fruits
Fruit juices
Meats
Milk, butter, and cheese
Nuts
Poultry
Salad dressings, fats, oils, and sauces
Sausage and sandwich meats
Seafood
Soups
Vegetables

Item	Measure	Calories
Beverages		
Coffee	1 cup, without cream or sugar	0
Chocolate milk, commercial	8 oz, ½ pint	185
Chocolate milk shake made with 8 oz milk, ice cream	1 regular fountain drink	420
Coca-Cola	1 can, 12 oz	160
Cider, sweet	1 glass, 8 oz	95
Egg nog, non-alcoholic	½ cup; 4 oz	170
Ginger ale	1 glass, 8 oz	80
Lemonade, fresh	1 large glass (1 oz lemon juice)	105
Lemonade, frozen	Approx 8 oz	
Pepsi-Cola	1 can, 12 oz	160
Root beer	1 small glass (4 oz)	50
Soda, ice cream, vanilla	1 regular fountain drink (approx 8 oz)	260
Tea	1 cup, without cream or sugar	0
Beverages, Alcoholic		
Ale, mild	1 bottle, 12 oz	150
Beer, malt (average 4% alcohol)	1 bottle, 12 oz	170
Brandy, Cognac or California (10.5% alcohol)	1 oz	75
Cider, fermented	6 oz	75
Daiquiri	1 cocktail	125
Gin, dry (80 proof)	1½ oz	105
Manhattan cocktail	1 cocktail glass (3½ oz)	165
Martini cocktail	1 cocktail glass (3½ oz)	140
Old Fashioned cocktail	1 cocktail glass (10 oz)	180
Pink Lady	1 cocktail	175
Rum	1 ½ oz	105
Scotch	1 oz	75
Tom Collins	1 regular bar drink (10 oz)	180
Vodka (90 proof)	1 oz	100
Whiskey, Bourbon, Irish, or rye	1½ oz	120
Whiskey, Scotch	1½ oz	110
Wine, red, white	3½ oz	75
Champagne	3½ oz	85
Port	3½ oz	160
Sauterne	3½ oz	85
Bread, Rolls, and Similar Products		
Boston brown bread	1 average slice, 3"×2/3"	105

Corn bread	2" square	115
Cracked wheat bread	1 slice	60
French or Vienna bread	1 average slice, approx 1 oz	75
Melba toast	1 slice, 4"×2"	15
Italian bread	1 slice, approx 1 oz	75
Raisin bread	1 slice, ½" thick	65
Rye bread (1/3 rye, 2/3 clear flour)	1 slice, ½" thick	55
White bread, enriched	1 slice, ½" thick	65
Whole wheat bread	1 slice, 1/2" thick	55
Biscuits, baking powder	1 biscuit, 2½" diameter	130
Bun, cinnamon	1	160
Bun, cinnamon with raisins	1	165
Coffee cake, iced with nuts	4½" diameter	240
Doughnut, yeast, plain, raised	3" diameter	125
Doughnut, yeast, jelly center, raised	3" diameter	225
Griddle cakes, buckwheat pancake mix	4" diameter	90
Griddle cakes, wheat flour	4" diameter	105
Muffins, bran	2-3/4" diameter (1 medium)	105
Muffin, corn meal	2-3/4" diameter (1 medium)	130
Muffin, white flour	2-3/4" diameter (1 medium)	120
Roll, sandwich	1 round or finger roll, 16 per lb	85
Roll, white, hard, no milk or butter	1	95
Roll, white, soft	1 cloverleaf	90
Roll, white	1	80
Tortilla (corn)	1	65
Tortilla (flour)	1	95
Waffle, made with enriched or unenriched flour	1 waffle, 4½"×5-5/8"×½"	215
Yeast	1 oz	24

Cereals and Cereal Products

Bran (almost wholly bran)	1 cup	145
Bran flakes (40% bran)	1 cup	105
Corn flakes	1 cup	95
Cheerios	1 cup	100
Cream of Wheat	¾ cup cooked	100
Farina, cooked	1 cup	105
Grape Nuts	¼ cup or 2 heaping tbsp (1 oz)	100
Hominy or grits, cooked	1 cup	120
Macaroni, cooked firm	1 cup	210
Macaroni, cooked tender	1 cup	150
Macaroni and cheese, baked	1 cup	465
Noodles, containing egg	½ cup cooked	105

391

Oatmeal, cooked	1 cup	150
Oat cereal, ready to eat	1 cup	100
Popcorn	1 cup	55
Puffed rice	1 cup	55
Rice, white, cooked	1 cup	165
Rice, wild	½ cup	297
Rice flakes	1 cup	120
Rice Krispies	1 cup	110
Shredded Wheat	1 biscuit	100
Puffed wheat	1 cup	43
Spaghetti, plain, cooked firm	1 cup	220
Spaghetti, plain, cooked tender	1 cup	165
Spaghetti, cooked tender with tomato sauce	1 cup with ½ cup canned tomato sauce	210
Spaghetti, cooked firm with tomato sauce	1 cup with ½ cup canned tomato sauce	265
Spaghetti, Italian style with tomato sauce, 2 meatballs, cheese 1 cup spaghetti, tender; ½ cup tomato sauce, canned; 3 oz meatballs; 2 tbsp Parmesan cheese		500
Wheat flakes, prepared cereal	1 cup	125
Wheaties	1 cup	105
Wheat, rolled, cooked	1 cup	180

Crackers, Pretzels, and Wafers

Graham crackers	4 small or 2 medium	55
Oyster crackers	10 crackers or 1 tbsp cracker meal	45
Ritz crackers	1 cracker	20
Saltines	2 crackers, 2" square	30
Soda crackers	2 crackers, 2½" square	60
Whole wheat crackers	1 cracker	15
Matzoh wafers	1 piece, 6" diameter	80
Pretzel sticks	5 small sticks	20
Pretzels	1 medium, 22 per lb	70
Ry-Krisp	1 double square wafer	20
Rye wafers	2 wafers, 1-7/8"×3-1/4"	45
Triscuits	2" square	25
Zwieback	1 piece, 60 per lb	30

Desserts

Apple Betty	1 cup	420
Brownies	2"×2"× ¾"	140
Angel cake	1/10 of large cake	145

Apple sauce cake	2" slice	200
Coconut cake with icing	1 average slice	150
Foundation cake, fudge icing	2" sector of 2-layer cake,	
	1/16 of cake 10" in diameter	420
Fruit cake, dark	2"×2"×½"	105
Plain cake	1 piece, 2"×3"×1½"	105
Plain cake, iced	2" sector of 2-layer cake,	
	1/16 of cake, 10" in diameter	320
Sponge cake	2" section, 1/12 of cake 8" in diameter	115
Chocolate fudge sauce	1 tbsp	50
Chocolate syrup	1 tbsp	100
Chocolate snap cookie, Sunshine	1	15
Chocolate chip cookie	1	75
Molasses cookie	1	70
Oatmeal cookie	3½" diameter	75
Plain cookie	1	70
Vanilla wafer	1	20
Cream puff with custard filling	1	245
Chocolate cupcake, fudge icing	1 medium cupcake	190
Vanilla cupcake, vanilla icing	1 medium cupcake	160
Custard, baked	½ cup	170
Éclair, chocolate icing, custard filled	1 average	315
Fudge	1 piece	116
Gelatin dessert, plain	½ cup	75
Gelatin dessert, fruit added	½ cup	85
Gingerbread	2"×2"×2"	205
Ice milk		55
Ice cream, vanilla	1/7 of quart brick	165
Vanilla	¼ pint, average serving	145
Ice, orange, water	Average serving, ½ cup	175
Sherbet, factory packed,		
based on 6–8 lb per gallon	Average serving, ½ cup	120

Pie

Apple pie	1/6 of 9" diameter pie	410
Apricot pie	4" slice	331
Blackberry pie	1/6 of 9" diameter pie	390
Blueberry pie	1/6 of 9" diameter pie	390
Cherry pie	1/6 of 9" diameter pie	420
Chocolate pie	1/6 of 9" diameter pie	295
Chocolate chiffon pie	1/6 of 9" diameter pie	525
Chocolate meringue pie	1/6 of 9" diameter pie	380
Coconut custard pie	1/6 of 9" diameter pie	365

Cream pie	1/6 of 9" diameter pie	300
Custard pie, plan	1/6 of 9" diameter pie	325
Lemon meringue pie	1/6 of 9" diameter pie	350
Mince pie	1/6 of 9" diameter pie	435
Pumpkin pie	1/6 of 9" diameter pie	305
Caramel pudding	½ cup	205
Chocolate pudding	½ cup	220
Vanilla pudding	½ cup	150
Bread pudding with raisins	½ cup	215
Rice pudding with raisins	½ cup	140
Tapioca pudding	½ cup	135
Shortcake, peach	1 peach on biscuit, no whipped cream, sweetened with 2 tbsp sugar	265
Shortcake, strawberry	1 cup berries on biscuit, no whipped cream, sweetened with 5 tbsp sugar	400

Eggs

Boiled or poached	1 medium-size egg	75
Fried	1 medium-size egg	105
Omelet	1-egg omelet	105
Scrambled with 1 tbsp milk, 1 tsp fat	1 medium-size egg	120
Egg white	From 1 medium-size egg	15
Egg yolk	From 1 medium-size egg	60

Fruits

Apple, raw	3" diameter	135
	2½" diameter	85
	2¼" diameter	60
Apple sauce, sweetened	½ cup	120
Apple sauce, unsweetened	½ cup	40
Apricots, raw	3 medium	55
Apricots, canned	4 medium halves and 2 tbsp syrup	95
Apricots, canned in water	½ cup, halves and liquid	40
Apricots, dried, cooked, sweetened	½ cup fruit and syrup	120
Apricots, dried, cooked, unsweetened	½ cup fruit and liquid	120
Apricots, frozen, sweetened	3 oz	70
Avocado, raw, peeled	½ avocado (3¼"×4")	170
Banana, raw	1 medium, 6"×1½" diameter	90
Banana, sliced	½ cup	70
Blackberries, raw	½ cup	40
Blackberries, canned in water	½ cup	50

Blackberries, canned in syrup	½ cup	110
Blueberries, raw	½ cup	40
Blueberries, syrup packed	½ cup	120
Blueberries, water packed	½ cup	45
Blueberries, frozen, no sugar	3 oz	50
Cantaloupe	¼ melon, 5" diameter	35
Cherries, raw	½ cup	45
Cherries, red, sour, pitted, canned (juice pack)	½ cup	60
Cherries, red, sour, pitted, syrup packed	½ cup	105
Coconut, fresh, shredded	½ cup	137
Cranberries	½ cup	22
Cranberry sauce, sweetened, canned or cooked	½ cup	202
Currants, red, raw	½ cup	30
Dates, "fresh" and dried, pitted	½ cup (6 dates)	240
Figs, raw	3 small (1½" diameter)	90
Figs, canned, syrup packed	3 medium figs, 2 tbsp syrup	85
Figs, dried	1 large, 2"×1"	55
Grapefruit, raw	½ medium, 4½" diameter, #64	40
Grapefruit, sections	½ cup, unsweetened	40
Grapefruit, canned in syrup	½ cup, solids and liquids	90
Grapes, raw (Concord, Delaware, Niagara)	½ cup	40
Grapes (Malaga, Muscat, Flame, Tokay)	½ cup	50
Honeydew melon, raw	2" wedge from 7" melon	50
Lemon	2" diameter	20
Lime	2" diameter	20
Loganberries	1/3 cup	30
Loganberries, canned in syrup	½ cup	90
Nectarine	1 fresh, large	100
Olive, manzanilla, green, bottled	1 small	7
Olive, pickled, green	1 "mammoth" size	7
Olive, pickled, ripe	1 mission variety	10
Orange, raw	3-3/8" diameter	105
Papaya, raw	1 cube (½" cube)	71
Peach, raw	2½" diameter	45
Peach, canned in syrup	2 halves, 2 tbsp juice	80
Peach, canned in water	2 halves, 1 tbsp juice	30
Peach, frozen (unsweetened)	4 oz	90
Pear, raw	1 large	95
Pear, canned in syrup	2 medium halves, 2 tbsp syrup	80

Pear, canned in water	½ cup or 2 halves with 2 tbsp liquid	35
Pineapple, raw	½ cup, diced	40
Pineapple, canned in syrup	2 small slices or 1 large slice plus 2 tbsp syrup	95
Pineapple, frozen, unsweetened	4 oz	104
Plum, raw	2" diameter	30
Plum, canned in syrup	3 plums without pits plus 2 tbsp juice	90
Prunes, dried, cooked with sugar	1/3 cup or approximately 6 medium with 2 tbsp liquid	160
Prunes, dried, cooked without sugar	1/3 cup or approximately 6 medium with 2 tbsp liquid	105
Prunes, dried, uncooked	4 medium prunes (50-60 per lb), ½"×1" x½"	75
Prunes, dried, uncooked	4 small, 70-80 per lb, 1-1/3" × 1"×½"	55
Raisins, cooked, sugar added	1 tbsp	35
Raisins, dried	1 tbsp	25
Raspberries, black, raw	½ cup	50
Raspberries, red, raw	½ cup	35
Raspberries, red, frozen	½ cup (unsweetened)	122
Strawberries, raw	½ cup	25
Strawberries, frozen	½ cup (sweetened)	117
Tangerine	2½" diameter	35
Watermelon	½ slice, ¾" thick	45

Fruit Juices

Apple juice, fresh or canned	4 oz	60
Grapefruit juice, fresh	4 oz	45
Grapefruit juice, canned, sweetened	4 oz	65
Grapefruit juice, canned, unsweetened	4 oz	45
Grapefruit-orange juice blend, canned, unsweetened	4 oz	65
Grape juice, bottled	4 oz	85
Lemon juice, fresh	4 oz	30
Lemon juice, canned, unsweetened	4 oz	30
Orange juice, fresh	4 oz	55
Orange juice, canned, unsweetened	4 oz	55
Orange juice, canned, sweetened	4 oz	65
Pineapple juice, canned	4 oz	60
Prune juice, canned	4 oz	85

Meat

Bacon, medium fat, broiled or fried	1 strip, 6" long, drained	50
Canadian bacon, cooked	1 slice, 2½" diameter × 3/16"	55

Beef, corned, canned has	1 small serving, ½ cup	200
Beef, dried or chipped	1 slice, 4"×5"	30
Beef, dried, creamed	½ cup, scant	210
Beef, hamburger, lean	1 patty, 3" diameter	150
Beef heart	4 per pound, 3 oz	265
Beef rib, roast or steak	2 slices, 2"×2¼ " × ¼", approx. 2 oz	190
Beef round, pan broiled	1 slice, 6"×3"×¼", approx 3½–4 oz	215
Beef steak, porterhouse, T-bone, or broiled	Small serving, approx 4"×3"×½ 3 oz	295
Beef tongue, boiled	1 slice, approx 1 oz	75
Beef sirloin, broiled	4"×2¼"× 1"	250
Beef prime rib	1 slice, lean	164
Beef stew with vegetables	1 cup	250
Chop suey, meat and vegetables	1 cup	200
Ham, boiled or baked	1 slice, 4¼"×4"×1/8", 3 oz	184
Lamb chop, rib, pan-broiled or broiled	1 medium chop, lean only, 3 oz	180
Lamb shoulder, pan-broiled or broiled	1 medium chop, 4"×3½" × ½"	215
Lamb, roast leg	2 slices, 3"×3¼" × 1/8"	205
Lamb, roast shoulder	2 slices, 3"×3½" × 1/8"	255
Liver, beef, pan-broiled	2 slices, 3"×2¼"× 3/8" (approx 2 oz)	170
Liver, calf, pan-broiled	2 slices, 3"×2¼"× 3/8´(approx 2 oz)	145
Meat croquette, beef	1 medium, 3¼"×1¾"	205
Meat loaf, beef or pork	1 slice, 4"×3"× 3/8"	265
Pork chop, pan-broiled or broiled	1 medium chop	235
Pork ham, fresh, roasted	1 slice, 4"×3"× ¼"	340
Pork loin, roasted	2 slices, 3½"×3"×¼"	265
Pork spare ribs, roasted	Meat from 6 average ribs	250
Veal, chop, loin, pan-broiled or broiled	1 medium to large chop	185
Veal cutlet, breaded	1 average cutlet, 4"×2¼"×½" (approx 2½ oz)	215
Veal leg, roasted	3 slices, 3"×3-3/8"×¼"	165

Milk, Butter, and Cheese

Butter	1 tbsp	100
Butter	1 pat or square, ½" thick	80
Cheese, blue	1 oz	105
Cheese, camembert	1 oz	85
Cheese, cheddar	1 oz	115
Cheese, cheddar (processed, American)	1 oz; 1 slice 3½" square × 1/8" thick	105
Cheese, cottage (from 2% fat milk)	1 oz or 2 level tbsp	25
Cheese, cream	1 oz	105
Cheese, cream, with pimiento	1 oz	65
Cheese, liederkranz	1 oz	85

Cheese, limburger	1 oz	95
Cheese, Parmesan	1 oz	110
Cheese, roquefort	1 oz	110
Cheese, Swiss	1 oz; 1 slice 3½" square × 1/8" thick	105
Cheese, Velveeta	1 oz	90
Cream (20% fat)	1 tbsp	30
Cream, heavy or whipping	1 tbsp	50
Cream, sour, heavy	1 tbsp	30
Milk, buttermilk, cultured	8 oz	85
Milk, evaporated	1 tbsp	25
Milk, condensed	1 tbsp	60
Milk, goat, whole	8 oz	65
Milk, cow, skim	8 oz	85
Milk, cow, whole	8 oz	165
Yogurt, part skim	8 oz	105
Yogurt, whole milk	8 oz	145

Nuts

Almonds, shelled, salted	12–15 nuts	95
Brazil nuts, shelled	1 small nut	25
Cashew nuts, roasted or cooked	6–8 medium nuts	90
Hickory nuts	15 nuts, small	105
Peanut brittle	1 piece, 2½"×2½"×3/8"	110
Peanuts, Virginia type, roasted	½ cup	400
Peanuts, Virginia type	8 nuts	45
Peanuts, Virginia type	1 tbsp chopped	50
Peanut butter	1 tbsp	90
Pecans	12 halves	105
Pecans	1 tbsp chopped	50
Walnuts, black	10 halves	95
Walnuts, English	12 halves	100
Walnuts, English	1 tbsp, chopped	50

Poultry

Chicken, canned, boned	3 oz; 1/3 cup	170
Chicken, broiler, fried	½ medium (margarine used)	465
Chicken, creamed	½ cup, scant	210
Chicken, roasted	2 slices, 6" ×2½"×¼"	200
Chicken, hen, stewed	½ breast or medium thigh	210
Chicken pie (peas, potato)	1 pie, 3¾" diameter	460
Chicken liver	1 small	50
Chicken salad	½ cup	200
Duck, roasted	2 slices, 3½"×3"×¼"	220

Turkey, roasted average for dark and light meat	2 slices, 6"×2½"×¼"	230

Salad Dressings, Fats, Oils, and Sauces

Butter	1 tbsp	100
Catsup, tomato	1 tbsp	15
Chili sauce	1 tbsp	15
Gravy, meat, brown	1 tbsp	40
Jams and jellies	1 tbsp	55
Lard	1 tbsp	125
Margarine	1 tbsp	100
Maple syrup, pure	1 tbsp	50
Mustard, prepared	1 tsp	4
Oils, salad or cooking	1 tbsp	125
Oils, olive	1 tbsp	125
Relish, India, Heinz	1 tbsp	25
Salad dressing, boiled	1 tbsp	30
Salad dressing, plain, commercial	1 tbsp	60
Salad dressing, French	1 tbsp	60
Salad dressing, Russian	1 tbsp	80
Salad dressing, Thousand Island	1 tbsp	65
Sauce, tartar	1 tbsp	95
Sauce, tomato, canned, Del Monte or Contadina	¼ cup	25
Sauce, white, medium	1 tbsp	30
Vinegar	1 tbsp	2

Sausage and Sandwich Meat

Bologna	1 oz	65
Frankfurter	1 frank, 5½" long, ¾" diameter	125
Liver sausage (liverwurst)	2 slices, 3" diameter × ¼" thick	150
Luncheon meat	1 slice, 4"×3½" × 1/8"	80
Sausage, Polish	1 slice, 1½" diameter × 1" long	85
Pork Sausage, cooked	1 link, 3" long × ½"	95
Pork Sausage, cooked	1 patty, 2" diameter (7 to lb)	185
Salami	1 slice, 3¾" diameter × ¼" thick	130
Vienna	1 sausage, 2" long × ¾" diameter	40

Sandwiches

1½ oz cheese

3 oz chicken

2 eggs

3 oz tuna

1 slice ham or other meat 350	2 slices bread with 2 tsp butter or mayonnaise

Seafood

Anchovies	3 thin fillets	20
Bluefish, broiled or baked	3 oz	125
Caviar, canned	1 tsp	30
Cod, fresh, raw	3"×3"×¾"	75
Codfish cake	2 balls or 1 large cake 2½" diameter	200
Clams, raw, long or round	4 medium	65
Crab meat, cooked or canned	1 cup	80
Crab, deviled	1 medium crab	185
Fish sticks, breaded, cooked	5 (4"×1"×½")	200
Flounder or sole, raw	3"×3"×3/8"	70
Frog legs, fried	3 large legs	210
Gefilte	½ cup	100
Haddock, fried	4"×2½"× ½"	210
Halibut, raw	3"×2"×1"	120
Lobster, broiled	1-pound lobster with 2 tbsp melted butter	245
Mackerel, canned (Pacific)	3 oz	154
Mackerel, raw (Atlantic)	4"×3"×½"	190
Oysters, meat only, raw	1 cup (13–19 medium)	150
Oysters, fried	6	400
Oysters, cocktail or on the half shell	6 medium oysters, 2 tbsp sauce prepared with chili sauce, catsup, horseradish, and Worcestershire sauce)	90
Salmon, baked	4 oz (3"×3"×½")	175
Salmon loaf	4½ oz	210
Sardines, canned, drained	5–7 small sardines, 3" long	175
Shad, baked or broiled	3"×3"×¾"	200
Shrimp, canned, drained	4 medium to large shrimp (60 per lb)	35
Shrimp cocktail	4 medium shrimp with 1 tbsp sauce prepared with chili sauce, catsup, horseradish, and Worcestershire sauce	50
Swordfish, broiled	3"×3"×¾"	140
Trout, brook	1 serving (5 oz cooked)	300
Tuna canned in oil, drained	3 oz (2/5 cup)	210
Tuna canned in water, drained	3 oz	108

Soups (canned)

Asparagus, cream of	7 oz	130
Bean	7 oz	161

Beans with pork	7 oz	135
Beef noodle	7 oz	70
Beef with vegetables	7 oz	60
Bouillon	7 oz	25
Celery, cream of	7 oz	145
Chicken, cream of	7 oz	140
Chicken Gumbo, Campbell's	7 oz	50
Chicken Noodle, Campbell's	7 oz	60
Chicken Rice, Heinz	7 oz	40
Clam Chowder, Heinz	7 oz	70
Consommé, Campbell's	7 oz	30
Gumbo Creole, Heinz	7 oz	65
Mushroom, Cream of, Campbell's	7 oz	185
Oxtail	7 oz	175
Pea, Green, Campbell's	7 oz	100
Pepper Pot, Campbell's	7 oz	90
Potato	7 oz	175
Tomato, cream of	7 oz	145
Tomato, cream of with water instead of milk	7 oz	75
Vegetable, Campbell's	7 oz	70
Vegetable Beef, Heinz	7 oz	80
Vegetable, Vegetarian, Campbell's	7 oz	65

Vegetables

Asparagus, fresh, cooked	½ cup cut spears	20
Asparagus, green or bleached, canned	6 spears, medium size, with 2 tbsp liquid	20
Beans, kidney, fresh, cooked or canned	½ cup	115
Beans, Navy, pea, and others, canned, baked with pork and molasses	½ cup	190
Beans, Navy, pea, and others, canned, baked with pork and tomato sauce	½ cup	145
Beans, Lima, fresh, cooked, or canned	½ cup	75
Beans, snap, green or yellow, fresh, cooked, or canned, drained	½ cup	15
Beets, fresh, cooked, or canned	½ cup diced or sliced	35
Beet greens, fresh, cooked	½ cup	20
Broccoli, fresh, cooked	½ cup or 2 stalks 5" long	20
Brussels sprouts, fresh, cooked	½ cup	25
Cabbage, raw	1 cup, shredded	25
Cabbage, cooked	½ cup	20
Cabbage salad (cole slaw) with boiled dressing	½ cup	40

Cabbage salad with cream and vinegar	½ cup	50
Carrots, raw	1 carrot, 5½"×1"; 25 thin strips	
	or ½ cup grated	20
Carrots, fresh, cooked, or canned	½ cup diced	20
Cauliflower, fresh, cooked	½ cup	15
Celery, raw	3 small inner stalks, 5" long	10
Celery, fresh, cooked	½ cup diced	10
Chard, leaves and stalks, fresh, cooked	½ cup	15
Collards, fresh, cooked	½ cup	30
Corn, sweet, white or yellow, fresh, cooked, or canned	½ cup	70
Cucumbers, raw	1 cucumber, 7½"×2"	25
Dandelion greens, fresh, cooked	½ cup	40
Eggplant	1 slice	15
Kale, fresh, cooked	½ cup	25
Kohlrabi, fresh, cooked	½ cup	25
Lettuce, loose leaf	1 head, 4" diameter	30
Lettuce, raw	2 large or 4 small leaves	7
Mushrooms, canned	½ cup, solids and liquids	14
Mustard greens, cooked	½ cup	15
Onions, whole, fresh, cooked	½ cup	40
Onions, green, young	6 small onions	25
Parsley, common, raw	1 tbsp, chopped	1
Parsnips, fresh, cooked	½ cup	65
Peas, green, immature, fresh, cooked	½ cup	55
Peas, green, canned	½ cup, drained	70
Peppers, green, raw	1 medium size	15
Pickles, dill or sour, cucumber	1 large, 4" long × 1¾" diameter	15
Pickles, sweet, cucumber or mixed	1 pickle, 2¾" long × ¾" diameter	20
Pickles, sweet, mixed	1 tbsp, chopped	15
Potatoes, white, baked, boiled, steamed, or pressure-cooked	1 medium, 2½" diameter	100
Potatoes, white, French fried	12 pieces, 2"×½"×½"	160
Potatoes, fried raw	½ cup	240
Potatoes, hash browned after holding overnight	½ cup	235
Potatoes, mashed, milk and butter added	½ cup	95
Potato chips	10 medium chips, 2" diameter	110
Pumpkin, canned	½ cup	40
Radishes, raw	4 small	4
Rutabagas, cooked	½ cup, cubed or sliced	25
Sauerkraut, canned	½ cup	15

Spinach, canned or fresh, cooked	½ cup	25
Squash, winter, boiled, mashed or canned	½ cup	45
Succotash	½ cup	95
Sweet potatoes, peeled, baked	1 sweet potato, 5"x2"	185
Sweet potatoes, candied	1 small, 3½"x2¼"	315
Tomatoes, raw	1 medium, 2"x2½"	30
Tomatoes, canned, or fresh, cooked	½ cup	25
Tomato juice, canned	½ cup	25
Tomato puree, canned	½ cup	45
Turnips, fresh, cooked	½ cup diced	20
Turnip greens, fresh, cooked, or canned	½ cup	20

APPENDIX 2

The Bray Diet Plan Menumax® Food Guide

C Appendix 2

The Bray Diet Plan Menumax® Food Guide

The following lists of foods are designed for the Menumax® system of menu planning. There are six lists:

List number	Food	Calories per unit
1	Bread and Cereals	70
2	Milk and Cheese	100
3	Fruits	50
4	Vegetables	50
5	Meat, fish, poultry, dry beans, eggs, nuts	75
6	Extras (fat, sugar, alcohol)	50

They can be used to plan meals that will provide good nutrition. This is done by using the grading system. Each food has been assigned a letter grade of A, B, C, or D, based on its overall nutritional quality. The foods with an A are most nutritious; those with a D are least nutritious. By selecting more foods with A or B than C or D, you will increase the yield of good nutrition in your diet.

List 1. Bread, Cereal, Rice, and Pasta
70 Calories per Serving
(range 60–80 calories)

Grade	Food	Serving size
Bread and Rolls		
A	Cracked wheat	1 slice
B	French or Vienna	1 average slice, approx 1 oz
B	Italian	1 slice, approx 1 oz
C	Raisin	1 slice
A	Rye or Pumpernickel (1/3 rye, 2/3 clear flour)	1 slice
B	White, enriched or not enriched	1 slice
A	Whole wheat	1 slice
	Bagel, small	½
C	Biscuits, baking powder, 2" diameter	¾ biscuit
D	Buns, cinnamon; cinnamon with raisin	½
D	Coffee cake, iced with nuts	3/10
B	Corn Bread (2' × 1½" × 1")	1 piece
B	Cornmeal, ground (dry)	2 tbsp
D	Doughnuts, yeast, plain (raised)	½
D	Doughnuts, yeast, jelly (raised)	3/10
	French toast (without syrup or butter) homemade	½ slice
	Griddle cakes, buckwheat pancake mix (4" diameter)	¾
	Melba toast	5 pieces
A	Muffins, bran	¾
A	Muffins, cornmeal	½
B	Muffins, white flour (English)	½ small
B	Pancake with milk (4" diameter)	¾
B	Roll, sandwich	1 round or finger roll
B	Rolls, white, hard, no milk or butter (higher in fat)	¾
B	Rolls, white, soft (cloverleaf)	¾
B	Rolls, white (frankfurter, hamburger)	½
	Tortillas, 6"	1
A	Waffle, made with enriched flour and milk (4" × ½")	½
A	Wheat germ	¼ cup
A	Yeast (compressed cake)	6 cakes
Cereals and Pasta		
A	Bran (almost wholly bran)	½ cup
A	Bran flakes (40% bran)	½ cup
A	Corn Flakes	¾ cup
A	Cheerios	¾ cup
B	Cream of Wheat (cooked)	¾ cup

B	Farina, cup	½ cup
B	Grape Nuts	3 tbsp
D	Hominy or grits, cooked	½ cup
B	Macaroni, cooked	½ cup
A	Macaroni and cheese, baked	3 tbsp
A	Noodles, containing egg	½ cup
A	Oatmeal, cooked	½ cup
A	Oat cereal, ready to eat	½ cup
D	Popcorn, no butter or fat	3 cups
B	Puffed rice (unfrosted)	1 cup
C	Rice, white, cooked	½ cup
B	Wild rice, cooked	1/6 cup
B	Rice flakes	¾ cup
B	Rice Krispies	¾ cup
A	Shredded Wheat	¾ biscuit
	Wheat, puffed, unfrosted	1 cup
A	Spaghetti noodles, plain, cooked	½ cup
A	Spaghetti, cooked, tomato sauce (canned tomato sauce)	1/3 cup with 3 tsp tomato sauce
A	Spaghetti, Italian style with tomato sauce, 2 meat balls, cheese	1/5 average serving
A	Wheat flakes, prepared cereal	2/3 cup
A	Wheaties	¾ cup
A	Wheat, rolled, cooked	½ cup

Crackers

C	Graham (2½" square)	2 squares
C	Oyster	20 crackers
C	Round butter type (Ritz)	4
C	Saltines (2" square)	6 crackers
C	Soda (2½" square)	2 crackers
C	Whole wheat	4 crackers
B	Matzoh wafers (6" × 4")	1 piece
C	Pretzel sticks (3-1/8 " × 1/8" diameter)	25 small sticks
C	Pretzels (22 per pound)	1½ medium
B	Ry-Krisp	5 double square wafers
B	Rye wafers (1-7/8" × 3¼ ")	4 wafers
C	Triscuits (2" square)	3 squares
B	Zwieback	2 pieces

List 2. Milk and Cheese Products,
100 Calories per Serving
(range 90–100 calories)

Grade	Food	Serving size
Cheese		
D	Blue	1 oz
D	Camembert	1-1/6 oz
C	Cheddar	7/8 oz
C	Cheddar (processed, American) 1" cube or 1 slice 3½" square × 1/8" thick)	1 oz
A	Cottage (from skim milk)	4 oz or 8 level tbsp
D	Cream cheese	7/8 oz
D	Liederkranz	1 oz
D	Limberger	1 oz
B	Parmesan	1 oz
D	Roquefort	1 oz
C	Swiss (slice, 3½" square × 1/8" thick)	1 oz
C	Velveeta	3 tbsp
D	Cream (20%)	3 tbsp
D	Cream, heavy or whipping	2 tbsp
D	Cream, sour, heavy	2 tbsp
Milk		
A	Buttermilk, cultured, 1¼ cups	10 oz
A	Low fat (2%; cow), ¾ cup	6 oz
A	Skim (cow), 1¼ cup	10 oz
C	Whole (3.5%; cow), ¾ cup	5 oz

List 3. Fruit and Fruit Juices
50 Calories per Serving
(range 40–60 calories)

Grade	Food	Serving size
D	Apples, unpared, 2" diameter	1
D	Apple juice	
D	Apple sauce, sweetened	¼ cup
	Apple sauce, unsweetened	½ cup
B	Apricots, raw	3 medium size
	Apricots, canned in water	4 medium halves
	Apricots, canned in heavy syrup	2 halves, no syrup
	Apricots, frozen	2 oz

407

D	Avocados, raw, 3½" diameter	1/8
C	Bananas, raw	½ medium (6" × 1½")
	Bananas, sliced	1/3 cup
C	Blackberries, raw	½ cup
C	Blackberries, canned in water	½ cup
D	Blackberries, canned in heavy syrup	¼ cup
C	Blueberries, raw	½ cup
C	Blueberries, water packed	½ cup
D	Blueberries, syrup packed	¼ cup
C	Blueberries, frozen, no sugar	3 oz
B	Cantaloupe, 5" diameter	½ melon
B	Cherries, raw	½ cup
B	Cherries, red, sour, pitted, canned (12)	½ cup
B	Cherries, red, sour, pitted, packed in heavy syrup	¼ cup
D	Coconut, fresh	1/8 cup
	Coconut, shredded, sweetened, dry	1/8 cup
C	Cranberries, raw	1 cup
D	Cranberry sauce, sweetened, canned or cooked	1/10 cup
C	Cranberries, raw	1 cup
D	Cranberry sauce, sweetened, canned or cooked	1/10 cup
C	Currants, red, raw	5/6 cup
D	Figs, raw (1½" diameter) canned in heavy syrup	2 small
B	Grapefruit, raw (4½" diameter)	½ medium
	Grapefruit sections, unsweetened	2/3 cup
	Grapefruit, canned in heavy syrup	1/3 cup solids and syrup
	Grapefruit juice, fresh	4 oz
	Grapefruit juice, canned, sweetened	3 oz
	Grapefruit juice, canned, unsweetened	4 oz
	Grapefruit-orange juice blend, canned sweetened	4 oz
D	Grapes, raw (Concord, Delaware, Niagara)	½ cup
D	Grapes (Malaya, Muscat, Flame, Tokay)	½ cup
D	Grape juice	¼ cup
C	Honeydew melon, raw (6" diameter)	¼
C	Lemons (2" diameter)	2
C	Limes (2" diameter)	2
D	Loganberries, canned in heavy syrup	1/3 cup
B	Nectarine	½ fresh
	Olives, manzanilla, green, bottled	7 small
	Olives, pickled, green	7 "mammoth" size
	Olives, pickled, ripe	5 "mission" variety
B	Oranges, raw (2½" diameter)	1
B	Orange juice	½ cup
B	Peaches, raw (2½" diameter)	1 piece

B	Peaches, canned in water	3 halves plus 1 tbsp liquid
D	Peaches canned in heavy syrup	1 half plus 2 tbsp syrup
B	Peaches, frozen, no sugar	2 oz
D	Pears, raw (3" diameter)	½ large
D	Pears, canned in water	2/3 cup or 3 halves and 2 tbsp liquid
D	Pears, canned in heavy syrup	1 medium half plus 2 tbsp syrup
B	Pineapple, raw (3½" × ¾" thick)	1 slice
	Pineapple, canned in syrup	1 small slice plus 2 tbsp syrup
B	Pineapple, frozen or canned in water	1½ small s lice
C	Plums, raw (2" diameter)	1½
	Plums, canned in heavy syrup	2 plums without pits plus 2 tbsp syrup
B	Prune juice	1/3 cup
C	Raspberries, black, raw	½ cup
	Raspberries, red, raw	2/3 cup
	Raspberries, red, frozen (sweet)	2 oz
B	Strawberries, raw	1 cup
B	Strawberries, frozen	1½ oz
B	Tangerines	1½" diameter
B	Watermelon (4" diameter × 1" thick)	1 slice

List 4. Vegetables
50 Calories per Serving
(range 40–60 Calories)

Grade	Food	Serving Size
A	Asparagus, freshly cooked	1¼ cup spears
A	Asparagus, green or bleached, canned	13-15 spears, medium size with 2 tbsp liquid
	Beans, kidney, freshly cooked or canned	¼ cup
A	Navy beans and others, canned and baked with pork and tomato sauce	1/6 cup
C	Lima beans, freshly cooked or canned	1/3 cup
B	Green snap beans, freshly cooked or canned, drained	2 cups
	Yellow snap beans, cooked or canned	2 cups
C	Beets, freshly cooked or canned (not Harvard beets)	¾ cup diced or sliced
A	Beet greens, freshly cooked	1½ cups
A	Broccoli, freshly cooked	1 cup or 5 stalks, 5" long
B	Brussels sprouts, freshly cooked	1 cup

C	Cabbage, raw	2 cups shredded
	Cabbage, cooked	1¼ cups
C	Cabbage salad with cream and vinegar	½ cup
C	Carrots, raw, 7" × 1"	2 carrots
	Carrots, freshly cooked or canned	1 cup diced
B	Cauliflower, freshly cooked	2 cups
B	Celery, raw	15 small inner stalks, 5" long
	Celery, freshly cooked	3 cups diced
A	Chard, leaves and stalks freshly cooked	1 cup
	Collards, freshly cooked	1 cup
D	Corn, sweet, white or yellow, 5" × 1¾" diameter	½ ear
	Corn, sweet, white or yellow, freshly cooked or canned	¼ cup
B	Cucumbers, raw	4 medium
	Dandelion greens, freshly cooked	1 cup
	Eggplant	3 slices
A	Kale, freshly cooked	1 cup
C	Kohlrabi, freshly cooked	1½ cups
A	Lettuce, raw	14 large or 28 small leaves
	Mushrooms, canned	1½ cups solids and liquids
A	Mustard greens, cooked	1½ cups
C	Onions, whole, freshly cooked	2¾ cups
	Onions, green, young	12 small onions
A	Parsley, common, raw	½ cup chopped
C	Parsnips, freshly cooked	½ cup
C	Peas, green, immature, freshly cooked	½ cup
C	Peas, green, canned	1/3 cup, drained, solids only
B	Peppers, green, raw (3" diam)	3 medium size
B	Pickles, dill or sour, cucumbers (4" × 1¾")	3 large
D	Pickles, sweet, cucumber or mixed (2¾" × ¾")	2 pickles
D	Pickles, sweet, mixed	3 tbsp, chopped
C	Potatoes, white, baked, boiled, steamed, or pressure-cooked (2½" diameter)	½ medium
D	Potatoes, white, French fried	4 pieces, 2" × ½" × ½"
D	Potatoes, fried, raw	1/10 cup
D	Potatoes, hash browned after overnight holding	1/10 cup
D	Potatoes, mashed, milk and butter added	¼ cup
C	Pumpkin, canned	2/3 cup
	Radishes, raw	30 small
C	Rutabagas, cooked, cubed, o sliced	2/3 cup
	Sauerkraut, canned	1½ cups
A	Spinach, canned or freshly cooked	1 cup
A	Squash, summer, freshly cooked	1-1/2 cups

410

	Squash, winter, boiled, mashed, or canned	½ cup
	Succotash	¼ cup
C	Sweet potatoes, peeled, backed (5" × 2")	1/3 sweet potato
C	Sweet potatoes, candied	1/6 small
A	Tomatoes, raw	1½ medium
A	Tomatoes, canned or freshly cooked	1 cup
B	Tomato juice, canned	1 cup
C	Turnips, freshly cooked, diced	1 cup
A	Turnip greens, freshly cooked or canned	1¼ cups

List 5. Meats, Fish, Poultry, Dry Beans, Eggs, and Nuts
75 Calories per Serving
(range 60–90 Calories)

Grade	Food	Serving Size
Meats		
D	Bacon, medium fat, broiled or fried	1½ strips, drained
B	Bacon, Canadian, cooked	1½ slices, 2½" diameter
D	Beef, corned, canned has	1/3 cup
	Beef, dried or chipped	2¼ slices, 4" × 5"
	Beef, dried, creamed	1/6 cup
	Beef, hamburger, lean round steak, broiled or pan broiled	1 patty, 2" diameter
D	Beef, rib, roast or steak, broiled	1 patty, approx 1 oz
B	Beef, round, pan broiled or broiled	1 slice, 6" × 3" × ¼" approx 1 oz
C	Beef tongue, broiled	1 oz
D	Beef steak, porterhouse, T-bone, or tenderloin, broiled	0.6 oz
D	Beef sirloin, broiled	1" × 2¼" × 1"
D	Beef, prime rib, roasted, lean	½ slice
B	Beef stew with vegetables	1/3 cup
	Chop suey, meat and vegetables	1/3 cup
A	Ham, boiled or baked	1 slice, 4¼" × 2" × 1/8"
D	Lamb chop, rib, pan broiled	½ medium chop
	Lamb shoulder, pan broiled or broiled	1 small chop
B	Lamb, roast leg	1 slice, 3" × 3" × 1/8"
A	Liver, beef, pan broiled	1 slice, 3" × 2" × 3/8"
	Liver, calf, pan broiled	1 slice, 3" × 2" × 3/8"
	Meat, croquette, beef	1 medium, 3" × ¾"
	Meat loaf, beef or pork	1 slice, 3½" × 1" × 3/8"
D	Pork chop, pan broiled or broiled	1 small chop
	Pork loin, roasted	1 slice, 3" × 2" × ¼"

	Pork spare ribs, roasted	Meat from 2 average ribs
B	Veal, chop, loin, pan broiled or broiled	½ medium chop
	Veal cutlet, breaded	1 average cutlet, 3" × 1" × ½"
A	Veal leg, roasted	1 slice, 3" × 4½" × ¼"

Sausage

D	Bologna	1oz
	Frankfurter	2/3 frankfurter, 5½" × ¾"
	Liver sausage (liverwurst)	1 slice, 3 "× ¼"
C	Luncheon meat	1 slice, 4" × 3½" × 1/3"
C	Polish style	1 slice, 1½" diam. × 1" long
D	Pork sausage, cooked	¾ link
	Pork sausage, cooked	½ patty
C	Salami	1 slice, 3¾" × 1/8"
	Vienna sausage	2 sausages, 2" × ¾"
A	Chicken, canned, boned	1½ oz; 1/6 cup
	Chicken, Creamed	1/6 cup
	Chicken, Roasted	1 slice, 3" × 3" × ¼"
B	Hen, stewed	1/5 breast or 1¼ oz
B	Chicken pie (peas, potatoes)	1/6 pie, 3¾" diameter
A	Chicken liver	1 medium liver
	Chicken salad	1/6 cup
C	Duck, roasted	1 slice, 3½ "× 1" × ¼"
B	Turkey, roasted average for dark and light meat	1 slice, 4" × 2½" × ¼"

Nuts

C	Almonds, shelled, salted	10-12 nuts
	Brazil nuts, shelled	3 small nuts
	Cashew nuts, roasted or cooked	5 medium nuts
	Hickory nuts	11 small nuts
A	Peanuts, Virginia type, roasted	1/10 cup
A	Peanuts, Virginia type	12 nuts
	Peanut butter	2½ tsp
	Pecans	8 halves
	Walnuts, black	8 halves
	Walnuts, English	9 halves

List 6. Fats, Sugar, Alcohol
50 calories per serving

Grade	Food	Serving Size
	Catsup, tomato	5 tbsp

412

Chili sauce	5 tbsp
Gravy, brown	2 tbsp
Margarine	2 tsp
Oils, salad or cooking	2 tsp
Salad dressing, French	4 tsp
Salad dressing, Russian	1 tbsp
Salad dressing, Thousand Island	1 tbsp
Mayonnaise	2 tsp
Tartar sauce	2 tsp
Tomato sauce, medium	¼ cup
White sauce, medium	8 tsp

Index of Subjects